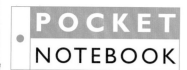

Pocket
PEDIATRICS

D1567794

Edited by

PARITOSH PRASAD, MD, DTM&H

The MassGeneral Hospital *for* Children™
Handbook *of* Pediatrics

Wolters Kluwer | Lippincott Williams & Wilkins
Health

Philadelphia · Baltimore · New York · London
Buenos Aires · Hong Kong · Sydney · Tokyo

Senior Executive Editor: Rebecca Gaertner
Managing Editor: Carly Hastie, Ashley Fischer
Project Manager: Priscilla Crater
Senior Manufacturing Manager: Benjamin Rivera
Marketing Manager: Kimberly Schonberger
Creative Director: Doug Smock
Production Service: Aptara, Inc.

© 2013 by **LIPPINCOTT WILLIAMS & WILKINS, a WOLTERS KLUWER business**
Two Commerce Square
2001 Market Street
Philadelphia, PA 19103 USA
LWW.com

Printed in China

Library of Congress Cataloging-in-Publication Data

Pocket pediatrics : the Massachusetts General Hospital for Children handbook of pediatrics / edited by Paritosh Prasad. – 2nd ed.
      p. ; cm. – (Pocket notebook)
  Includes bibliographical references and index.
  ISBN 978-1-4511-5152-7 (pbk.)
  I. Prasad, Paritosh.   II. Massachusetts General Hospital for Children.
III. Series: Pocket notebook.
  [DNLM: 1. Pediatrics–methods–Handbooks. WS 39]
  LC classification not assigned
  618.92–dc23

                                                        2012035868

Care has been taken to confirm the accuracy of the information presented and to describe generally accepted practices. However, the authors, editors, and publisher are not responsible for errors or omissions or for any consequences from application of the information in this book and make no warranty, expressed or implied, with respect to the currency, completeness, or accuracy of the contents of the publication. Application of the information in a particular situation remains the professional responsibility of the practitioner.

The authors, editors, and publisher have exerted every effort to ensure that drug selection and dosage set forth in this text are in accordance with current recommendations and practice at the time of publication. However, in view of ongoing research, changes in government regulations, and the constant flow of information relating to drug therapy and drug reactions, the reader is urged to check the package insert for each drug for any change in indications and dosage and for added warnings and precautions. This is particularly important when the recommended agent is a new or infrequently employed drug.

Some drugs and medical devices presented in the publication have Food and Drug Administration (FDA) clearance for limited use in restricted research settings. It is the responsibility of the health care provider to ascertain the FDA status of each drug or device planned for use in their clinical practice.

To purchase additional copies of this book, call our customer service department at (800) 638-3030 or fax orders to (301) 223-2320. International customers should call (301) 223-2300.

Visit Lippincott Williams & Wilkins on the Internet: at LWW.com. Lippincott Williams & Wilkins customer service representatives are available from 8:30 am to 6 pm, EST.

10 9 8 7 6 5

CONTRIBUTORS

Jeffrey A. Biller, MD
Attending, MassGeneral Hospital for Children

Sarabeth Broder-Fingert, MD
Resident, Massachusetts General Hospital Pediatric Residency

Harmony Caton, MD, MPH
Resident, Harvard Associated Medicine and Pediatrics Residency

Verne S. Caviness, MD, DPhil
Attending, MassGeneral Hospital for Children

Joseph H. Chou, MD, PhD
Attending, MassGeneral Hospital for Children

Rebecca Cook, MD
Resident, Harvard Associated Medicine and Pediatrics Residency

Brian M. Cummings, MD
Attending, MassGeneral Hospital for Children

Sophia Delano, MD
Resident, Massachusetts General Hospital Pediatric Residency

Dominica P. Donnal, MD
Resident, Massachusetts General Hospital Pediatric Residency

Fei J. Dy, MD
Resident, Massachusetts General Hospital Pediatric Residency

Meredith Eicken, MD
Resident, Massachusetts General Hospital Pediatric Residency

Ashley A. Ferullo, MD
Resident, Massachusetts General Hospital Pediatric Residency

Alison Friedmann, MD, MSc
Attending, MassGeneral Hospital for Children

Nina L. Gluchowski, MD
Resident, Massachusetts General Hospital Pediatric Residency

Eric F. Grabowski, MD, DrSci
Attending, MassGeneral Hospital for Children

Elena K. Grant, MBChB
Resident, Massachusetts General Hospital Pediatric Residency

Lynne L. Levitsky, MD
Attending, MassGeneral Hospital for Children

Kristen A. Lindgren, MD, PhD
Resident, Massachusetts General Hospital Pediatric Residency

David A. Lyczkowski, MD
Resident, Harvard Associated Medicine and Pediatrics Residency

Hasan S. Merali, MD
Resident, Massachusetts General Hospital Pediatric Residency

Natan Noviski
Attending, MassGeneral Hospital for Children

Aura Obando, MD
Resident, Harvard Associated Medicine and Pediatrics Residency

Casey Olm-Shipman, MD
Clinical Fellow, MassGeneral Hospital for Children

Deepak Palakshappa, MD
Chief Resident, Massachusetts General Hospital Pediatric Residency

Paritosh Prasad, MD, DTM&H
Clinical Fellow, Massachusetts General Hospital

Sylvia Romm, MD
Resident, Massachusetts General Hospital Pediatric Residency

Ana Maria Rosales, MD
Attending, MassGeneral Hospital for Children

Olga Rose, MD, MAS
Resident, Massachusetts General Hospital Pediatric Residency

Holly Rothermel, MD
Attending, MassGeneral Hospital for Children

Emily B. Rubin, MD
Resident, Harvard Associated Medicine and Pediatrics Residency

Chadi M. El Saleeby, MD, MS
Attending, MassGeneral Hospital for Children

Matan Setton, MD
Resident, Harvard Associated Medicine and Pediatrics Residency

Manasi Sinha, MD, MPH
Clinical Fellow, MassGeneral Hospital for Children

Elizabeth C. TePas, MD, MS
Attending, MassGeneral Hospital for Children

Anna Tien Labowsky, MD
Clinical Fellow, MassGeneral Hospital for Children

Avram Traum, MD
Attending, MassGeneral Hospital for Children

Sze Man Tse, MD, MDCM
Clinical Fellow, MassGeneral Hospital for Children

Julia Elisabeth von Oettingen, MD, Dr. med.
Resident, Massachusetts General Hospital Pediatric Residency

Melissa A. Walker, MD, PhD
Resident, Massachusetts General Hospital Pediatric Residency

Linda T. Wang, MD
Attending, MassGeneral Hospital for Children

Abigail R. Woodhead, MD
Resident, Massachusetts General Hospital Pediatric Residency

Lael Yonker, MD
Clinical Fellow, MassGeneral Hospital for Children

Young-Ho Yoon, MD
Attending, MassGeneral Hospital for Children

Mary Zelime Ward, MD
Clinical Fellow, MassGeneral Hospital for Children

FOREWORD

Physicians in training face many challenges every day. Among the most pressing of these is the need to provide clinical care while at the same time adding to their knowledge base for how best to provide that care. Thus, this imperative to "learn on the job" requires ready access to current, accurate, evidence-based medical information that can be used to support their experiential learning.

This handbook is a superb example of trainees teaching other trainees. It has been carefully assembled by a group of outstanding residents and fellows, working together with mentors for each relevant discipline. It is organized the same way in which residents and fellows encounter medical conditions needing their attention: by hospital or outpatient location and by organ system. It is clearly meant to be an evolving resource and it reflects the increasing body of evidence that frames the standard of care for pediatric medicine. Dr. Prasad and his fellow trainees have done an extraordinary job weaving the science that underpins the practice of pediatric medicine into a very valuable manual of pediatric practice. This handbook will have a permanent residence in my jacket pocket. I doubt it will spend much time there.

RONALD E. KLEINMAN, MD
Physician in Chief, MassGeneral Hospital for Children
Chair, Department of Pediatrics
Chief, Pediatric Gastrointestinal and Nutrition Unit
Massachusetts General Hospital
Charles Wilder Professor of Pediatrics
Harvard Medical School

PREFACE

In the two years since its publication, the *MGHfC Pocket Pediatrics hand-book* has been put to the test by a new generation of interns and residents. Their input and insight has resulted in this, the 2nd edition of the *MGHfC Pocket Pediatrics* handbook. As ever, we remain committed to creating a highly portable rapid reference for the pediatric health care practitioner in training with a specific emphasis on high-yield information and evidence-based practice.

To that end, this new edition has been heavily revised, trimmed in some areas and expanded in others with multiple new sections, including chemotherapeutics and their associated adverse effects, the evaluation and management of ADHD, and schematic diagrams of congenital heart disease to name only a few. We have even added an entirely new chapter of Clinical Images in Pediatric Dermatology.

As before, this handbook is not meant to be a comprehensive treatment of the whole of pediatrics, or even an exhaustive treatment of the specific topics treated within its pages. The topics were chosen because they are believed to represent the core knowledge one would wish to have at one's disposal. The information collected on each topic was selected and organized to present a high-yield overview of each subject by currently training residents and fellows and revised by active pediatric attendings. Each section has been re-reviewed with an eye to presenting the most up-to-date evidence-based practices and society and association guidelines, with the addition of well in excess of one hundred new citations to point interested readers in the direction of more complete treatments of each topic. Where evidence is lacking, we have included accepted best practices as well as the opinions of our experts at the Massachusetts General Hospital for Children.

As in the prior edition, great care has been taken to formulate every reference in such a way that each can be typed directly as provided into the search bar of www.pubmed.gov and should directly take the searcher to the article in question. (For Cochrane reviews, the two letter, six digit locator #'s are provided).

We acknowledge as well that this handbook will forever be a work in progress, as our understanding of pediatrics continues to grow and as, day by day, new knowledge about disease processes, new laboratory tests and procedures, and new evidence-based practice guidelines are added to our collective armamentarium. We have endeavored to make the following text as current as possible, but it should never take the place of clinical experience and clinical judgment.

PARITOSH PRASAD, MD, DTM&H

ABBREVIATIONS

AA – abdominal aorta
Ab – antibody
abd – abdomen
ABG – arterial blood gas
abn – abnormal
Absorp – absorption
Abx – antibiotics
accel – accelerate
accum – accumulation
ACEI – angiotensin converting enzyme inhibitors
Acq – acquired
adenoCa – adenocarcinoma
adj – adjacent
adol – adolescent
adolesc – adolescent
Afib – atrial fibrillation
Aflutter – atrial flutter
Ag – antigen
alk phos – alkaline phosphatase
Amp – amplitude or ampicillin depending on context
amt – amount
Amy – amylase
ANA – anti-nuclear antibody
ANC – activated neutrophil count
anom – anomalous
antag – antagonist
anter – anterior
antichol – anticholinergic
AR – aortic regurgitation
ARB – angiotensin receptor blocker
AS – aortic stenosis
ASA – aspirin
ASD – atrial septal defect
assoc – associated
asym – asymmetric
avg – average
Azithro – azithromycin

bact – bacterial
BB – beta blocker
b/c – because
bld – blood
BNP – brain natueretic peptide
BP – blood pressure
bpm – beats per minute
brady – bradycardia
btw – between
BUN – blood urea nitrogen
bx – biopsy

carbs – carbohydrates
cath – catheterization
CBC – complete blood count
c/b – complicated by
CCB – calcium channel blocker
CDH – congenital diaphragmatic hernia
CF – cystic fibrosis
CHD – congenital heart disease
chemo – chemotherapy
CHF – congestive heart failure
chorio – chorioamnionitis

chromo – chromosome
chrono – chronological
Cipro – ciprofloxacin
circ – circumcision
CKD – chronic kidney disease
clinda – clindamycin
CMV – cytomegalovirus
coags – coagulation studies
coarct – coarctation
colo – coloscopy
communic – communication
compens – compensation
conc – concentration
congen – congenital
conj – conjugated
constip – constipation
consump – consumption
Cort – corticosteroid
Cr – creatinine
CrCl – creatinine clearance
cres-decres – crescendo-decrescendo
crit – criteria
CTA – clear to auscultation
CTD – connective tissue disease
CTX – chest x-ray or ceftriaxone
cx – cultures
CXR – chest x-ray

d/c – discontinue
DCM – dilated cardiomyopathy
Ddx – differential diagnosis
dec – decrease
decomp – decompression
degen – degenerative
dehyd – dehydration
deliv – delivery
depol – depolarized
depriv – deprivation
Derm – dermatology
desc – descending
dev – development
Dex – dexamethasone
diff – differential
dig – digoxin
discrep – discrepancy
dissem – disseminated
DM – diabetes mellitus
d/o – disorder
DOL – day of life
dsDNA – double-stranded DNA
DTR – deep tendon reflex
dx – diagnosis
dysfxn – dysfunction
dz – disease

EBV – Epstein–Barr virus
ED – emergency department
EMG – electro myelograph
eos – eosinophils
epi – epinephrine
epo – epoetin alfa
Erythro – erythromycin
esoph – esophageal

esp – especially
ESR – erythrocyte sedimentation rate
essent – essential
EtOH – alcohol
eval – evaluation
evid – evidence
exacerb – exacerbate
exp – expiratory
explan – explanation
ext – extremity

FB – foreign body
FHx – family history
FMF – familial Mediterranean fever
func – function
f/u – follow up
fx – fracture or function depending
fxn – function

GAS – group A Streptococcus
Gastro – gastroenteritis
GERD – gastro-esophageal reflux disease
gest – gestation
gluc – glucose
GVHD – graft versus host disease
Gyn – gynecology

HA – headache
Hct – hematocrit
Hib – Haemophilus influenza B
HIV – human immunodeficiency virus
HoNa – hyponatremia
HoTN – hypotension
H&P – history and physical
HR – heart rate
HSM – hepatosplenomegaly
HTN – hypertension
Hx – history
hyperaldo – hyperaldosteronism
HyperCa – hypercalcemia
hypercoag – hypercoagulability
hyperK – hyperkalemia
HyperNa – hypernatremia
hyperphos – hyperphosphatemia
hypervent – hyperventilation
HypoCa – hypocalcemia
HypoNa – hyponatremia
hypophos – hypophosphatemia
hypoplast – hypoplastic

Ig – immunoglobulin
immunocomp – immunocompromised
imperf – imperforate
improv – improvement
inadeq – inadequate
inc – increase
incid – incidence
incomp – incompatibility
inflamm – inflammatory
infxn – infection
ing – ingestion
inhib – inhibitor
innomin – innominate
inpts – inpatients

insig – insignificant
insp – inspiratory
insuff – insufficient
intracard – intracardiac
intravag – intravaginal
inv – inverted
irreg – irregular
IVF – intravenous fluids
IVIG – intravenous immunoglobulin
jnts – joints

JVD – jugular venous distension
JVP – jugular venous pressure

LA – left arm
LAD – lymphadenopathy
Leuks – leukocytes
Levo – Levofloxacin
LFT – liver function tests
LL – left leg
LLSB – left lower sternal border
LN – lymph nodes
LOC – loss of consciousness
LUSB – left upper sternal border
LV – left ventricle
LVH – left ventricular hypertrophy
lymphoprolif – lymphoproliferative

maint – maintenance
Malfxn – malfunction
malig – malignancy/malignant
malnut – malnutrition
mat – maternal
max – maximum
M. cat – Moraxella catarrhalis
mec – meconium
mech – mechanism
meds – medications
mgmt – management
MI – myocardial infarction
Mineralocort – mineralocorticoid
Mitoc – mitochondrial
mod – moderate
monit – monitor
MR – mitral regurgitation
MS – mitral stenosis
multi – multiple
musc – muscular
mut – mutation
MV – mitral valve
mvmt – movement
MVP – mitral valve prolapse

nec – necrotizing
NEC – necrotizing enterocolitis
neonat – neonatal
NHL – Non-Hodgkin lymphoma
NICU – neonatal intensive care unit
NKCs – natural killer cells
nml – normal
N. mening – Neisseria meningitidis
nontyp – nontypeable
norepi – norepinephrine
NSAID – non-steroidal anti-inflammatory drug
N/V – nausea/vomiting

obst – obstruction
occ – occasionally
OCP – oral contraceptive pills
optho – ophthalmology
OTC – over the counter
outpt – outpatient

PA – pulmonary artery
palp's – palpitations
PALS – pediatric advanced life support
Pancr – pancreatic
parasymp – parasympathetic
PCN – penicillin
PCR – polymerase chain reaction
PDA – patent ductus arteriosus
PE – pulmonary embolism
peds – pediatrics
periph – peripheral
PFT – pulmonary function test
Phenobarb – phenobarbital
pheo – pheochromocytoma
pHTN – pulmonary hypertension
Plts – platelets
PMI – point of maximal impulse
PMNs – polymorphonuclear cells
PNA – pneumonia
PO – per oral
polyartic – polyarticular
pop – population
poss – possible
post – posterior
PPI – proton pump inhibitor
pRBCs – packed red blood cells
predom – predominant
Preg – pregnancy
pres – pressure
prev – previous
PRN – per requested need
prog – prognosis
progest – progestin
prophy/ppx – prophylaxis
prot – protein
prox – proximal
PS – pulmonic stenosis
pt – patient
PTX – pneumothorax
pulm – pulmonary
PVM – pulmonary venous markings
PVR – pulmonary vascular resistance
p/w – presents with
pyelo – pyelonephritis

RA – right arm
RAD – reactive airway disease
RAE – right atrial enlargement
RBBB – right bundle branch block
RCT – randomized controlled trial
rec – recommendation
refrac – refractory
regurg – regurgitation
renovasc – renovascular
req – required
resp – response
resusc – resuscitation
resxn – resection
retic – reticulocyte

RF – rheumatoid factor
rhabdo – rhabdomyolysis
rpt – repeat
RSV – respiratory syncytial virus
RV – right ventricle
RVH – right ventricular hypertrophy
RVOT – right ventricular outflow tract
Rx – treatment
rxn – reaction

sat – saturation
SBI – spontaneous bacterial infection
SBP – systolic blood pressure
SEM – systolic ejection murmur
sens – sensitivity
sev – severe
sign – significant
signif – significant
sinopulm – sinopulmonary
SOB – shortness of breath
spec – specificity
S. pneumo – Streptococcus pneumoniae
spont – spontaneous
SSRI – selective serotonin reuptake inhibitor
Staph/S. aureus – Staphylococcus aureus
std – standard
STI – sexually transmitted infection
subclav – subclavian
subseq – subsequent
suff – sufficient
sugg – suggests
suppl – supplementation
supravent – supraventricular
Surg – surgery
SVR – systemic vascular resistance
SVT – supra-ventricular tachycardia
sx – symptoms
symp – sympathetic
syn – syndrome
sz – seizure
szr – seizure

tachy – tachycardia
TB – tuberculosis
thal – thalassemia
tol – tolerance
tox – toxicity
TR – tricuspid regurgitation
TS – tricuspid stenosis
TV – tricuspid valve

uncirc – uncircumcised
Uncomp – uncomplicated
univ – universal
unk – unknown
URI – upper respiratory infection
Uro – urology
US – ultrasound
U/S – ultrasound
UTI – urinary tract infection

Vanco – vancomycin
ventric – ventricle
Vfib – ventricular fibrillation
Vit – vitamin

ABBREVIATIONS ×

vol – volume
VSD – ventriculoseptal defect
VT – ventricular tachycardia
Vz/vac – vaccine
VZV – varicella zoster virus

w/ – with
w/i – with in
w/o – with out
wnl – within normal limits

WPW – Wolf–Parkinson–White
w/u – work up

xfer – transfer
xfusion – transfusion
xplant – transplant
XRT – radiation therapy

yo – years old

CONTENTS

INFECTIOUS DISEASE
Rebecca Cook, Emily B. Rubin, Sophia Delano, and Chadi M. El Saleeby

GENETIC AND METABOLISM
Paritosh Prasad

NEUROLOGY
Kristen A. Lindgren, Mary Zelime Ward, Casey Olm-Shipman, and
Verne S. Caviness

	Heart Rate	Respiratory Rate	BP (SBP/DBP)
Premature	120–170	40–70	75–55/45–35
0–3 mo	100–150	35–55	85–65/55–45
3–6 mo	90–120	30–45	90–70/65–50
6–12 mo	80–120	25–40	100–80/65–55
1–3 yr	70–110	20–30	105–90/70–55
3–6 yr	65–110	20–25	110–95/75–60
6–12 yr	60–95	14–22	120–100/75–60
12+ yr	55–85	12–18	135–110/85–65

Reproduced from *Nelson Textbook of Pediatrics.* 18th ed. Saunders; 2007:70–74, 677, 2434.

• A recent systematic review of 69 observational studies suggests that previously published reference ranges for HR & RR may require updating. These centile charts & an interactive calculator available at http://madox.org/tools-and-resources (Lancet 2011;377:1011)

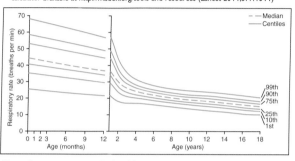

Above: Respiratory rate centiles for children from birth to 18 yr

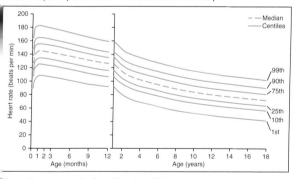

Above: Heart rate centiles for children from birth to 18 yr

DEVELOPMENTAL MILESTONES

Bright Futures Guidelines for Health Supervision of Infants, Children, and Adolescents. 3rd ed. 008:39; Pediatr Rev 2010;31:267; Pediatr Rev 2010;31:364; Pediatr Rev 2011;32:533)

Age	Gross Motor	Fine Motor	Cognition and Communication	Social–Emotional & Self-help
1 mo	• Lifts chin when prone • Turns head when supine	• Hands tightly fisted • Hands to mouth	• Throaty noises • Startles to sounds	• **Fixates on faces (should do by 2 mo)** • Discriminates parent's voice
2 mo	• Lifts chin when prone • Head bobs if held sitting	• **Tracks past midline (by 4 mo)** • Hands unfisted ¹/₂ of time, holds hands together	• Coos • Alerts to voice & sounds	• **Social smile (by 6 mo)** • Recognizes parent
4 mo	• Props on wrists when prone • **No head lag when pulled to sit** • Rolls front to back	• Tracks to 180° • Shakes rattle • Mouths objects • Reaching for objects	• **Orients to voice (by 6 mo)** • Alt vocalization w/ speaker; "converses" • Repeats actions if results are interesting	• Laughs out loud • Enjoys looking around • Smiles spontaneously
6 mo	• **Sits unsupported (by 9 mo)** • Commando crawls (8 mo)	• Reaches w/ one hand • Transfers hand to hand • Raking grasp	• Babbles "dada" • **Listens, then vocalizes when speaker stops (by 9 mo)**	• Recognizes strangers
9 mo	• Pulls to stand • Cruises • Crawls	• Pincer grasp (9–12 mo) • Bangs blocks together	• **Babbles "mama" (by 12 mo)** • Imitates sounds • **Responds to name (by 12 mo)**	• Waves "bye-bye" • **Reciprocates gestures (by 12 mo)** • Uses sound to get attention • Stranger anxiety
12 mo	• Stands alone • **Walks few steps alone (by 18 mo)**	• Primitive marks on paper • Finger feeds part of meal	• 1 word • Immature jargon	• Proto-imperative pointing • Pat-a-cake • Imitates • Follows 1-step command w/ gesture
15 mo	• Walks carrying objects • Stoops & recovers • Climbs on furniture	• Scribbles in imitation • Stacks 3–4 cubes • Turns pages • Uses spoon, cup	• **3–6 words (by 24 mo)** • Says no correctly	• Follows single-step command w/o gesture • **Proto-declarative pointing**
18 mo	• Walks up steps with hand held • Runs well • Throws ball	• Scribbles spontaneously • 4-cube tower	• 10–25 words • Points to people and 3 body parts when named • **Spoken language/ gesture combos**	• Helps in house • Removes clothing • **Imaginative play**
2 yr	• Walks down steps using rail • Throws ball overhand, kicks ball	• Lines cubes up as train • Imitates circle and/or line	• >50 words 50% intelligible • **2-word phrases**	• Follows series of 2 independent commands • Takes off clothing • Parallel play
2.5 yr	• Jumps • Walks on toes • Alternates feet going up stairs	• Turns paper pages in book • 8-cube tower	• Uses pronouns • Recites parts of known books	• Washes & dries hands • Puts on clothing • Imitates adult activities

3 yr	• Balance on each foot for 3 sec • Pedals tricycle • Heel–toe walk • Catches ball	• Copies a circle • Strings beads • Unbuttons clothes	• >200 words • **3-word sentences** • Speech 75% intelligible • Uses plurals	• Brushes teeth w/ help • Names friends • Imaginative play • Begins sharing • Knows name, age, sex • Toilet trained
4 yr	• Hops on one foot • Gallops	• Copies a cross and square • Draws 4–6-part person • Buttons	• Follows 3-step commands • 100% intelligible • Knows colors • Has memorized songs • Understands adjectives	• Tells tall tales • Interactive play (elaborate fantasy) • Group play • 1 close friend
5 yr	• Skips	• Copies a triangle • Cuts w/ scissors • Writes first name	• Identifies most letters, numbers out of order • Counts to 10 • Future tense • Reads 25 words	• Has group of friends • Apologizes for mistakes
6 yr	• Tandem walk	• Ties shoes • Draws diamond • Writes first & last names, short sentences	• 8–10 word sentences • Knows days of the week • Reads 250 words	• Same-sex best friend • Distinguishes fantasy from reality

Bolded milestones are *red flags* if missed by age specified in parentheses.

Red Flags
- Missed milestones (particularly bolded ones) or loss of previously acquired milestones should prompt further developmental & medical assessment
- Persistent fisting at 3 mo may represent earliest indication of neuromotor dysfxn
- Rolling <3 mo, pulling directly to stand (rather than sit) at 4 mo, W-sitting, bunny hopping, and toe-walking may indicate spasticity
- Primitive reflexes (Moro, asymmetric tonic neck) disappear btw 4–6 mo; persistence at 9 mo may indicate neuromotor dysfxn
- Protective postural reflexes (righting, protection, equilibrium) appear btw 6–9 mo; if not present, will lead to difficulty sitting and standing
- Due to Back to Sleep campaign, tummy time important for reaching milestones
- Hand dominance before 18 mo may indicate contralateral weakness
- Failure to alert to environmental stimuli may indicate visual or auditory deficits

HEALTHCARE MAINTENANCE

Bright Futures Guidelines for Health Supervision of Infants, Children, and Adolescents. 3rd ed.; 2008:39; Pocket Guide)

Age	Anticipatory Guidance	Screening
New-born	• Weight gain, feeding • Crib safety (own crib in parents' room, narrow slats with sides up, back to bed, no loose bedding) • Rear-facing car seat in back seat[a] • Home safety (smoke detectors, water temp <120°, no smoking) • Emergency phone numbers, CPR	• Newborn genetic screen • Hearing (if not done in hospital) • Postpartum depression • *Vision, BP (if risk factors/concerns)*
1 mo	• Start supervised "tummy time" • Develop routines, recognizing cues • Calm baby by rocking, talking, swaddling, never shake • Toy safety (caution w/ loops, strings, cords)	• Maternal postpartum depression • *TB (if risk factors)*

2 mo	• Strategies for increased fussiness • Plan for return to school/work • Keep small objects, plastic bags out of reach • Always supervise when on high place or in tub	• Verify hearing screening and rescreen if needed
4 mo	• Put to bed when awake but drowsy, can sleep in crib in own room (lower mattress before begins sitting) • Introduce cereal if child ready • Avoid bottle in bed	• Anemia (if preterm/ LBW, not on iron-fortified formula)
6 mo	• Support increases in language and cognitive development, read aloud • Introduce single-ingredient soft foods if ready; limit juice • Clean teeth with washcloth/soft brush & water • Home safety (block stairs, cleaning products, heaters, outlet covers, window guards; lock weapons; avoid infant walkers)	• Oral health risk assessment • Lead (if risk factors) • TB (if risk factors)
9 mo	• Discipline (+ reinforcement, distraction, limit use of "no") • Anticipate changing sleep pattern • Be aware of new social skills & separation anxiety • Limit or avoid TV, videos, computers • Provide 3 meals, 2–3 snacks/d; ↑ texture & variety of table foods, introduce cup • Water safety (always be w/i arm's length)	• Structured developmental screen • Oral health risk assessment
12 mo	• Discipline (time out, praise, distraction) • Est. bedtime routine w/reading, 1 nap/d • Supervise tooth brushing bid w/ fluoride, only bottled water • Encourage self-feeding (avoid small, hard food; choking) • Lock medications, know poison control num	• Anemia, lead
15 mo	• Maintain consistent routine. Present child with options, speak in simple clear language • Avoid bottle in bed • Fire safety (lock matches, lighters)	
18 mo	• Support independence but set limits • Daily playtime, read, sing • Anticipate anxiety in new situations • Toilet training (when dry for 2 hr at a time, knows wet/dry/bowel movement, pulls pants up/down)	• Structured developmental screen • Autism-specific screen
2 yr	• Switch to forward-facing car seat w/ harness[a] • Help child express feelings • Encourage play w/ others • Teach personal hygiene, toilet training (above) • Encourage active play: Use bike helmet, supervise outdoor play, cross street w/ adult • Switch to fat-free milk[b]	• Autism screen • Lead screen • Dyslipidemia (if risk factors)
2.5 yr	• Repeat speech with correct grammar • Establish family routine including exercise	• Developmental screen (structured)
3 yr	• Encourage storytelling, imaginative play • Limit media exposure to <2 hr/d, no TV in bedroom[b] • Move furniture away from windows	• Visual acuity measurement
4 yr	• Consider structured learning programs (pre-school, museum trips), encourage reading • Teach safety around adults (abuse prev) • Answer ?'s about body parts using appropriate terms	• Visual acuity measurement • Audiometry
5–6 yr	• Discuss school experiences • Eat breakfast, fruits, and vegetables • 2 cups low-fat milk/dairy per d • 60 min mod to vigorous physical activity per d[b] • Begin flossing daily • Water safety, swimming lessons • Use safety equipment with sports	• Visual acuity measurement • Audiometry (6 yr)

7–8 yr	• Once 4'9", can stop using booster seat in car; must use lap and shoulder belt[a] • Ask teacher for evaluation if any concerns • Encourage independence • Discuss rules and consequences • Note and discuss early pubertal changes • Supervise computer use	• Snellen test (8 yr) • Audiometry (8 yr)
9–10 yr	• Encourage self-responsibility, assign chores • Know child's friends and ensure adequate supervision, discuss bullying • Puberty, body image • Counsel about sexual activity • Counsel about avoiding tob, alcohol, drugs • Limit non-academic screen time to 2 hr/d	• Snellen test (10 yr) • Audiometry (10 yr) • Universal lipid screening
11–14 yr	• Begin speaking w/ child alone at clinic visits • 3+ servings low fat milk/daily per d • Coping with stress, mood changes, non-violent conflict resolution • Secure alcohol and prescription medications • 13 yo may sit in front seat of car • Caution with drivers using any alcohol/drugs	• Snellen (once during time period) • STI screening (if sexually active) • Substance use • Lipid screening (if abn b/w 9–11 yo or new risk factors)
15–17 yr	• Driving safety: Limit night driving, teen driving; always wear seat belt • Encourage responsibility, comm involvement • Violence prev, sexual activity, substance use	• Snellen (once during time period) • Screening
18–21 yr	• Planning for the future • Continue discussions regarding violence prevention, sexual activity, substance use	• Snellen (once during time period) • Fasting lipid profile

[a]Car Safety Seats: A Guide for Families 2012, AAP.
[b]Pediatrics 2011;128:S213.

Basic Concepts

• Assess parent–child interaction during visits
• Review age-appropriate vital signs and growth curves at each visit
• Unintentional injuries are the primary cause of death in children over age 1 yr, so focus should be placed on injury prevention during HCM visits. AAP has policy updates regarding specific recommendations (Pediatrics 2007;119:202)

Attention Deficit Hyperactivity Disorder
Pediatrics 2011;128:1007; Pediatr Rev 2003;24:92)

AAP recommends eval in pts 4–18 yo w/ hyperactivity, inattention, impulsivity, & academic or behavior concerns
Dx requires meeting DSM-IV criteria & requires observation from caregivers or teachers regarding duration & severity of symptoms & degree of impairment
ADHD rating scales can be helpful in making the diagnosis
Should assess for comorbid psychiatric or medical conditions
Rx varies based upon age & severity. May need referral to additional specialists

Cholesterol Screening (Pediatrics 2011;128:S213)

Evidence supports early identification & Rx of dyslipidemia to reduce CVD risk
Obtain fasting lipid panel (FLP) twice btw 2–8 yr & avg results if +FH for early CVD (men <55 yo, women <65 yo), parents w/ dyslipidemia, or child w/ other risk factors or high-risk condition (Table 9-5 in Guideline)
Universal lipid screening between 9–11 yr (FLP or non-fasting non-HDL chol)
Ages 12–17 yo, recheck FLP twice if new risk factors
Repeat universal lipid screening btw 18–21 yr as lipid levels ↓10–20% w/ puberty
Manage per algorithms if abnormal

IMMUNIZATIONS

Basics

Guide for parents: http://www.cdc.gov/vaccines/parents/index.html
VISs are available at: http://www.cdc.gov/vaccines/pubs/vis/default.htm
Up-to-date schedules available at http://www.cdc.gov/vaccines/schedules/index.html

Vaccine Safety

- Vaccine Adverse Event Reporting System (VAERS): http://www.vaers.hhs.gov
- Unexpected or clinically significant event after vaccine admin should be documented in medical record and VAERS form should be completed
- Reportable adverse events: Anaphylaxis, anaphylactic shock, brachial neuritis, encephalopathy or encephalitis, chronic arthritis, TTP, vaccine-strain measles viral infxn, paralytic polio, intussusception, death, or any adverse reaction that would be contraindication to future administration
- National Vaccine Injury Compensation Program: Provides compensation for people who have suffered injury 2/2 a covered vaccine: www.hrsa.gov/vaccinecompensation

Thimerosal (N Engl J Med 2007;357:1281; Pediatrics 2004;114:793)

- Mercury-containing preservative w/ antibacterial and antifungal properties
- All routinely recommended vaccines are thimerosal-free except some multi-dose vial flu vaccines and antivenoms
- IVIG and Rho immune globulin do not contain thimerosal
- Multi studies do not support assoc btw thimerosal exposure and neuro-psych deficits

Contraindications (J Allergy Clin Immunol 2004;114:1010)

- To any vaccine: Anaphylaxis after a previous vaccine dose or component
- Live attenuated vaccines should be administered together or at least 28 d apart
- **DTap, Tdap:** Encephalopathy w/i 7 d of admin of previous dose
  - Defer vaccine in pts w/ progressive neurologic disorder (infantile spasms, uncontrolled epilepsy, encephalopathy) until neurologic status clarified
  - Freq boosters may result in Arthus-like rxn; painful swelling shoulder to elbow
- **Hepatitis B vaccine:** Caution in pts w/ severe yeast allergy, allergic rxn rarely occur
- **Influenza (live-attenuated):** Pregnancy, known severe immunodeficiency, certain medical conditions, anaphylactic allergy to eggs
- **Influenza (inactivated):** Anaphylactic allergy to eggs
- **IPV:** Contains trace amounts of streptomycin, neomycin, and polymyxin-B
- **MMR:** Pregnancy, known severe immunodeficiency; contains trace amt neomycin
- **Varicella:** Pregnancy, known severe immunodeficiency; contains trace amt neomycin, precaution if received antibody-containing product w/i 11 mo
- **Rotavirus:** SCID
- **Zoster:** Suppression of cellular immunity, pregnancy

NOT Contraindications to Vaccinations

- Mild acute or convalescent illness with low-grade fever in an otherwise well child
- On antimicrobial therapy
- Nonspecific allergies or relatives with vaccine allergies
- Prior rxn to vaccine that included soreness, redness, or swelling at the injection site
- Prematurity — vaccines should be given according to birth age, not corrected age
- Immunosuppression of household contact (inactivated flu vaccine preferred)
- Pregnancy in a household contact or if breast-feeding
- FHx of seizures, SIDS, or of an adverse event following vaccination

OVERVIEW OF GROWTH

(Nelson Textbook of Pediatrics. 18th ed. Saunders; 2007:70–74, 677, 2434; Pediatr Rev 2006;27:e1; Pediatr Rev 2011;32:404)

- Term infants lose up to 10% of BW, then regain by 2 wk
- Avg infant BW doubles by 4 mo and triples by 1 yr; height doubles by age 3–4
- Exclusively breast-fed infants gain wt faster than formula-fed for first few mo, then more slowly after 3 mo; resolves by 1 yr
- Growth during puberty accounts for nearly 1/5 of height. Girls achieve peak height at Sexual Maturity Rating 2–3 compared with boys at Rating 3–4
- **Anterior fontanelle:** Normal size 20 ± 10 mm; closes at 9–18 mo
- **Posterior fontanelle:** Closes by 2 mo
- Excessively large fontanelle: IUGR, hypothyroid, prematurity, Trisomy 13/18/21, hydrocephalus, achondroplasia, Apert syndrome, cleidocranial dysostosis, cong. rubella, Hallermann–Streiff syndrome, hypophos, Kenny syndrome, osteogenesis imperfecta, pyknodysostosis, Russell–Silver syndrome, Vit D def rickets
- Excessively small fontanelles: Microcephaly, craniosynostosis, hyperthyroidism
- Average growth and caloric requirements (Adapted from Nelson Textbook of Pediatrics

Age	Average Weight Gain (g/d)	Length (cm/mo)	Head Circumference (cm/mo)	Daily Caloric Allowance (kcal/kg/d)
Birth–3 mo	25–30	3.5	2	115
3–6 mo	20	2	1	110
6–9 mo	15	1.5	0.5	100
9–12 mo	12	1.2	0.5	100
1–3 yr	8	1	0.25	100
4–6 yr	6	3 cm/yr	1 cm/yr	90–100

Midparental Height

- Boys: (Paternal height in in. + maternal height in in. + 5)/2 +/– 3 in.
- Girls: (Parental height in in. + maternal height in in. – 5)/2 +/– 3 in.

Growth Charts (Am Fam Physician 2003;68:879) (Growth charts at www.cdc.gov/growthcharts)

- CDC recommends using WHO charts for ages 0–2 yr and CDC charts after 2 yr (MMWR Recomm Rep 2010;59(RR-9):1–15)
- WHO charts developed based on predominantly breast-feeding children in environments supporting optimal growth and are considered "ideal" growth charts compared with CDC charts representing "actual" growth patterns
- Length should be measured via length-board (<2 yo); height measured via stadiometer
- Head circ measured just above eyebrow and ears, across most prominent part occiput
- Special growth charts available for: Trisomy 21, Prader–Willi, Williams syndrome, Cornelia de Lange syndrome, Turner syndrome, Rubinstein–Taybi syndrome, Marfan syndrome, achondroplasia, and low and very low BW preterm infants <1,500 g (use Infant Health and Developmental Program [IHDP] growth curves)

FAILURE TO THRIVE

Pediatr Rev 2000;21:257; Am Fam Physician 2003;68:879; Clin Fam Pr 2003;5:293; Pediatr Rev 2006;27:e1; Pediatr Rev 2011;32:100)

Introduction

No standard dx criteria exist; failure to thrive (FTT) most commonly defined as decel growth across 2 major percentile lines, or weight for age less than 5th percentile
Challenging to interpret: Crossing 2 major percentile curves (either ↑ or ↓) found to be common btw birth to 6 mo of age (32–39% of Californian infants), less common btw 6–24 mo (6–15%), & least common btw 24–60 mo (1–10%). Shifts in weight-for-height occurred nearly twice as frequently (Pediatrics 2004;113:e617)
1° etiology is malnutrition, 2/2 multi medical, behavioral, psychosocial, & environ causes
Malnourishment 1st decreases weight, then height, then head circumference
Decreased height growth suggests congenital, genetic, or endocrine abnormality
Proportional decrease in height and weight suggests underlying chronic medical condition

Etiology

Inadequate caloric intake

- Incorrect formula prep or breast-feeding challenges, difficulty transitioning to table food, excessive juice intake
- Mech feeding diff (anatomic, oral lesions), motor diff (oromotor dysfxn, CNS dz)
- Familial dysfxn, disturbed parent–child relationship (neglect or hypervigilance)
- Poverty and food insecurity

Inadequate absorption

- Milk protein allergy, GERD, vit or mineral (acrodermatitis enteropathica, scurvy)
- CF, Celiac disease, IBD, biliary atresia, or liver disease
- Chronic toddler diarrhea, infectious diarrhea
- Necrotizing enterocolitis or short-gut syndrome

Increased metabolic demand

- Hyperthyroidism, growth hormone deficiency, hypercortisolism, pituitary insufficiency, diencephalic syndrome, insulin resistance (IUGR)
- Hypoxemia (congenital heart disease, chronic lung disease, tonsillar hypertrophy)
- Chronic infection (TORCH, HIV, TB, immunodeficiency)
- Malignancy or renal disease
- Genetic abn (Trisomy 21, 18, 13, Russell–Silver, Prader–Willi, Cornelia de Lange)
- Metabolic disorders (storage diseases, amino acid disorders)

Clinical Manifestations
- Plot weight, height, and head circumference at every visit; assess trend
- Detailed history: Diet, types of foods, & eating behaviors
  - PMH: Birth history (premature, SGA, IUGR, short gut), newborn genetic screen
  - FHx: Stature of family members, FTT, mental illness, eating disorders, resp or GI dz
  - SHx: Caregivers, family support, stressors (economic, intrafamilial, major life events), substance abuse, child protective service involvement
- PE: Dysmorphic features, evid. of underlying dz, signs of abuse/neglect
  - Assess severity of malnutrition
- Observe interactions between parent and child, especially during feeding

Diagnostic Studies
- Review 3 d food diary
- Consider referrals (GI, nutrition, feeding eval, OT, PT, SW, psych, genetics)
- No routine lab tests are indicated, unless suggested by the history or physical exam
- General tests to consider include CBC, Chem20, U/A, fecal fat, stool guaiac, sweat chloride test, celiac testing (total IgA, Tissue Transglutaminase (TTG) IgA)

Management
- Outpatient: Dependent upon etiology of FTT
  - Feeding behavior mod w/ high-calorie diet (catch-up growth)
    - 120 kcal/kg × (median weight in kg/current weight in kg) = kcal needed
    - Usually 1.5–2× recom daily caloric intake; catch-up weight precedes height
  - Suppl cals w/ conc. formulas, high-cal milk drinks (PediaSure), calorie-rich foods
  - MVI w/ iron and zinc
  - Structure mealtime
- Inpatient: Pts w/ severe malnutrition (weight <60% of ideal, hypothermia, bradycardia, or HoTN), electrolyte abn, dehydration, failure to achieve catch-up growth w/ outpt mgmt, or if concern for child safety
- Most children resume growth w/ intervention within wks to mos, may require supplemental enteral feeds to increase rapidity of growth

OVERWEIGHT AND OBESITY

(Pediatrics 2007;120:S164; Pediatrics 2007;120:S193; Pediatrics 2007;120:S229; Pediatrics 2007;120:S254)

Definition
- Calculation of body mass index (BMI) = ([weight (kg)]/[height (m)]^2) recommended for screening d/t ease of calculation and correspondence with adult measures
- Age- and sex-specific BMI charts established by CDC in 2000
- BMI categories from the 2007 AAP Expert Committee report
  - <5th percentile: Underweight; 5th–84th percentile: Healthy weight; 85th–94th percentile: Overweight; ≥95th percentile: Obese; ≥99th percentile: Severely obese (cutoff points for ≥99th percentile available at Pediatrics 2007;120:S164)

Prevalence & Epidemiology (JAMA 2006;295:1549; Pediatrics 2010;125:361)
- 33.6% children 2–19 yo overweight [NHANES 2003–2004] and 12–18% of 2–19 yo pts are obese, a three- to six-fold increase from 1970s
- Increased risk among African American and Hispanic populations

Selected Complications of Obesity
- **Respiratory:** Asthma exacerbation, OSA, cardiopulmonary deconditioning
- **Cardiovascular:** HTN, dyslipidemia, pulm HTN and cor pulmonale, inc risk of corona heart disease as adult if still overweight/obese (N Engl J Med 2007;357:2329)
- **GI:** GERD, constipation, gallbladder disease, nonalcoholic fatty liver disease
- **Endocrine:** DM2, PCOS, metabolic syndrome (↑ waist circ + 2 of following: ↑ triglycerid ↓ HDL, HTN, insulin resistance) (Pediatrics 2005;116:473)
- **Orthopedic:** Slipped capital femoral epiphysis, Blount's disease, musculoskeletal stre
- **Dermatologic:** Intertrigo, acanthosis nigricans
- **Neurologic:** Pseudotumor cerebri (idiopathic intracranial hypertension)
- **Psychiatric:** Depression
- Premature death

Clinic Assessment
- USPSTF recommends screening all children >6 yo for obesity using BMI
- Risk factors: SGA at birth, mat gest DM, parental obesity, FHx of DM2/HL/HTN

- Assess diet and physical activity; always check BP
- Labs
  - **Fasting lipids:** See Healthcare Maintenance section
  - **Fasting plasma glucose:** (ADA recs [Diabetes Care 2012;34:S11])
    - <10 yo and prepubertal: No routine screening
    - At onset of puberty if <10 yo or starting at 10 yo: BMI >85th% (or >85% wt for height or wt >120% ideal for height) and any 2 of following: FHx of T2DM in 1st- or 2nd-degree relative; Native American, African American, Latino, or Asian/Pacific Islander ethnicity; signs of or risk for insulin resistance (acanthosis nigricans, HTN, dyslipidemia, PCOS, birth wt was SGA), or maternal diabetes or GDM during child's gestation. Screen q3yr
  - **Transaminases:** Biannually for all pts >95th %ile for BMI or >85th %ile w/ additional risk factors per AAP Expert Committee recs (Pediatrics 2007;120:S164), ALT more important per Endocrine Society recs (J Clin Endo Met 2008;93:4576)

Prevention (Adv Nutr 2012;3:56)

- Diet: Limit sugar-sweetened drinks, encourage fruits and veg, eat QD breakfast, limit eating out, limit portion size, encourage family meals
- Physical activity: Limit TV time ≤2 hr/d, no TV in bedroom, USDA/AAP/CDC recommendation is ≥60 min mod–vigorous physical activity QD, ↓ sedentary activities.

Treatment

- Stages of Rx per AAP Expert Committee recs
  - **Stage 1:** Prevention plus – prev counseling as above w/ qmo f/u 3–6 mo
  - **Stage 2:** Structured weight mgmt – dietitian referral, freq monitoring q3–6 mo
  - **Stage 3:** Comprehensive multidisciplinary intervention – involvement of behavioral counselor and exercise specialist; qwk visits for 8–12 wk
  - **Stage 4:** Tertiary care intervention – very low-cal diets, meds, and/or bariatric surgery for adolescents
- USPSTF recommends referral to intensive weight mgmt program (dietary, physical activity, and behavioral interventions) (Pediatrics 2010;125:361)
- Increased cardiovascular risk from childhood overweight/obesity is not permanent! Data from 4 cohorts demonstrated that non-obese adults who were overweight or obese as children had reduced risks for Type 2 DM, HTN, dyslipidemia, and atherosclerosis similar to those who had been never overweight or obese (N Engl J Med 2011;365:1876)

BREAST-FEEDING

Breast-feeding Rates United States, 2001 (CDC National Immunization Survey 8/1/11; accessed January 2012)

- 74.5% initiate, 44.3% at 6 mo, 23.8% at 1 yr of age
- Goal for Healthy People 2020: 82% initiate, 60.6% at 6 mo, 34.1% at 1 yo

Infant Benefits (Pediatr Rev 2011;32:267; Pediatrics 2012;129:e827)

- Colostrum known as "first immunization" containing high concentrations of antibodies
- ↑ immunity: ↓ AOM, GI infections, hospitalizations for lower respiratory infections, NEC. Effect of maternal immunoglobulins in human milk at mucosal level in mouth, nasopharynx, and GI by blocking entry of microbes; also has anti-inflammatory and anti-oxidant properties, and probiotics that limit growth of intestinal pathogens
- All benefits magnified in pre-term infants and in the developing world
- Long-term benefits: ↓ SIDS, food allergies, atopic dermatitis, asthma, celiac dz, IBD, obesity, DMII, leukemia, and lymphoma; improved neurodevelopmental outcomes, visual and auditory acuity, intelligence scores, teachers ratings

Maternal Benefits

- ↓ risk of breast and ovarian CA, DMII (if no history of gestational diabetes); cumulative breast-feeding >12 mo: ↓ risk for RA, HTN, hyperlipidemia, CV dz
- May facilitate return to pre-pregnancy weight and reduce osteoporosis and postpartum depression but data less clear
- Benefits for infant and mother correlate with dose and duration of breast-feeding

Contraindications

- Infant with classic galactosemia (galactose 1-phosphate uridyltransferase deficiency), maple syrup urine disease, phenylketonuria
- Certain medications: Search function available on LactMed: http://toxnet.nlm.nih.gov/cgi-bin/sis/htmlgen?LACT

- Mother receiving radioactive isotopes until cleared, antimetabolites or chemotherapeutic agents, or those using drugs of abuse. If stable on methadone maintenance OK to BF
- Bacterial mastitis: Allow for maternal comfort and 24 hr of effective antibiotic rx
- HSV, varicella–zoster lesions of the breast (may use other breast if unaffected), consider anti-viral ppx in infant along with anti-viral rx of mother
- HIV infection in developed world (exclusive BFing may provide survival benefit in places where there is lack of clean water, poor availability of formula, and high rate of dehydrating illness)
- Mother w/ HTLV 1 or 2, active untreated pulmonary TB (until infant on INH or mother treated for 2 wk), untreated brucellosis
- Maternal CMV in pre-term or LBW infants: Poss assoc w/ late onset sepsis-like syndrome; antiviral rx may be indicated

NOT Contraindicated
- Maternal Hep B surface antigen positive, Hep C infection (unless co-infected w/ HIV)
- Maternal carriage of CMV for term infants, isolated maternal fever
- Candidal infection of breast; treat both mother and infant and continue BFing

Selected AAP Breast-feeding Recommendations
- Baby Friendly Hospital Initiative (by WHO–UNICEF) endorsed by AAP, promotes 10 steps to successful breast-feeding
- Vitamin D supplementation
  - Begin from birth; 400 IU daily
  - D/c when daily consumption of Vitamin D-fortified formula or milk >500 mL
- Frequency of feeding
  - 8–12 times daily during initiation; 6–8 times daily when well established
- No water needed under 6 mo; no cow's milk until age 1 yr
- Introduced complementary iron-rich foods at 4–6 mo (AAP recs 6 mo for exclusively breast-fed infants), otherwise supplement 1 mg/kg/d iron starting at 4 mo until then
- Follow-up visits
  - Check weight and breast-feeding at 3–5 d and 10–14 d

Breast-feeding Support
- Lactation consultant www.ilca.org, La Leche League www.llli.org

---

COW'S MILK PROTEIN ALLERGY

See Allergy section.

REFLUX

See GI section.

SUDDEN INFANT DEATH SYNDROME (SIDS)

Definition (Pediatrics 2011;128:e1341; Pediatr Rev 2007;28:209)
- Cause assigned to unexplained death of infant <1 yo after thorough eval including scene investigation, autopsy, and review of clinical history. Infant usually previously healthy
- Comprises majority of SUID (sudden unexpected infant death), which is term for all such deaths, whether cause identified or not

Epidemiology
- 2,327 infants in 2006 in US: 3:2 – ♂:♀, Black and American-Indian infant rates double that of white infants. Asian and Hispanic infants rate half of white infants
- Rate ↓ from 1.2 deaths per 1,000 live births in 1992 to 0.57 in 2001, stable since then. AAP issued recs on supine sleeping in 1992, "Back to Sleep" education campaign began in 1994. Changes since 1999 may be related to reclassification of other causes of SUID
- Similarly, prevalence of supine sleep positioning stable since 2001 at 75%
- Third leading cause of death in infancy, top cause of death in 1–12 mo-old age group

Risk Factors
- Prone and side sleeping positions (↑ risk of re-breathing expired gasses), soft bedding, overheating. Risk higher in side sleeping than in prone position
- Maternal smoking during pregnancy and environmental tobacco smoke
- Inadequate prenatal care, young maternal age, prematurity or low birth weight
- Family with one SIDS death has 2–6% risk of a second SIDS death

- **Pathophysiology: Proposed Mechanisms**
  - Convergence of exogenous stressor (i.e., prone position), critical period of development (i.e., immature cardio-respiratory/arousal systems), & vulnerable infant (i.e., LBW) lead to progressive asphyxia, bradycardia, HoTN, met acidosis, ineffectual gasping, and death
  - Re-breathing theory: Prone infants trap exhaled CO_2 around face, ↓ arousal. Some SIDS infants w/ brainstem w/ 5HT-R abn at ventral medulla; ↓ arousal resp to hypercarbia & hypoxia
  - In utero nicotine exposure alters expression of nicotinic acetylcholine receptor in brainstem areas that control autonomic function, depresses recovery from hypoxia, and impairs arousal patterns
  - Some SIDS infants w/ polymorphisms in 5HT transporter gene w/ ↓ [5HT] at synapse
  - Other genes related to QT prolongation and autonomic nervous system development

Differential Diagnosis
- Sepsis, PNA, cardiomyopathy, congenital heart dz, arrhythmia, prolonged QT, accidental or non-accidental trauma, suffocation, and inherited metabolic disorders

Risk Reduction
- Supine sleep position at all times (remind 2° caregivers)
- Firm crib mattress covered w/ single fitted sheet; avoid blankets but if used, should be tucked in 3 sides, not covering the face/head
- Breast-feeding (may reduce risk of SIDS by 50%)
- Avoidance of tobacco, smoke, alcohol, and illicit drug exposure
- Pacifier use confers protection (50–60% ↓ risk). Begin after breastfeeding established
- Room sharing without bed sharing (can reduce risk of SIDS by 50%). No evidence that in-bed co-sleepers reduce risk of SIDS & are not recommended by AAP. Avoid co-bedding of twins and multiples
- Routine immunization (may reduce risk of SIDS by 50%)
- Avoid overheating. (Risk of SIDS may be reduced in well-ventilated rooms, possibly with use of fan)

SKULL DEFORMITIES

Positional skull deformity (Pediatrics 2011;128:136; Clin Pediatr (Phila) 2007;46:292)
- **Etiology:** Limited or selective head rotation + supine position + flat resting surface + rapid skull growth + gravity = positional skull deformity
- **Basic types**
  - Plagiocephaly: From Greek "plagios" for oblique or slanting and "kephalos" for head, asymmetric flattening of occiput w/ anterior displacement of ipsilateral ear, forehead, & cheek; resulting in shape similar to parallelogram; ~70% right sided, not related to handedness
  - Scaphocephaly/dolichocephaly: From Greek "skaphe" for boat or skiff, ↑'d anterior–posterior relative to biparietal diameter, often develops in premies
  - Brachycephaly: From Greek "brakus" for short, ↑'d biparietal relative to AP diameter, can result from symmetric flattening of occiput; more common in Asia
- **Epidemiology:** Depends on criteria used, seems to have ↑'d significantly since AAP's "Back to Sleep" campaign started, likely btw 13–48% of infants under 1 yo
- **Risk factors**
  - Assoc w/ supine pos, male gender, firstborn status, motor delay or ↓ time on abd, ↑ use of car seats/carriers, unvaried feed position "head positional preference"
  - Skull deformity may be present at birth, related to intrauterine constraint (multiples, oligohydramnios, breech), forceps or vacuum use at delivery, prematurity
  - Can also result from or be exacerbated by torticollis or visual deficits
- **Clinical presentation**
  - Vast majority of parents report no flattening of head at birth
  - Flattening noted, worsens between 0–4 mo; typically stabilizes 4–6 mo; becomes less noticeable after 6 mo
  - Flattening of occiput, anterior displacement of ipsilateral ear, forehead, and cheek
  - Head takes on a parallelogram shape
- **Differential:** Lambdoid craniosynostosis presents similarly; rare: Incidence 3 in 100,000
  - In contrast to DP, ear posteriorly displaced ("if the ear is near, steer clear", and refer); head takes on a trapezoidal shape
  - Palpable bony ridge at lambdoid suture, between occipital and parietal bones
- **Diagnosis, prevention, and treatment**
  - Note risk factors, evaluate head shape at each well visit
  - Imaging not needed; assess for torticollis or visual defects

- Prevention: "Tummy time" while awake and observed; alternate position of head (right vs. left occiput) while sleeping supine, as well as feeding position; minimize time in car seat and other supine seating
- Initial Rx: Infant head positioning w/ rounded/non-flattened side against mattress or car seat while sleeping or sitting supine (consider Δ position of infant orientation in crib so that items of visual interest are on non-flattened side), ↑ tummy time
- Physical therapy: Neck stretching if torticollis present (may be underdiagnosed), refer if not improved by 2–3 mo
- Helmet therapy: If deformation severe or no improvement by 4–6 mo with above interventions; may be expensive. Also useful for brachycephaly (symmetric decrease in AP diameter, increase in biparietal diameter) related to supine positioning
- Formal criteria for helmet involve differences in transcranial diagonal diameters
- Decision to refer: Assessment tool available at www.cranialtech.com

Craniosynostosis (Pediatr Clin North Am 2004;51:359; Pediatr Ann 2006;35:365)
- **Etiology:** Premature closure of sutures causing skull deformity
- **Epidemiology:** Uncommon, average incidence of 1 in 2,000
- **Clinical presentation:** Frequently has history of abnormal head shape since birth
  - Head shape depends upon which sutures fuse prematurely (sagittal most common, then coronal, then metopic, then lambdoid; in 13% multiple sutures involved)
  - Head growth restricted in direction perpendicular to prematurely fused suture while compensatory growth occurs parallel to affected suture (Virchow's law)
  - Resulting restriction can lead to ↑ ICP, cognitive, and neurologic deficits
  - Lambdoid craniosynostosis presents similarly to deformational plagiocephaly
    - Rare: Incidence 3 in 100,000
    - In contrast to DP, ear posteriorly displaced ("If the ear is near, steer clear" and refer); head takes on a trapezoidal shape
  - Sagittal craniosynostosis results in scaphalocephaly
    - Most common single suture synostosis, 1 in 5,000, 80% males
    - May cause frontal bossing and prominent occiput
  - Coronal craniosynostosis leads to plagiocephaly if unilateral, brachycephaly if bilateral
    - Most common synostosis assoc with syndrome (Alagille, Apert, Cornelia de Lange, Crouzon, Treacher Collins), typically bilateral
    - Unilateral 60% ♀; freq assoc w/ DDH, micrognathia torticollis; plagiocephaly is anterior, rather than posterior as in positional or lambdoid synostosis
- **Diagnosis and treatment**
  - Immediate referral to neurosurgeon before imaging is appropriate if suspected
  - Treatment is with helmet and/or surgery

NEONATAL JAUNDICE

Introduction (Pediatr Rev 2011;32:341; Pediatrics 2004;114:297)
- Jaundice = yellowing of skin, sclera, and mucous membranes 2/2 deposition of bilirubin, which is produced from the breakdown of hemoglobin (Hgb)
  - Occurs in 2/3 of healthy FT infants; 10% develop severe jaundice (>17 mg/dL)
  - Cephalocaudal progression with increasing bilirubin level (face to trunk to palms and soles): Estimate of level from visual assessment; face = 5 mg/dL, chest = 10 mg/dL, abdomen = 12 mg/dL, and palms/soles >15 mg/dL. Not visible if <4 mg/dL. If above nipple line, level likely <12 mg/dL
  - Need confirmation via transcutaneous or serum bilirubin measurement
- Acute bilirubin encephalopathy (ABE) is the acute manifestation of bilirubin toxicity during the first postnatal weeks
  - Phase 1 (early, first few d): Lethargy, poor feeding, high-pitched cry, hypotonia
  - Phase 2 (intermed, first wk) irritability alternat w/ lethargy; high pitched cry; may see ↑'d extensor tone; backward arching of neck (retrocollis) & trunk (opisthotonos); fever
  - Phase 3 (advanced, after first wk): Stupor to coma; no feeding; shrill cry; hypertonia; retrocollis–opisthotonos; apnea; fever; seizures
- Kernicterus: Chronic/permanent sequelae of bili deposition in basal ganglia & brainstem
  - Athetoid CP, upward gaze paralysis, hi-freq hearing loss/deafness, enamel dysplasia

Bilirubin Metabolism (Pediatr Rev 2006;27:443)

- Reticuloendothelial system: Hgb degraded by heme oxygenase and biliverdin reductase to unconj bilirubin, which binds albumin. Unconj bili fat soluble; able to cross the blood–brain barrier, can be neurotoxic
- Liver: Uridine diphosphate glucuronosyltransferase (UGT 1A1) convert unconj bili to conj bilirubin, conj bile excreted into bile, water soluble, does not cross blood–brain barrier
- Intestine: Much of conj bili hydrolyzed back to unconj form and absorbed into enterohepatic circulation (EH), rest is excreted in stool. Intestinal bacteria reduce conj bili to urobilinogen, reducing EH circulation but newborn gut initially sterile

Pathophysiology (Pediatr Rev 2006;27:443; Pediatr Rev 2011;32:341)

- Hyperbilirubinemia 2/2 ↑ production, ↓ conjugation, or impaired excretion of bilirubin
- ↑ **Bili production** (unconjugated)
  - **Hemolytic** (>6% reticulocyte count, hemoglobin < 13, hepatosplenomegaly)
    - Coombs (+): ABO, Rh, and minor antigen incompatibility
    - Coombs (−): RBC memb defects (spherocytosis), enzyme def (pyruvate kinase, G6PD), Hgb defects (SCD, thal), drugs (streptomycin, Vit K)
  - **Nonhemolytic** (normal reticulocyte count and hemoglobin)
    - Extravascular blood: Cephalohematoma, bruising, CNS bleed
    - Intravascular blood = polycythemia (high Hb/HCT): 2/2 delayed cord clamping, fetal–maternal xfusion, twin–twin xfusion, maternal DM or smoking, high altitude
    - Intestinal = ↑ EH circ; ↓ stooling, CF, Hirschsprung, pyloric stenosis, obstruct
- ↓ **bili conj** (unconj): Breast milk jaundice, hypothyroid, Gilbert and Crigler–Najjar
- **Impaired bilirubin excretion** (conjugated)
  - Biliary obstruction: Biliary atresia, choledochal cyst, 1° sclerosing cholangitis, gallstones, Dubin–Johnson, and Rotor syndromes
  - Metabolic disease: α-1 antitrypsin def, CF, galactosemia, glycogen storage dz, Gaucher, Wilson, Niemann–Pick, genetic dz, Trisomy 21 and 18, Turner
  - Infection: UTI, sepsis, idiopathic neonatal hepatitis, Hep B, TORCH
- ↓ Albumin binding (unconj): Low albumin, meds (CTX, sulfa, steroids), acidosis

Physiologic Jaundice (Pediatr Rev 2006;27:443; Pediatr Rev 2011;32:341)

- Transient elevation of unconj bili after 24 hr of life but w/i first wk 2/2 multi factors
  - Newborn relatively polycythemic, which is resolved by hemolysis
  - Neonatal erythrocytes larger w/ shorter lifespan (70–90 vs. 120 d for adult)
  - Immature liver: ↓ glucuronyl transferase activity and ↓ uptake of unconj bilirubin
  - ↑ EH circ: Sterile neonatal gut does not degrade conj bili, reverts and is reabsorbed
  - Colostrum: Small vol leads to weight loss and slow passage of bili-rich meconium
- Breast-feeding jaundice
  - Early onset; peaks DOL 3–5: 2/2 relative caloric depriv, mild dehyd, and delayed passage of mec; Rx: Inc freq feeds (10×/d w/ formula suppl as needed)
- Breast milk jaundice ("human milk jaundice")
  - Late onset; peaks DOL 6–14; can persist 1–3 mo
  - 2/2 breast milk substances (B-glucuronidases and non-esterified fatty acids), which inhibit normal bilirubin metabolism; actual causal substance unknown
  - Rx: Can interrupt breast-feeding ~2 d (to ↓ bili level, pump in btw), then resume

Pathologic Jaundice (Pediatrics 2004;114:297; Pediatr Rev 2011;32:341)

- Any jaundice w/i 1st 24 hr of life or beyond 21 d, rapid rise Tbili (crossing percentiles in risk nomogram below), Tbili >17 mg/dL in FT newborns, or any evidence of underlying illness should prompt further evaluation

Risk Factors for Development of Severe Hyperbilirubinemia (Pediatrics 2004;114:297; Pediatrics 2009;124:1193)

- Major: Predischarge bili level in high-risk zone (see nomogram below), jaundice in 1st 24 hr, isoimmune or other hemolytic dz, GA <37 wk, prev sibling Rx'd w/ phototherapy (PTX), cephalohematoma/bruising, exclusive breast-feeding, East Asian race
- Minor: Predischarge bili high intermediate-risk, GA 37–38 wk, jaundice seen before discharge, prev sib w/ jaundice, macrosomic infant of diabetic mother, mother >25 yo
- Nomogram for designation of risk (Pediatrics 1999;103:6)

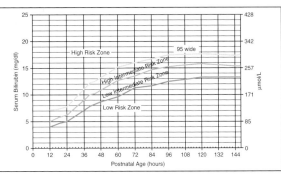

Hyperbilirubinemia Neurotoxicity Risk Factors (Pediatrics 2004;114:297; Pediatrics 2009;124:1193)

- Isoimmune hemolytic dz, G6PD def, asphyxia, sepsis, acidosis, albumin <3mg/dL (gestational age considered separately)
- These risk factors, plus sig lethargy or temp instability, used in determining indications for treatment of hyperbilirubinemia (referred to as "risk factors" in PTX and exchange transfusion figures below)

Evaluation (Pediatr Rev 2011;32:341; Pediatrics 2004;114:297)

- Physical exam
  - Assess for jaundice (cephalocaudal progression)
  - Bruises, pallor, petechiae, hepatosplenomegaly, weight loss, and dehydration
- Labs: Tbili/Dbili, blood type, direct Ab test (Coomb), CBC/diff/smear
  - Consider retic count, G6PD, ETCO2, CF screen, albumin
  - If ↑ conj bili; U/A and cx, consider sepsis eval (blood cx and LP, as well)
  - Persistent hyperbili (>3 wk): Tbili/Dbili review thyroid & galactosemia screen results, eval infant for clinical evidence of hypothyroidism
  - Can use online calculators using Bhutani nomogram; www.bilitool.org

Rx of Unconjugated Hyperbili (N Engl J Med 2008;358:920; Pediatrics 2004;114:297)

- **Phototherapy (PTX):** Light in blue–green spectrum (wavelength 430–490 nm) convert unconj bili to more water-soluble form excreted in bile and urine w/o conjugation
  - Congenital or family history of porphyria is absolute contraindication to PTX
  - If bili does not fall or continues to rise despite PTX, hemolysis is likely
  - Serum albumin <3 lowers threshold to start PTX
  - Can stop PTX when bili is <13–14 mg/dL
  - No need to delay discharge to check rebound bilirubin level (J Pediatr 1998;133:705; Arch Pediatr Adolesc Med 2002;156:669). Check 24 hr after d/c in cases of hemolytic dz, prematurity, or PTX started <72 hr of life (Arch Dis 2006;91:31)

Guidelines for Phototherapy in Hospitalized Infants ≥35 Wk (AAP Guidelines 2004)

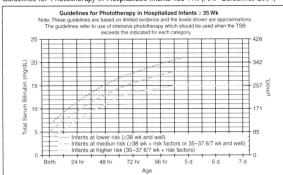

- **Exchange transfusion:** Removes bilirubin and damaged erythrocytes from circulation
  - Reaching exchange transfusion levels (bili ≥25 mg/dL) is a medical emergency
  - In isoimmune hemolytic dz, may avoid exchange transfusion rx w/ IVIG (0.5–1 g/kg over 2 hr), should give if bili is rising despite intensive PTX or if bili level is w/i 2–3 mg/dL of the appropriate exchange level (see below), can repeat dose in 12 hr
  - Immediate exchange transfusion if bili >5 mg/dL above these lines or infant has ABE, also if bili reaches these levels despite intensive PTX
  - Consider exchange if T bili remains above exchange level after 6 hr of intensive PTX
  - Can calculate "bilirubin/albumin" ratio to help determine need for exchange transfusion along w/ other risk factors
    - Infants ≥38 wk: 8; if higher then concerning
    - Infants 35–37.9 wk and well, or ≥38 wk if higher risk or hemolytic dz: 7.2
    - Infants 35–37.9 wk and higher risk, or hemolytic disease: 6.8

Guidelines for Exchange Transfusion in Infants ≥35 Wk (AAP Guidelines 2004)

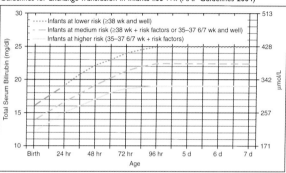

- Pharmacology
  - Phenobarbital and ursodeoxycholic acid lower bili levels by facilitating bile flow
  - Tin-mesoporphyrin – inhibits production of heme oxygenase (not FDA approved)

COLIC

See GI section.

AUTISM SPECTRUM DISORDER (ASD)

(Pediatrics 2007;120:1183; Pediatr Rev 2008;29:86; BMJ 2011;343:d6238)

Introduction
- Neurodevelopmental condition with criteria currently undergoing revision; see below
- ASD includes autistic disorder, Asperger disorder, and pervasive developmental disorder – not otherwise specified – these, plus childhood-disintegrative disorder, likely to be merged into single category of ASD. Rett syndrome would be separate
- CDC: 1 in 88 US children identified, male:female ratio <5:1 (www.cdc.gov/autism)
- Etiology unknown; apparent genetic and nongenetic risk factors include affected parent or sibling, ↑ parental age, genetic/chromosomal conditions like fragile X or tuberous sclerosis; in utero exposure to meds like valproate and SSRIs; prematurity and LBW
- Associated medical problems: Seizures in 20–35%, pica, constipation, feeding problems, and sleep disturbances (BMJ 2011;343:d6238)
- AAP recs early ID (Pediatrics 2007;120:1183)
  - Early intervention improves outcomes (Pediatrics 2010;125(1):e17)
  - Comprehensive eval for identifiable etiology: See below
  - Genetic counseling for parents: ≥4–7% recurrence risk in younger/future sib

Criteria for Dx of Autism (DSM-IV-TR 2000.75) (*Criteria applicable to pt <3 yo)
- Impairment in reciprocal social interaction
  - *Impaired nonverbal behavior (eye contact, facial express, posture, and gestures)
  - *Absent seeking interaction (no pointing, showing, or bringing objects of interest)

- *Lack of social or emotional reciprocity
- Lack of peer relationships
- Impairment in communication
  - *Delay or lack of spoken language (w/o compensation via gestures)
  - If w/ adeq speech, inability to initiate or sustain a conversation
  - Stereotyped and repetitive use of language; lack of make-believe or imitative play
- Repetitive patterns of behavior, interest, and activities
  - Intense preocc w/ stereotyped interest; persistent preocc w/ parts of objects
  - Inflexible adherence to specific routines or ritual's
  - Repetitive motor mannerisms (hand-flapping, whole-body movements)

Proposed DSM-V Revisions: Must meet criteria from A, B, C, and D
(www.dsm5.org/ProposedRevision/Pages/proposedrevision.aspx?rid=94)

- Persistent deficits in social communication & interaction, manifest by all 3
  - Deficits in social-emotion reciprocity (annml social approach, failure of nml back & forth conversation, lack of initiation of social interaction)
  - Deficits in nonverbal communicative behaviors used for interaction (poorly integrated verbal/nonverbal communication, abnml eye contact & body language, deficits in understanding/use of nonverbal comm, lack of facial expression/gesture)
  - Deficits in developing/maintaining relationships (difficulties with adjusting behavior to social context, difficulties in sharing imaginative play, lack of interest in people)
- Restricted, repetitive patterns of behavior, interests, or activities, manifest by 2 of
  - Stereotyped or repetitive speech, motor movements, use of objects
  - Excess adherence to routines, ritualized patterns of behavior, resistance to change
  - Highly restricted fixated interests that are abnml in intensity and focus
  - Hyper-/hyporeactivity to sensory input or fascination with sensory aspects of env
- Symptoms must be present in early childhood
- Symptoms limit and impair everyday functioning
- DSM 5 likely to include all 3 diagnoses under ASD only, subdivided into severity levels

Surveillance and Screening (Pediatrics 2007;120:1183)

- AAP recs surveillance at each well visit (risk factors include sib with autism, pediatrician concern, and parental or other caregiver concern), also screening at 18 and 24 mo with autism-specific screening tool (i.e., M-CHAT for toddlers, SCQ for children >4 yo)
- If autism suspected (two or more risk factors, positive or concerning results on autism screening tool or eval of communication and social skills), refer to autism dx clinic, early intervention (<3 yo) or education services/program (>3 yo), and audiology
- Absolute indications for immed eval: **"Red Flags"** (Neurology 2000;55:468)
  - No babbling, pointing, or other gestures by 12 mo; no single words by 16 mo
  - No 2-word spontaneous phrases (not just echolalia) by 24 mo
  - Any loss of any language or social skills at any age
  - Siblings of children with ASD should undergo heightened surveillance as above

Diagnostic Studies (Pediatrics 2007;120:1183; BMJ 2011;343:d6238)

- Hearing tests (behav audiometrics, middle ear fxn, and electrophys procedures)
- Lead level, Hgb (periodic screening if pica)
- Detailed history (esp family), physical for dysmorphisms, Wood's lamp exam
- Genetic testing (karyotype – either high res or with microarray; chromosomal microarray) and DNA testing for fragile X if pt has GDD/MR, MECP2 testing in girls if concern for Rett
- Targeted studies (selective metabolic testing, EEG, MRI) considered if cyclic vomiting, lethargy, seizures, dysmorphic or coarse facial features, MR, hypopigmented macules, or if newborn screening is inadequate or unavailable
- Consider referral to neurology, genetics, child psych or developmental pediatrician as indicated. Include speech therapists, OT, special ed/IEP, SW
- Ddx includes Down, CHARGE assoc, fragile X, tuberous sclerosis, PKU, fetal alcohol syndrome, Angelman, Rett, and Smith–Lemli–Opitz syndromes

Treatment Approaches: Early initiation is imperative, best outcomes

- Educational approaches: Early start Denver model and TEACCH (improve cognitive performance, language skills, adaptive behavior skills)
- Disruptive behavior best targeted with functional behavioral assessment (IDs modifiable behaviors & teaches new skills and desirable behaviors)
- Speech/language tx (promote functional communication), social skill instruction, occupational therapy
- Tx of psychiatric comorbidities – best data for risperidone, aripiprazole, methylphenidate
  - No 2-word spontaneous phrases (not just echolalia) by 24 mo
  - Any loss of any language or social skills at any age
  - Siblings of children with ASD should undergo heightened surveillance as above

Diagnostic Studies
- Hearing tests (behav audiometrics, middle ear fxn, and electrophys procedures)
- Lead level, Hgb (periodic screening if pica)
- Genetic testing (karyotype) and DNA analysis for fragile X if parents w/ MR, MECP2 testing in young girls if concern for Rett
- Targeted studies (selective metabolic testing, EEG, MRI) considered if cyclic vomiting, lethargy, seizures, dysmorphic or coarse facial features, MR, hypopigmented macules, or if newborn screening is inadequate or unavailable
- Consider referral to neurology, genetics, child psych, or a developmental pediatrician. Include speech therapists, OT, special ed/IEP, SW
- Ddx includes Down, CHARGE assoc, fragile X, tuberous sclerosis, PKU, fetal alcohol syndrome, Angelman, Rett, and Smith–Lemli–Opitz syndromes

Treatment Approaches: Early initiation is imperative for best outcomes
- Educational approaches: Early start Denver model and TEACCH (improve cognitive performance, language skills, adaptive behavior skills)
- Disruptive behavior best targeted with functional behavioral assessment (IDs modifiable behaviors & teaches new skills and desirable behaviors)
- Speech/language tx (promote functional communication), social skill instruction, occupational therapy
- Tx of psychiatric comorbidities – best data for risperidone, aripiprazole, methylphenidate

LEAD SCREENING AND TOXICITY

(Pediatr Rev 2010;31:399; Pediatrics 2005;116:1036; NEJM 2003;348:1517;
Environ Health Perspect 2005;113:894; Pediatrics 2007;120:e1285;
Pediatr Clin North Am 2007;54:271)

Sources of Lead
- Lead paint (banned in US in 1977) chips or dust, contaminated soil or household dust (from exterior paint or prior use of leaded gasoline from nearby traffic)
- Air: Historically important until leaded gas phased out 1973–1986 with >96% reduction in lead levels 1980–2005, now most comes from industrial emissions, esp lead smelters
- Water from lead pipes and solder, also brass fittings; worse if standing/stagnant or hot
- Imported or antique toys, cookware, ceramics
- Imported folk/ethnic/herbal remedies, cosmetics, foods, and spices
- Occupational: Ceramic/glass work, auto/ship repair, plumbing, painting, mining, soldering
- Transplacental (infant lead levels approximate maternal levels)

Lead Screening
- Most at risk: African-American children, pts on Medicaid, lower SES or urban areas, recent immigrants, developmental delays, and repetitive oral behaviors, those w/ siblings with elev lead levels
- Begin 6 mo, assess pt risk (pre-1950 home w/ peeling paint; pre-1978 w/ renovating; sibling or friend w/ toxicity; household adult in high-risk occupation; high-risk home location)
- Children w/ gov assistance (Medicaid, WIC) screen btw 9–12 mo and again at 24 mo
- Non-Medicaid eligible pts, selective screening according to state recs. Screen at age 3 to 6 yo if not screened previously
- Immigrants, refugees, and international adoptees screened upon arrival to US
- Consider screening in all pts w/ PDD, pica, or those who are neglected or abused

Pathogenesis
- Toxic to CNS and PNS, hematopoiesis, kidneys, liver, and endocrine systems; children at inc risk b/c immature blood–brain barrier. Lead interferes with neurotransmission and disrupts cell migration during brain development
- Inhibits enzymes in heme synthesis δ-aminolevulinic acid dehydratase (ALA) and ferrochelatase (resulting in ↑ protoporphyrin levels)
- Inhibits pyrimidine 5' nucleotidase (results in basophilic stippling [BS])

Clinical Symptoms
- **Neuro:** Dev delay, cogn deficits, ADHD, aggression, delinquency, hearing loss, periph neuropathy, encephalopathy (Δ MS, szr, ataxia, papilledema/cerebral edema, coma)
  - IQ decline of 3.9 for levels 2.4–10 mcg/dL, by 1.9 for levels 10–20 mcg/dL, and by 1.1 for levels of 20–30 mcg/dL (Environ Health Perspect 2005;113:894)
  - Relationship nonlinear 2/2 differential lead saturation pathways (highest <10 mcg/dL)

- **Heme:** Microcytic hypochromic anemia, hemolysis (↓ RBC lifespan), BS, inhibits T-cell fxn
- **Renal:** Proximal tubular dysfunction (aminoaciduria, glycosuria, hyperphosphaturia/hypophosphatemia), ↑ risk for adult-onset HTN and CKD
- **GI:** Abd colic, anorexia, vomiting, constipation, lead lines at interface teeth and gingiva
- **Endocrine:** Delayed puberty, growth failure, vitamin D deficiency/osteopenia
- **Ortho:** Lead lines on long-bone radiographs, dental caries, spontaneous abortion, impairs cartilage mineralization

Diagnostic Studies
- Venous lead level (VLL) >10 mcg/dL = + (if capillary >10 mcg/dL need venous confirmation)
  - If lead level is elevated, screen all siblings, housemates, and friends
  - Blood lead levels peak at 18–30 mo, then gradually decline
- Free erythrocyte protoporphyrin or zinc-chelated protoporphyrin: ↑ w/ iron def & lead poisoning (VLLs >30 mcg/dL), may help assess chronicity & response to rxs
- CBC, retic count, iron level, TIBC, ferritin level; if hx ingestion/pica, obtain KUB
- For chelation, check Chem20 and U/A; if w/ dimercaprol or succimer, check G6PD

Management
- No RCTs that chelation improves neurocognitive outcomes; protocols based on clinical judgment and experience

Recommendations for Confirmed Venous Lead Levels	
Level mg/dL	**Recommendations**
Any level	Obtain environmental history; provide risk-reduction and nutrition education. Calcium and iron supplements (prevent lead absorption). Vitamin C (encourages renal excretion of lead); consider zinc therapy. Rearing in nurturing and stimulating env may dec severity of neurotoxicity. Any level >10 must be reported to local department of public health
<10	**Consider retesting within 3 mo**
10–14	**Repeat lead level within 1 mo**
15–19	**Repeat w/i 1 mo.** If the lead level remains 15–19 mcg/dL × 3 mo, proceed according to recs for 20–44 mcg/dL range. Consult w/ Lead Poisoning Prevention Programs (LPPPs) for home investigation and services
20–44	**Repeat w/i 1 wk.** Obtain lead eval: (H&P, env hx, dev assess, eval for iron def anemia, KUB and abd decontam if indicated. Consult w/ LPPPs for home investigation and services) Consider chelation therapy
45–69	**Rpt w/i 24–48 hr.** Refer for chelation w/in 48 hr; relocate to lead-safe environ during chelation. Administer oral succimer (DMSA) at 10 mg/kg q8h × 5 d followed by 10 mg/kg q12h × 14 d. Free erythrocyte or zinc protoporphyrin testing to assess response to tx. **Obtain lead eval**
>70	Immediate hospitalization and chelation. Repeat STAT lead level. Administer dimercaprol 25 mg/kg qd IM divided in 6 doses for min of 72 hr, plus Ca Na2 EDTA for a total of 5 d. Free erythrocyte or zinc protoporphyrin levels. **Obtain lead eval** as above
Never	Test hair, teeth, fingernails for lead; obtain imaging of long bones

Environmental abatement information: www.epa.gov/lead

- **Pharmacologic therapy**
  - Calcium disodium ethylenediaminetetraacetate (EDTA)
    - Indication: VLL 45 mcg/dL or encephalopathy
    - Side effects: Renal dysfunction, hypokalemia; monitoring: For hydration Chem10, UA, and telemetry
    - Contraindications: Anuria
    - If encephalopathic, separate infusion of EDTA and BAL by >4 hr
  - Succimer (DMSA); indication: VLL 45–69 mcg/dL
    - Side effects: Hypersensitivity reactions, GI sx, transient transaminitis, ↓ hemoglobin, reversible neutropenia; monitoring: LFTs and CBC
  - Dimercaprol (BAL = "British anti-Lewisite"): Indication: VLL 70 mcg/dL or lead encephalopathy
    - Side effects: Pain, hemolysis in G6PD, toxic complexes if given w/ iron, HTN, N/V, fever, lacrimation, paresthesia, renal dysfunction, zinc depletion, headache, leucopenia, tachycardia, hyperpyrexia
    - Contraindications: G6PD, hepatic disease, peanut allergy
    - Monitoring: CV and mental status; alkalinize urine during tx

CONTRACEPTION

(Pediatrics 2007;120:1135; Pediatr Rev 2008;29:386)

The Oral Contraceptive Pill (OCP)

- Either combo synthetic estrogen (ethinyl estradiol [EE] or mestranol pro-drug) and progestin (of varying potency) or a progestin only pill (POP)
- Estrogen suppresses gonadotropin surge → prevention of ovulation
- Progestins thicken cervical mucus, alter tubal peristalsis, and create endometrial atrophy → deter sperm motility, egg fertilization, and implantation
- Theoretical failure rate ~0.3%; **typical use failure rate: ~8%**, 2/2 poor adherence
- "Estrogen-dominant" (full-figured, significant menstrual symptoms) pts may benefit from less estrogenic or more potently androgenic pill. "Androgen-dominant" (hirsute, acne, PCOS) pts may benefit from more estrogenic vs. less androgenic
- Generics have equivalent tolerability and efficacy; often significantly more affordable
- New extended-cycle formulations (w/ 1–4 withdrawal bleeds/yr) have good efficacy and can reduce effects of hormone w/drawal
- Benefits: Help tx DUB, dysmenorrheal, acne, hirsutism, PCOS, and dec risk of uterine and ovarian cancers
- Initiate with either monophasic or multiphasic but at low dose estrogen (20–35 mcg) and titrate up as needed after 3-mo trial. Initiate on d 1 of menstrual cycle or on Sunday after menstrual cycle begins; take pill same time every day. Encourage condoms in conjunction with OCPs. F/up 6 wk to 2 mo after initiation

OCP Side Effects, Monitoring, and Contraindications

- Estrogen side effects include blood clots, irregular menses, breast tenderness, fluid retention, nausea, increased appetite, headache, and hypertension (can trial pill containing lower estrogen dose)
- Progestin effects include menstrual Δ, bloating, mood Δ, HA, nausea, weight gain. Drospirenone (in Yasmin) has diuretic and antiandrogenic activity; caution in pts at risk of hyperK+ or with renal insufficiency
- Androgenic side effects (less common; incl acne, hirsutism, male pattern hair loss)
- Class IV contraindications: H/o DVT, PE, CVA, AMI, Factor V Leiden or other thrombophilia, migraine w/ aura or neurologic changes. (Refer to complete WHO guidelines at http://www.who.int/reproductive-health/publications/mec/3_cocs.pdf)

Other Options

- **Vaginal rings:** (NuvaRing®) Combined hormone-containing silicone ring, hormones absorbed vaginally, avoids 1st-pass metab. Intravaginal 3 wk, ↑ rate of pt satisfaction
- **Transdermal:** Absorb E&P through skin; less effective in pts >90 kg, avoids 1st-pass metab
  - Each patch should be worn for 7 d before replacing, on a new site each time
  - FDA warning: 60% more total estrogen in patients' blood c/w 35 mcg OCP
- **Injectable:** Depot medroxyprogesterone acetate (progestin only, Depo-Provera) IM q3mo, ↓ reliance on pt adherence
  - High discontinuation 2/2 side effects (menstrual irreg, wt gain, ↓ in bone density)
  - Fertility can take up to 10 mo to return
  - Combined injectable contraceptives injected q1mo and offer advantage of both improved adherence w/o side effect profile of progestin only injections
- **Subdermal contraceptive implants:** Progestin-only rod (Implanon) inserted below the skin, effective for up to 3 yr. Fertility returns promptly after removal
  - Irregular bleeding is a common side effect, but diminishes with continued use
- **Intrauterine devices (IUD)**
  - The levonorgestrel-releasing IUD has been approved for up to 5 yr of use
  - Copper-containing IUD acts via a local inflammatory response
  - Chance of ectopic pregnancy is <1:1,000 women yr of use
  - Causes reduction in bleeding (amenorrhea by 1 yr in many users)
  - Recommended in parous women with no h/o PID or ectopic preg, in monogamous relationships

Emergency Contraception (EC)

- POPs (Plan B), combined OCPs, mifepristone (not available in US)
- Methods interfere w/ : Ovulation, follicular development, and corpus luteum maturation. No evidence of effect on implantation or postovulatory events
- The sooner the better. In general, EC initiated w/i 72 hr of unprotected intercourse ↓ risk of pregnancy by ≥75%. Effectiveness shown for up to 120 hr after unprotected sex
- Plan B (OTC) consists of 2 × 0.75 mg tabs of LNG q12 hr. Single dose (1.5 mg) administration has similar effectiveness (Cochrane Database Syst Rev 2008;16;(2))

- "Yuzpe regime": Uses OCPs as EC (less effective, large # pills, ↑ side effects)
- Patients may experience vaginal spotting, nausea/vomiting after use of EC

GYNECOLOGIC EXAM

(Pediatrics 2010;126(3):583)

Background
- External genital exam should be conducted at all annual exams. No speculum/bimanual exam required prior to rx of hormonal contraception (can test urine hCG and STIs)
- STI testing now urine or vaginal swab based; does not require speculum exam
- Current guidelines for Pap test: At age 21, unless HIV+ or immune suppressed for which paps initiated at onset of sexual activity
- Despite high exposure to HPV, most sexually active adolescents clear infection without intervention; avoids potential pregnancy complications in future
- Low grade lesions and ASCUS followed by repeat Pap at 1 yr intervals; colpo only for persistent abnormality or high grade lesion over 2 yr period

Indications for Pelvic Exam
- Persistent vaginal discharge, dysuria in sexually active teen, dysmenorrheal unresponsive to NSAIDs, amenorrhea, abnml vaginal bleeding, lower abdominal pain, IUD or diaphragm placement, suspected rape/sexual abuse, pregnancy, pap test

EATING DISORDERS

(Pediatr Rev 2011;32:508; Pediatr Rev 2006;27:5)

Definition

Criterion	DSM-IV Anorexia Nervosa
Body weight	Refusal to maintain wt ≥85% expected for ht/age (DSM-V proposed change: Restriction of caloric intake leading to signif low body wt). Restrictive and binge/purging types
Menstruation	Absence of 3 consecutive menstrual cycles in postmenarchal females (DSM-V likely excludes this criterion)
Fear of wt gain	Intense fear of (DSM-V: OR persistent behavior to avoid) wt gain though underweight (DSM-V: Significant low-weight)
Body image	Disturbance in way or body shape is experience; denial of seriousness of condition; undue influence of wt/shape in self-perception (DSM-V: No change)
Criterion	DSM-IV Bulimia Nervosa
Binge eating	Eating large amounts in discrete period (2 hr), larger than average
Compensatory behavior	Recurrent self-induced vomiting, laxative use, diuretics, enemas, fasting, or excess exercise to prevent wt gain
Frequency	Binging/compensatory behavior at least 2×/wk for 3 mo (DSM-V: binge/compen behav on avg ≥1×/wk for 3 mo
Self-evaluation	Overly influenced by body shape/weight

- **Eating disorder NOS:** Pts meet some, not all of diagnostic criteria for above EDs, includes binge eating disorder (lack compensatory behaviors)
- **Female athlete triad:** Hypothalamic amenorrhea, osteoporosis, low energy availability (+/- eating disorder) in female athlete. Low body fat → ↓estrogen → amenorrhea and low bone mineral density
- Approximation of IBW ♀: 100 lb for 60 in., + 5 lb each added in.; ♂: 106 lb for 60 in., + 6 lb for each in. (Pediatr Rev 2006;27:5)
- Expected wt (kg) for adolescent: (Height in meters)^2 × 50th percentile BMI for age and sex

Epidemiology
- AN: 0.9% of ♀, 0.3% of ♂. BN: 1.5% ♀, 0.5% of ♂. EDNOS: 3.5% in ♀, 2% of ♂
- Caucasian and Asian females > African-American and Latino
- Evidence for moderate to substantial heritability. Risk factors: Obese girls or early puberty, perfectionism, concerns over self-control, low self-esteem, past hx of abuse, certain sports (cheerleading, gymnastics, running)
- Suicidality and cardiac complications are leading causes of death

Evaluation: Eating Disorders Examination-Questionnaire (http://www.psychiatry.ox.ac.uk/research/researchunits/credo/assessment-measures-pdf-files/EDE-Q6.pdf)

- Hx obtain past, current, and ideal body weight; eating patterns, binge/purge, restrictive and other behaviors, exercise hx, body image concerns, menstrual hx; confirmation from family as patients may be manipulative
- ROS and PMH assess sx of malnutrition (i.e., constipation, feeling cold or faint), vomiting (chest pain, hematemesis)
- Assess for comorbid mental illness: Major depression, anxiety disorders, OCD, anxiety disorder, social phobia, other mood disorders, substance use, high-risk sexual behavior; ask about **suicidality**
- Labs: CBC, CMP, TSH, amy/lipase, ESR, hCG. Consider LH/FSH, estradiol, prolactin
- ECG if electrolyte abn, cardiac symptoms, significant weight loss, or bulimia
- Radiographic studies (upper or lower GI, abd, and/or head imaging) when indicated
- DEXA recommended if amenorrhea >6 mo, annually if amenorrhea persists

Medical Complications/Physical Findings

- Derm/orofacial: Erosion of tooth enamel/cavities, parotid gland hypertrophy, calluses on knuckles (Russell sign), hypercarotenemia, alopecia, acne, lanugo, halitosis
- Metabolic derangements: **Hypernatremia** 2/2 restricted intake; **hyponatremia** 2/2 water loading; **hypokalemic, hypochloremic metabolic alkalosis** 2/2 vomiting, and diuretics; **hypophosphatemia** as part of **refeeding syndrome** in rx phase
- Cardiac: **Bradycardia**, HoTN, orthostasis, **arrhythmia**, prolonged QT, MV prolapse/murmur, pericardial effusion, cardiomyopathy and CHF, sudden cardiac death
- Pulmonary: Aspiration PNA and PTX from forceful vomiting, pulm edema 2/2 refeeding
- GI: Vague abn pain, constipation, delayed gastric emptying, esophageal irritation and chest pain, hematemesis 2/2 Mallory–Weiss tears/esoph rupture, gallstones, rectal prolapse, SMA syndrome, LFT abn, usually nml albumin (if ↓, eval for other dx)
- GU: Renal stones, atrophic vaginitis, atrophy of genitalia
- Neuro: Szr (hypoNa), peripheral neuropathy, brain atrophy, long-term neurocog abn
- Endocrine: ↓LH/FSH and estrogen, amenorrhea, **osteopenia, and osteoporosis (fractures);** ↓ thyroid fxn (hypothermia), often sick euthyroid
- Heme/immuno: Mild anemia (folate or iron def), ↓ ESR, WBC, plt count, altered immunologic markers

Treatment: Requires multidisciplinary team; use of eating disorder protocol with privileges as incentives. Often stabilized inpatient, transferred to residential tx center.

- Monitoring and rx of electrolyte disarray, sudden death may occur from hypoK
- Cautious nutritional support in severely malnourished (<30% below IBW) to avert **refeeding syndrome** (hypoPhos, fluid and electrolyte shifts, edema, CHF, arrhythmia, stupor, hemolysis, ATN, coma). Start w/ 1,000–1,600 kcal/d, ↑ by 200–400 kcal daily, monitor and supplement phosphorous. Goal wt gain ~1/2 lb/d. May require NGT or PN feedings
- **Criteria to hospitalize in AN:** <75% IBW or refractory weight loss despite intensive mgmt, refusal to eat, body fat <10%, HR <50 bpm AM, <45 bpm PM, SBP <90 mm Hg, orthostatic by HR (>20 bpm) or BP (>10 mm Hg), T < 96° F (35.6°C), arrhythmia, electrolytes abnml, suicidality
- **Criteria to hospitalize in bulimia:** Syncope, K < 3.2 mEq/L, Cl < 88 mEq/L, esophageal tears, arrhythmia or ↑QTc, hypothermia, suicidality/cutting, intractable vomiting, hematemesis, failure to respond to outpatient treatment
  Psych mgmt w/ therapy (CBT, psychotherapy, family therapy) and/or medications (i.e., SSRIs – fluoxetine in particular in bulimia)
  Rx MVI with 400–800 IU Vit D and 1,200 mg Calcium, PPI if GERD, toothpaste with sodium bicarb if vomiting. No data to support use of OCPs to prevent bone loss

Prognosis

Recovery in 46% of AN patients, 45% of bulimia pts; 20 and 23% respectively, had chronic course. Mortality: 5% in AN and 0.32–3.9% for bulimia, 5.2% for EDNOS

(For more information, see specific sections in other chapters.)

Asthma (guidelines at http://www.nhlbi.nih.gov/guidelines/asthma/index.htm.)

(See PICU and Pulmonary chapters for further management)

- Management based on respiratory rate, retractions, ability to speak or cry, oxygen sat, FEV_1, peak flow (FEV_1, peak flow not practical for most settings)
- Use results to determine single neb vs. 3 stacked doses of albuterol & ipratropium
  - Evidence shows equiv of nebs and MDI w/ spacer (Pediatr Emerg Care 1996;12:263; J Pediatr 2004;145:172), in practice most ERs administer nebs. (Keep HR <200)
  - Prednisone/prednisolone IV/PO 1–2 mg/kg. (Guidelines for Diagnosis and Management of Asthma, NIH 2007 at website above)
    - IV preferred if severely ill, or if unable to PO
    - Max dosing is 60 mg PO/IV
  - O_2 to keep SpO_2 >92%; further treatment based on response to initial management
- Risk factors for asthma-related death: ICU admit, intubation, 2 hospitalizations or 3 ER visits in the past yr, low SES, inner city, high routine use albuterol, illicit drug use, psych dz
- **Management** (EPR3: Guidelines for Diagnosis and Management of Asthma, NIH 2007)
  - **See figure in the next page**

Supraventricular Tachycardia (Pediatric Advanced Life Support, 2010; Pediatr Emerg Care 2007;23:176)

(See PICU and Cardiology chapters for further management)

- Suspected when HR >180 in children, >220 in infants
- Incidence of 1–4 per 1,000
- Distinguishing SVT from sinus tachycardia:

	ST	SVT
HR	Infants <220 Children <180	Infants >220 Children >180
Beat-to-beat interval	Variable	Fixed
P waves	Visible, normal axis	Abn axis; often hidden in QRS/ST
Onset	Gradual	Abrupt
Vagal maneuver	Gradual slowing, then returns	Abrupt termination
Cardioversion response	None	Abrupt conversion
Fever	Strongly associated	2–3% of patients have fever

- **Management** (continuous EKG monitoring recommended)
  - Immediate assessment of hemodynamic status and obtain an EKG
  - Obtain large bore IV access as close to central circulation as possible
  - **Unstable** (i.e., poor perfusion, low BP, respiratory distress, ΔMS)
    - Synchronized cardioversion: 0.5–1 J/kg in synch mode (if narrow complex)
      - If ineffective, can ↑ to 2 J/kg. Consider sedation & analgesia when possible
    - Can attempt vagal maneuvers or adenosine while preparing for cardioversion
  - **Stable** (i.e., nml cap refill, BP, mental status, and no evidence of respiratory distress/CHF)
    - Attempt **vagal maneuvers**
      - Infants: Ice water on forehead, eyes, nose for 10–15 sec (33–62% effective)
      - Children: Valsalva for 15 sec while supine (blow into occluded straw; thumb)
        – OR –
    - **Adenosine** 0.1 mg/kg IV (max 6 mg initial dose) infused as fast as possible a a site closest to central circ, followed by flush (72–77% effective)
      - If no effect, ↑ 0.2 mg/kg then 0.3 mg/kg q1–2min until effect or max dose (12 mg); if administered in central line, use $^1/_2$ dose
        – OR –
    - **Synchronized cardioversion:** 0.5–1 J/kg. If ineffective, can ↑ to 2 J/kg. Consider sedation and analgesia whenever possible
  - **Refractory SVT (stable patient).** Obtain cardiology consult and consider:
    - **Amiodarone** 5 mg/kg IV/IO load over 20–60 min. Max dose 300 mg. May repeat up to 15 mg/kg (max daily dose). Alternatively 5 mg/kg IV loading dos in incremental doses of 1 mg/kg IV for 5–10 min
      – OR –
    - **Procainamide** 15 mg/kg IV over 30–60 min. Do not use routinely with amiodarone

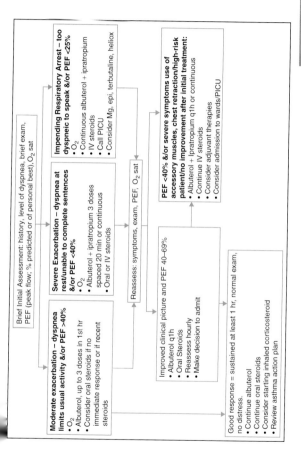

ED-Asthma 2-2

Brief Initial Assessment: history, level of dyspnea, brief exam, PEF (peak flow; % predicted or of personal best), O₂ sat

Moderate exacerbation – dyspnea limits usual activity &/or PEF >40%
• O₂
• Albuterol, up to 3 doses in 1st hr
• Consider oral steroids if no immediate response or if recent steroids

Severe Exacerbation – dyspnea at rest/unable to complete sentences &/or PEF <40%
• O₂
• Albuterol + ipratropium 3 doses spaced 20 min or continuous
• Oral or IV steroids

Impending Respiratory Arrest – too dyspneic to speak &/or PEF <25%
• O₂
• Continuous albuterol + ipratropium
• IV steroids
• Call PICU
• Consider Mg, epi, terbutaline, heliox

Reassess: symptoms, exam, PEF, O₂ sat

Improved clinical picture and PEF 40-69%
• Albuterol q1h
• Oral Steroids
• Reassess hourly
• Make decision to admit

PEF <40% &/or severe symptoms use of accessory muscles, chest retraction/high-risk patient/no improvement after initial treatment:
• Albuterol + ipratropium q1h or continuous
• Continue IV steroids
• Consider adjuvant therapies
• Consider admission to wards/PICU

Good response = sustained at least 1 hr, normal exam, no distress.
• Continue albuterol
• Continue oral steroids
• Consider starting inhaled corticosteroid
• Review asthma action plan

Shock/Hypotension (Pediatr Rev 2010;31:311)

(See PICU chapter for further management)

- Shock is a state w/ inadeq delivery of O_2 and nutrients to meet the demand, best assessed by end-organ fxn and perfusion (mental status, UOP, capillary refill) (*Pediatric Emergency Medicine*, 2nd ed. McGraw-Hill 2002:60)
- Final common pathway of multiple dz processes (sepsis, anaphylaxis, dehydration, etc.)
  - Preterm babies on DOL # 1, MAP should be equal to gestational age
  - Lower limit SBP in full-term babies: At 1–2 kg 50 mm Hg, at 3–10 kg 60 mm Hg
  - Lower limit SBP in infant/child ≥10 kg 70 mm Hg (+ 2× age in yr, when age ≤10)
  - **Clinical manifestations:** Hx volume loss (vomiting, diarrhea, polyuria, or trauma w/ blood loss), febrile illness (sepsis), exposure to antigen (allergy), spinal trauma
  - Exam w/ early ↑HR and often ↑RR (metabolic acidosis compensation), SBP may be preserved 2/2 significant peripheral vasoconstriction (w/ cap refill >2 sec). Later w/ obtundation and poor periph pulses
- Tachycardia is often the earliest and most sensitive sign of early shock but it is nonspecific; hypotension itself is often a late and ominous finding

	Specific HX and Exam	Cardiac Output	Peripheral (systemic) Vasoconstriction	Management
Hypovolemic	Volume loss (diarrhea, vomiting, polyuria, blood loss)	↓	↑	Volume replacement (NS bolus 20 cc/kg × 3, then RBC transfusion)
Septic – Early – Late	Fever, infectious source (indwelling lines, PNA, etc.)	↑ ↓	↓ (warm) ↑ (cold)	Initially w/ volume, then Abx and pressors (see PICU chapter)
Cardiogenic	Hx of congenital heart dz, sweats w/ feeds, etc.	↓	↑	Eval for pulm edema; if no rx w/ volume; cards consult
Distributive	Spinal cord trauma Allergic exposure (w/ assoc rash, etc.) Toxin (drug) related	↑	↓	Initially w/ volume – Epinephrine w/ anaphylaxis – Pressors for neurogenic shock

- Also consider **obstructive shock** 2/2 tamponade, massive PE, tension PTX; if present treat underlying etiology
- **Diagnostic studies:** Consider stat CBC, glucose, K, Ca, lactate, ABG, SvO_2
- **Management:** Obtain large bore IV access and give NS 20 cc/kg bolus, repeat up to 3×, then consider blood products. If unable to obtain IV access, obtain IO access
  - Patient may need ventilatory support to ensure adequate oxygenation
  - Pressors: Often dopamine 2–20 mcg/kg/m (can use peripherally) (see PICU chapter)
    - Ensure pt is euvolemic before initiation of pressors
    - In pts who are volume & pressor unresponsive, consider IV stress dose steroids
    - In pts w/ evidence of anaphylaxis (urticarial rash, airway involv) use epinephrine
    - Central access is required for the use of most pressors

Seizures (Emerg Med Clin North Am 2007;25:1061)

(See PICU and Neurology chapters for further management)

- **Etiology:** Infectious (febrile, meningitis, brain abscess), neurologic (hypoxic-ischemic encephalopathy, VP shunt malfxn, neurocutaneous syn), metabolic (electrolyte abn, hypoglycemia, hypoxia, inborn errors of metab), trauma (abuse, ICH), tox, neoplasm
- **Febrile seizure:** Seizure w/ febrile illness in pt aged 6 mo–5 yo
  - Simple if <15 min, single episode and generalized seizure, non-focal neuro exam
  - Complex if >15 min, recurs within 24 hr or focal seizure
- **Partial szr** arises in 1 hemisphere, is focal, and classified as simple if consciousness is not impaired (just motor or sensory effect) and complex if consciousness is altered
- **Generalized szr** both hemispheres; consciousness depressed; convulsive or nonconvulsive
- **Status epilepticus:** Continuous seizure >30 min or >1 seizures w/o return to baseline
- **Evaluation and Management:**
  - ABCs (support as needed), check finger stick glucose and temperature, pertinent history: h/o szr, anti-epileptics, family history, medications and toxins, recent illness, trauma, obtain IV or IO access, recheck ABCs

- If febrile, treat fever & infectious w/u based on age. If afebrile, call neurology
- Lorazepam 0.05–0.1 mg/kg IV (max 4 mg); rpt q5min to max total dose 10 mg in 20 min; place patient on their side to avoid aspiration
  - Reassess ABCs and need for airway support after each dose
  - Diazepam, (2–5 yr 0.5 mg/kg; 6–11 yr 0.3 mg/kg; >11 0.2 mg/kg PR; max 5–10 mg), less effective and leads to more respiratory depression than lorazepam
- After 2 doses of lorazepam; consider fosphenytoin 20 PE/kg IV; after fosphenytoin consider levetiracetam 25–50 mg/kg IV (Pediatr Neurol 2009;41:37)

STRIDOR

STRIDOR 2-4

Definition
- High-pitched sound of turbulent airflow in upper airway indicates airway obstruction
  - Inspiratory stridor usually indicates obstruction above the vocal cords
  - Expiratory stridor usually indicates obstruction below the vocal cords

Differential Diagnosis
- Causes include croup, epiglottitis, and bacterial tracheitis (BT may be the most freq life-threatening upper airway infection currently) (Pediatrics 2006;118:1418)
- Consider differential diagnosis anatomically based on inspiratory or expiratory stridor
- **Nose:** Inspiratory stridor, snoring; in neonates consider choanal atresia
- **Pharynx:** Gurgling/muffled voice
  - Afebrile: Macroglossia, micrognathia, tonsil/adenoid hypertrophy
  - Febrile: Retropharyngeal/peritonsillar abscess
- **Larynx:** High-pitched inspiratory stridor, voice change, hoarseness
  - **Afebrile:** Laryngomalacia, laryngeal web, cyst, vocal cord paralysis, laryngotracheal stenosis, intubation, foreign body, cystic hygroma, subglottic hemangioma, laryngospasm, psychogenic stridor, vocal cord paralysis
  - **Febrile:** Croup, epiglottitis
- **Trachea:** Insp & exp stridor: Tracheomalacia, bact tracheitis, external compression, TEF

Croup (Laryngotracheobronchitis)
- Characterized by barking cough, +/– inspiratory stridor, +/– respiratory distress
  - Peak incidence 1–2 yo, Sept to Dec, M > F. Parainfluenza virus accounts for >50%, the next most common cause is RSV (Pediatrics 1983;71:871)
- **Mild:** Dexamethasone 0.6 mg/kg PO/IM ↓ rpt visits, length of sx, and parental stress, and ↑ sleep (N Engl J Med 2004;351:1306). Also consider cool mist, hydration, & antipyretics
- Can use oral prednisolone 1–2 mg/kg PO; $t_{1/2}$ of prednisolone 24 hr; $t_{1/2}$ of Dex 32 hr
- **Moderate to severe:**
  - Mist tent or humidified oxygen near child's face (not supported by Cochrane review)
  - Dexamethasone 0.6 mg/kg PO/IM/IV (N Engl J Med 1998;339:498; meta-analysis in BMJ 1999;319:595)
    - Equivalence of PO vs. IM dosing shown in study of moderate croup. (Pediatrics 2000;106:1344)
  - Racemic epi (2.25%) 0.05 mL/kg/dose in 3 mL NS (max 0.5 mL) q15 min up to 3× PRN, watch HR (Pediatrics 1992;89:302)
    - Cochrane review (CD006619) supported benefit at 30 min post-nebulized epi but not at 2 hr and 6 hr post though decreased rate of hospitalization
    - If epi given, need obs (effects wears off in 2 hr). Obs in ED for min 4–6 hr
    - Decrease epi dose for known cardiac disease

Epiglottitis
Usually 2/2 Hib. Incidence of Hib ↓ by >99% since intro of conj vaccine in 1998 (MMWR 2002;51:234). P/w toxic child, drooling, sitting forward, stridor
True emergency requiring immediate intubation in controlled environment (if possible), any manipulation of child may cause full obstruction
Give O_2 as accepted by child, allow parent to accompany child to allay anxiety
Summon senior pediatrician, anesthesiologist, and ENT or pediatric surgeon
If **unstable,** intubate emergently; bag-mask w/ high pres, may need to disable pop-off
If **stable** with **high suspicion** (toxic, febrile, leaning forward, audible stridor, uncertain vaccination record) escort pt to OR for laryngoscopy/intubation

- If **moderate/low suspicion,** obtain lat neck x-ray (thumbprint sign), will agitate them
- Once **airway is secure,** check CBC/diff, cx of blood and epiglottis, start Abx (such as ceftriaxone) covering Hib, S. pneumo, and Grp A strep

Bacterial Tracheitis (Pediatrics 2006;118:1418; Emerg Med Clin North Am 2007;25:961)

- Commonly seen in fall/winter, 6 mo–8 yr
- **Presentation:** Viral prodrome followed by acute onset of toxic appearance, high fever (mean 101.8°F/38.8°C), cough, resp distress. Unlikely to drool, may be able to lie flat
- **Management:** To OR for endoscopy to obtain sample for GS and cultures and intubation. If intubating in ER consider smaller ETT than usual because of airway edema
  - Abx to cover S. aureus, S. pneumo, M. catarrhalis, H. flu, and alpha-hemolytic strep
  - CXRs usually normal or similar to croup (steeple sign), blood cx usually negative

Lemierre's Disease (Pediatr Crit Care Med 2003;4:107; Am J Otolaryngol 2010;31:38; J Emerg Med 2010;39:436; J Clin Microbiol 2003;41:3445)

- Jugular vein suppurative thrombosis preceded by pharyngitis or dental infections; internal jugular vein thrombophlebitis leads to metastatic complications; most commonly caused by Fusobacterium necrophorum; may present with respiratory distress
- Criteria for diagnosis:
  - Previous oropharyngeal infection
  - Septicemia following oropharyngeal infection
  - Swelling or unilateral tenderness of the neck, jaw
  - Metastatic abscesses to the lung, liver, kidneys, or joints
  - Fusobacterium necrophorum isolated from blood cultures or abscess aspiration
  - Rapid progression
- Diagnostic procedures: Blood culture, ultrasound, CT neck with contrast
- Treatment: ABCs, antibiotics, e.g., ampicillin–sulbactam and metronidazole. Consider surgery and anticoagulation

Diagnostic Studies for Stridor in General

- Initial eval w/ CXR lat/AP neck film; ENT (direct laryngoscopy), consider fluoro if available. Determine cause: Start initial management, but etiology can define specific treatments

ANAPHYLAXIS

(Pediatr Emerg Care 2007;23:49; J Allergy Clin Immunol 2010;126:477)

Definition (Pediatrics 2000;106:762; J Allergy Clin Immunol 2006;117:391)

- Anaphylaxis is a serious systemic reaction, which is rapid in onset and may cause death
  - IgE hypersensitivity 2/2 systemic mediator from sensitized mast cells & basophils
  - **Uniphasic reaction** occurs immediately after exposure
  - **Biphasic reaction** includes a recurrence of sx that develops after resolution of initial reaction. 1–20% of anaphylaxis episodes & occur btw 8–72 hr after initial reaction
  - **Protracted reaction:** Any anaphylaxis episode lasting for hrs to d beyond initial rxn

Symptoms of Anaphylaxis

Skin	Diaphoresis, flushing, pruritus, urticaria, warm sensation, angioedema
Respiratory	Oropharynx/lip tingling or itching, throat/chest tightness, hoarseness, stridor, wheezing, dyspnea, respiratory failure
GI	Nausea, diarrhea, vomiting, cramps
CV	Arrhythmias, hypotension, shock, arrest
Neuro	Dizziness, visual changes, tremor, disorientation, syncope, seizures
Others	Impending sense of doom, metallic taste, rhinorrhea, tearing

Criteria for Anaphylaxis

- Highly likely when any 1 of the following 3 criteria is fulfilled:
  - Acute onset (min to hrs) involving skin &/or mucosal tissue & ≥1 of following:
    - Respiratory compromise (e.g., dyspnea, wheeze, stridor, hypoxemia)
    - Reduced SBP or assoc sx of end-organ hypo-perfusion (syncope, hypotension)

- ≥2 of the following occurring rapidly (min to several hrs) after exposure to allergen
  - Skin &/or mucosal involv (hives, itching, flushing, & swollen lips, tongue, or uvula)
  - Reduced SBP or associated symptoms of end-organ hypo-perfusion
  - Respiratory compromise
  - Persistent GI symptoms
- Reduced SBP after exposure to a **known** allergen for that pt (min to several hrs)

Management

- Remove allergen. ABCs; CVR/O₂ monitor, continuous BP monitor. Place patient in recumbent position with the lower extremities elevated if tolerated
  - IM epinephrine is first line treatment (1:1,000 solution, 0.01 mg/kg [0.01 mL/kg] max 0.3 mg [0.3 mL])
    - Repeat q5–15min as needed
    - Consider epinephrine infusion for persistent hypotension
  - Supplemental oxygen
  - Obtain IV/IO access: Aggressive volume resuscitation, start with 20 cc/kg and repeat for orthostasis, hypotension or incomplete response to IM epinephrine
  - Inhaled β₂-agonists for wheeze
  - H₁ blocker: Diphenhydramine IV (1.25 mg/kg/dose, up to 50 mg/dose); works for urticaria and pruritis, will not help with respiratory symptoms, GI symptoms, or shock
  - H₂ blocker: Ranitidine IV (0.5–1 mg/kg, up to 50 mg/dose)
  - Corticosteroids:
    - Methylprednisolone IV 1–2 mg/kg up to 125 mg/dose
- **Observation:** Usual observation is 6–8 hr
- Tryptase level: Consider sending within 4–6 hr of presentation for unclear cases to improve diagnostic accuracy Tryptase levels can be normal during food anaphylaxis. Remember that tryptase levels will not help you in the acute setting
- **Therapy for patient at discharge:**
  - First line therapy EpiPen (0.3 mg) for pts >30 kg and EpiPenJr (0.15 mg) for pts 15–30 kg. Consider EpiPenJr for pts <10 kg. (Visit www.epipen.com for helpful information.) If used as outpatient, must return to the ED
  - Second line therapy:
    - Corticosteroids: Prednisone daily for 2–3 d
    - H₁ blocker: Diphenhydramine: Every 6 hr for 2–3 d
    - H₂ blocker: Ranitidine: Twice a d for 2–3 d
    - Avoidance of allergen
    - Follow-up with primary care physician and consider referral to allergist

ALTE 2-6

APPARENT LIFE-THREATENING EVENT (ALTE)

Definition (Pediatr Clin North Am 2005;52:1127)
- Described as an event frightening to the observer and including any of the following:
  - **Apnea:** Central (no resp effort) or obstructive (breath w/ paradox inverse motion of chest/abd and ↓ O₂ sat by 3%). Apnea >20 sec or shorter w/ ↓ HR or hypotonia
    - CHIME study (1,079 infants on home card-resp monitors) – 43% w/ apnea and bradycardia >20 sec w/o diff in freq btw "healthy" infants and those w/ Hx idiopathic ALTE requiring vigor stim and CPR. # events >30 sec similar in both groups (Pediatr Rev 2007;28:203)
  - **Change in color:** Central cyanosis (>5 g/dL deoxy-hgb) w/ bluish lips or tongue
    - Distinguished from acrocyanosis (bluish color of hands and feet) & circumoral cyanosis; both of which are benign in the absence of other signs of shock or sepsis
  - **Change in muscle tone**
  - **Coughing or gagging**
  May or may not require stimulation to resolve (includes being picked up by caregiver)
  Uncomplicated ALTEs not related to SIDS (in fact, ALTEs and SIDS have different risk factors. Campaigns that have dec rates of SIDS have had no impact on ALTEs)

Incidence (Am Fam Physician 2005;71:2301; Pediatr Clin North Am 2005;52:1127)
0.01–0.5%; by definition <1 yo (most <10 wk); though limited data
Etiology determined in 77% of cases in 1 meta-analysis (though ranging from 9–83% among the studies evaluated) (Arch Dis Child 2004;89:1043)
Risk factors: Repeated apnea, pallor, Hx of cyanosis, feeding difficulties, prematurity

Diagnostic Studies
- Review of 239 cases; 17.7% of tests + 5.9% contributed to dx (Pediatrics 2005;115:885)
- **High-yield testing:** Suggested by H&P. If nothing is suggested, consider U/A and Ucx, WBC, GERD screen (pH probe), neuroimaging, pneumogram, nasal washing (esp RSV and *B. pertussis*) (Curr Opin Pediatr 2007;19:288) toxicology (not looked at in this study)
- **Low-yield testing:** Lytes, ABG, full septic w/u, EKG, EEG, lat neck films, CXR, barium swallow, "milk scan" (contrast scintigraphy), CVR monitoring o/n

Ddx	GI (reflux, colic, gastroenteritis) 31–33% in collected series Idiopathic 23–28% in collected series CNS (seizure, head trauma, perinatal hypoxic-ischemic encephalopathy, congenital, central hypoventilation) 11–15% in collected series Respiratory (RSV, RAD, PNA, pertussis, foreign body) 8–11% in collected series ENT 4% (laryngomalacia, laryngeal/subglottic stenosis, OSA) Abuse (shaken baby syndrome, Münchhausen-by-proxy) Breath-holding, periodic breathing Other infections (sepsis, botulism, meningoencephalitis) Metabolic (HypoNa/Ca/glycemia, CAH, acidosis) Congenital (vascular ring) Cardiac (CHD, cardiomyopathy, arrhythmia) Toxic (ingestion) Anemia
Useful history	Recent illness, relation to sleep/feeding/position, birth history, appearance (color, tone), duration, sequelae, response to stim, h/o seizures, fitful sleeping, snoring, mouth breathing, location of event (parents bed, 1st d in day care), position found (prone)

Management
- **Admission:** Study (59 infants) w/ use of high-risk criteria (age <30 d old and multi-ALTEs in 24 hr) predicted w/ 100% sens all cases needing hospitalization (Pediatrics 2007;119:679). Also high risk if premature or <43 wk corrected (J Pediatr 2008; 154:332)
  - Proposes that nontoxic full term pts w/ nml exam & >30 do p/w 1st ALTE w/ likely breath-holding spell safe to discharge home (Pediatrics 2007;120:448)
  - Criteria for breath-holding spells
    - Physically healthy pt btw the ages of 6 and 24 mo
    - Spell follows orderly tetrad of provocative emotional stimulus, expiratory apnea & cyanosis, opisthotonic rigidity, & then stupor
    - Entire sequence of events up to stupor phase lasts a few minutes. Stupor can last a variable length of time
    - Child may have many attacks per day or only a few at irregular intervals
    - FHx often discloses breath-holding spells, particularly if grandparents are questioned
    - PE, including careful cardiac evaluation, is normal
    - EEG, ECG & MRI nml, if obtained; generally Hx establishes dx w/o these tests
- Consider social work consult
- Consider admission if complex resuscitation required, abn PE, lab test, or social concerns
- **Other:** Consider CPR training for parents
  - Home monitoring appt in preterm at-risk, high-risk recurrent apnea, bradycardia, and hypoxemia following discharge or w/ infants who are equipment dependent, have conditions affecting resp reg, or those w/ unstable airways (Pediatrics 2005;115:885)

Prognosis
- No developmental diff in f/u studies at 10 yr, some ↑ breath-holding at 3 yr. ↑ risk o subsequent SIDS, only if recurrent episodes require CPR

These guidelines DO NOT replace clinical judgment. If in doubt, always err on the side of conservative management. Close follow-up continues to be the most important tool for evaluating children with fever. Caretakers of febrile children under 36 mo old should be in daily contact with a medical provider.

Epidemiology (Curr Opin Pediatr 2008;20:96)
- Etiology of bacterial infection is changing in children w/ advent of vaccines
- Hib and PCV7 vaccines have resulted in sign ↓ rates of Haemophilus and Strep infxn
- Following implementation of the above vacs, incidence of true bacteremia ↓ to 1%
- **All studies evaluating approach to fever w/o source exclude patients w/ immune compromise (sickle cell, cancer, long-term steroid use), indwelling devices (VP shunts, venous catheters), concurrent Abx rx, or fever >5 d**

Clinical Manifestations (MGH Pediatric ED guidelines; Emerg Med Clin North Am 2007;25:1087)
- If a child appears toxic, warrants complete eval, empiric management, and admit
  - Blood culture, Abx, Ucx, CSF cx.
- Of children >3 mo w/ fever >40°C; ~38% found to have severe bacterial infxn (SBI)
- Duration of fever does not predict bacteremia
- Hx of fever per parents at home (rectal temp) in afebrile patient in office warrants further eval (1 study 6/63 afebrile pts w/ Hx of fever as above found to have SBI)
- Multiple studies evaluated low-risk criteria and institutional practices vary

Identified Sources & Diagnostic Evaluation (Ann Emerg Med 2000;36:602) (i.e., what counts as "identified source" of fever that eliminates or modifies the workup?)

<28 d old
Identified Source
- Nothing counts as a source, pt needs full sepsis workup
  - **Definition: Rectal temp ≥100.4°F/38°C**
  - For newborns, refer to "sepsis eval in the newborn" in the NICU chapter
  - Of pts <28 do p/w fever >38°C to ED ~12% w/ SBI (Emerg Med Clin North Am 2007;25:1087)
  - Most common bacterial infxns are UTIs and occult bacteremia
  - RSV+ is not a source; consider CXR if resp symptoms are present
  - Neonatal HSV (1:3,200) deliveries; the 1st 2 wk of life and only minority w/ fever
    - Add acyclovir 20 mg/kg IV if risk factors present
    - Risk factors: 1° maternal infection (esp w/ vaginal delivery), PROM, use of fetal scalp electrodes, skin, eye or mouth lesions, seizures, CSF pleocytosis

Diagnosis/Evaluation/Management
Labs: Bcx, CBC/diff, Sterile Ucx (cath or bladder tap)/UA, LP, CXR (if resp sx, chest findings or O₂ sat <95%), stool cx if Hx of diarrhea
Admit for 48 hr r/o sepsis on Amp/Gent (Abx doses in NICU section)
Consider Vanco and/or acyclovir/HSV PCR if abn LP (esp if risk factors for exposure to resistant organisms and/or HSV risk factors as described above)

9–90 d
Identified Source
RSV+ infants aged 1–3 mo are at a lower risk for a serious bacterial infection; though concurrent UTI still a significant concern in infants with bronchiolitis. (Pediatrics 2004;113:1662)

Diagnosis/Evaluation/Management
Fever w/o identified source in infants 29–90 d: Rectal temp ≥100.4°F/38°C
Low-risk criteria for febrile infants 29–90 d
- **Clinical criteria:** Previously healthy FT w/ uncomp course. Nontoxic, well appearing, no suspicion of meningitis (i.e., fussiness, lethargy, poor feeding) Reliable access to f/u care (no language, financial, etc. barrier)

- **Laboratory criteria:**
  - WBC count 5–15,000/mm^3
  - Urine: Neg GS unspun (best), or neg UA (Leukocyte esterase and nitrite neg), or <5 WBC per HPF
  - If diarrhea is present: <5 WBCs per HPF in stool and guaiac neg
  - CSF: <8 WBC/mm^3, no polys, neg GS and nml protein/glucose for age, non-bloody tap (applies to option 1 below only)
- If **NOT "low risk,"** pt needs full sepsis eval w/ LP. Admit on IV Abx as "No" column

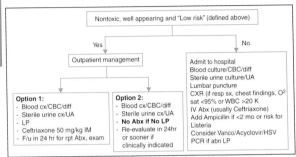

90 d–36 mo
Identified Source
- Rapid influenza positive
- PNA on CXR (obtain Bcx before Abx, consider LP, esp w/ young pts and, high fever)
- Cellulitis (need Bcx before Abx and consider LP, esp w/ young pt, high fever)
- Clinical evidence of bronchiolitis and RSV positive rapid antigen
  - Viral infxn (enterococcus, RSV, rotavirus, HSV) in pts < 3 mo ↓ risk concurrent SBI from 12.3% (w/o source) to 4.2%; for just RSV+ ↓ risk concurrent SBI from 11.7% to 5.5% (Emerg Med Clin North Am 2007;25:1087)
  - Still need to obtain urine as at least 5% FWS 2/2 UTI; general recs are U/A & Ucx in girls <24 mo, uncirc males <24 mo, circ males <6 mo (Pediatr Ann 2008;37:673)
    - Recent AAP guidelines w/ prediction rules for U/A & UCx can be avoided in pts 2–24 mo (Pediatrics 2011;128:e595); these are not regularly used
    - Girls 2 mo–24 mo w/ ≤2 of following; <12 mo, fever >2 d, temp >39.0°C, Caucasian race, in the absence of alternative source have ≤2% chance of UTI
    - UTI in males: Risk factors are nonblack race, temp ≥39.0°C, fever >1 d
      - Circ males w ≤3 RF have <2% UTI. Uncirc males always have >2% risk
  - Some would do full sepsis eval, especially in younger infants or higher fever

Diagnosis/Evaluation/Management
- Clinical evidence of bronchiolitis or rapid influenza positive
- Focal PNA on exam or by CXR (Bcx before Abx, esp w/ young pt, high fever)
- Cellulitis (consider Bcx before Abx, esp in young infants or high fever)
- Otitis media ("a little red" does not count. TM immobile, bulging, etc.)
  - Consider sterile Ucx/UA if Hx of multi "ear infections" or frequent antibiotic use
- Gastroenteritis: To consider a source, it needs to be (1) multi-episodes of both vomiting and diarrhea, (2) dx should be "in season", and (3) +/− rotavirus test if possible
  - Guaiac stool: If positive, send for stool cx and obtain CBC and blood cx
  - Consider GS for WBC (stool leuks). If >5 WBC in stool, send stool and blood cx. Abx not indicated before stool cx results, unless child is toxic
- Rapid strep+ (not very common in this age group)
- URI: Can coexist w/ bacteremia, cannot be considered sole source in children <1 yc
- Identifiable viral exanthem or mucosal findings, such as Coxsackie and Varicella
- **Fever without an identified source in 90 d–36 mo olds** (see the following table)

Full sepsis evaluation
Admit on IV antibiotics

← Yes — Toxic appearing? — No → Rectal temperature >39°C (102°F) — No →

↓ Yes

↓ (under Rectal temperature path "No"):

- No blood tests
- Consider screening urine
- No Antibiotics
- Antipyretics*
- Daily contact w/ PCP (phone or visit) as long as febrile
- Return to PCP if fever >2 d or condition worsens

*For Ibuprofen use in >6 mo, patients should be well-hydrated prior to use

(under Toxic appearing "No" / temperature path):

1. Sterile urine culture/UA:
   - Obtain sterile urine in the presence of ≥1 risk factors: Girls: white race, age <12 mo, temp ≥39°C, fever ≥2 d. Boys: Nonblack race, temp ≥39°C, fever >24 hr, uncircumcised
   - Consider sterile Ucx/UA in all pts <36 mo, esp Hx of multi "ear infxns", freqAbx use (missed UTIs), or nonspec GI sx (vomiting, diarrhea)
   - If UA +, rx w/ outpt Abx (if well appearing); f/u Ucx
   - If starting Abx, consider blood cx, esp in younger infants.
2. Infants/toddlers who did not receive Strep pneumovac at 2, 4 and 6 mo (Need adequate proof of immunity against pneumococcus. E.g., Doc in blue immunization book; Med record; Parent states child received shots at 2, 4, and 6 mo; or from PCP. (Pediatr Infect Dis J 2000;19:187; Pediatr Infect Dis J 2001;20:1105; Pediatrics 2001;108:835; Pediatrics 2004;113:443)
   - CBC/diff & blood culture
   - If WBC count >15,000, give ceftriaxone 50 mg/kg IM (up to 1 g)
   - Follow up at 24 hr for repeat ceftriaxone
   - If WBC count >15,000, chest findings, O2 sat <95% or WBC >20,000
3. CXR if resp sx, chest findings, O2 sat <95% or WBC >20,000
4. Consider LP if concerned about partially treated meningitis
5. Antipyretics*
6. Return or see PCP if fever persists >48 hr or condition deteriorates

APPENDICITIS

- Inflammation of the appendix 2/2 outlet obstruction (w/ fecalith, 2/2 lymphoid hyperplasia, etc.), fills w/ mucus under pressure w/ vascular/lymphatic stasis of appendiceal wall. This can result in inflammation of surrounding structures and/or rupture

Epidemiology (BMJ 2006;333:530; N Engl J Med 2003;348:236)
- Most common surgical abd emergency in peds; most common in teen yr, slightly M > F
- ~20% of pts undergoing ex lap for appendectomy have normal appendix

Differential Diagnosis
- Same as for acute abdomen; specifically consider other RLQ structures (nephrolithiasis, testicular or ovarian torsion, ovarian cyst, ectopic pregnancy, PID, intussusception, IBD, UTI, or pyelonephritis)

Clinical Manifestations (JAMA 2007;298:438)
- Only 50% patients have classic symptoms described by Murphy w/ colicky periumbilical abdominal pain, followed by N/V, anorexia, and subsequent migration of pain to RLQ
  - Can also (but may not) see diarrhea, constipation, fever, bilious emesis, etc.
- Generally w/ pain progressing from central to RLQ w/i 24 hr
- More difficult to ascertain Hx in younger pts; w/ increased time to diagnosis and higher risk of perforation (delay in rx of >36 hr results in perforation rate of ~65%)
- Abdominal exam for guarding and rebound (evidence of peritonitis), localization of pain (usually RLQ but can vary in small children w/ retrocecal or pelvic appendix)
  - **McBurney point:** 2/3 down along line from umbilicus to anterior superior iliac spine; classically point of maximal tenderness in simple appendicitis (BMJ 2006;333:530)
  - **Rovsing sign:** Palpation of LLQ w/ pain in RLQ; sens 30%, spec 84%
  - **Psoas sign:** Pain w/ straight leg extension at R leg while lying on R side; inflamed appendix lying on R psoas muscle. Sens 26–36%, spec 86–87%
  - **Obturator sign:** Pain w/ flexion and internal rotation at R hip; inflamed appendix in contact w/ obturator internus muscle. Sens 28%, spec 87%
- Complete PE (including pelvic or testicular exam) as lobar PNA, testicular or ovarian torsion or ectopic pregnancy can all mimic appendicitis
- W/ perforation, pain initially crescendos then improves w/ subsequent worsening clinical status, progression to frank peritonitis and shock
- PAS & Alvarado scoring systems do not have adequate predictive values. (Am J Emerg Med 2011;29:972); though modified Alvarado may ↓ CT use (Arch Surg 2011;146:64)

Diagnostic Studies (JAMA 2007;298:438; Pediatr Ann 2008;37:433; Radiology 2006;241:83)
- Evaluate w/ CBC diff. Based on history and PE, consider electrolytes w/ LFTs (esp sexually active female), amy, lipase, type & screen, U/A, Bcx and Ucx, CRP/ESR
- Inc WBC w/ sens 67% and spec 80%. Low/nml WBC NPV 92%. Left shift sens 59%, spec 90%. High WBC & left shift combined sens 79%, spec 80% (Pediatr Emerg Care 2007;23:69)
- Abd U/S – no radiation; assess for noncompressible, fluid-filled, blind tube >6 mm in diameter in RLQ. Limited by body habitus and inter-operator variability. In pediatric patients, sens 88% (95% CI: 86%, 90%) and spec 94% (95% CI: 92%, 95%)
- Abd imaging is often obtained; studies are equivocal w/ regard to ↓ time to OR and ↓ false + rate abd CT in pediatric patients (I+/O+, often w/ rectal contrast) – very sensitive 94% (95% CI: 92%, 97%), spec 95% (95% CI: 94%, 97%) and high PPV; w/ dilated (>7 mm) fluid-filled appendix w/ thickened walls, failure of contrast to fill appendix and fat stranding or can show other etiologies for pain
- Young children <10 yo tend to have limited fat which decreases visualization rate of appendix and can lead to equivocal studies (AJR Am J Roentgenol 2001;176:497)

Management and Complications (BMJ 2006;333:530)
- Managed w/ surgical removal of appendix, very low rates of surgical complications
- The most common complication is appendiceal rupture prior to OR w/ subsequent peritonitis
  - Risk of perforation w/ >36 hr from sx onset 16–36%, inc 5% every 12 hr thereaft
  - Lower SES confers ↑ risk for rupture to school-aged children (JAMA 2004;292:197
  - Mgmt w/ triple Abx (amp/gent/Flagyl) and surgical clean out once inflammation quie now single-agent rx w/ pip/tazo shown to be equivalent (Pediatrics 2007;119:905)

INTUSSUSCEPTION

- Telescoping of 1 segment of bowel onto adjacent section leading to vascular insufficiency, bowel wall edema, & possibly infarct. Most common at ileocecal junction
- Can be assoc w/ a "lead point" (3–10%); mass, lymphoid tissue, Meckel diverticulum, etc.

Epidemiology (Pediatrics 2011;127:e296)
- Most common cause of intestinal obstruction in infants and young children. Most common age 5–9 mo but can occur at any age. 67% occur by 1 yo
- ↑ risk w/ age >5 mo, males and those who p/w lethargy, bilious vomiting, and no diarrhea
- Prior rotavirus vaccine (RotaShield) withdrawn 2/2 concern for assoc w/ intussusceptions
  - RotaTeq (pentavalent) and Rotarix (monovalent) vaccines w/ good safety/efficacy profiles in large trials; no ↑ risk of intussusception w/ use of these new vaccines

Clinical Manifestations (Arch Pediatr Adolesc Med 2000;154:250)
- Classically p/w intermittent abd pain (pulling legs up to abd), abd mass (classically sausage-shaped mass in RLQ) and bloody stool (classically currant jelly stools); in reality this triad seen in <50% of patients
- Can p/w just lethargy, usually late in course, but can be early, especially w/ infants
- Often w/ Hx of recent viral infection and higher incidence in spring and autumn

Diagnostic Studies and Management (Clin Radiol 2005;60:39; Pediatr Radiol 2009;39:S140)
- Primarily dx'd on radiography, but need high index of suspicion, check stool guaiac
- Plain abdominal radiographs: May be nml or may show frank obstruction w/ dilated loops, rarely (if perforated) free air. May see **"target" sign** (intussusceptus) over R kidney or **"crescent" sign** (intestinal gas trapped btw two intussuscepted surfaces). Absence of bowel gas in ascending colon is very specific. If plain film positive, proceed to ultrasound or air enema. If negative, age >5 mo, absence of bilious emesis, and presence of diarrhea → can be observed
- Ultrasound: w/ 98–100% sensitivity and 88–100% specificity in experienced hands
  - May see **"target" sign** or **"pseudokidney"** sign w/ several concentric rings; can be operator dependent though. Also Doppler blood flow does not correlate w/ necrosis
- Contrast (barium or H_2O soluble agent) or air enema: Diagnostic and therapeutic but w/ small risk (0–3%) perforation (lower w/ air); discuss w/ pediatric surgery if available
- Contrast or air enema results in reduction of intussusception 55–95%; if not, need surgery

BURNS

(Pediatr Emerg Care 2005;21:449; Crit Care Med 2002;30:S500; Crit Care Med 2009;37:2819)

Burns (Pediatric Emergency Medicine, 2nd ed. McGraw-Hill. 2002;692)
- Severity of burn related to duration of exposure and temperature to which exposed
- Accidental scalding is the most common burn in peds; highest mortality w/ house fire w/ inhalation injury
- Always consider the possibility of intentional burns as a form of abuse

Degree of Burns	
Degree	**Description**
First Degree	Only epidermis involved, painful and erythematous
Second Degree	Epidermis and dermis involved, but dermal appendages spared. Any blistering qualifies as 2nd degree. Deep 2nd-degree burns may be white and painless, require grafting, and progress to full thickness with wound healing
Third degree	Full-thickness burns involving epidermis and all of dermis, including dermal appendages. Leathery and painless; require grafting
Fourth degree	Full thickness involving muscle, bone, or fascia. Evaluate for compartment syndrome

- If electrical injury suspected, can have rhabdomyolysis w/ myoglobinuria, also can have cardiac arrhythmias as well as injury at distal sites

Assessment of Burn Surface Area					
% BSA	<1 yr	1–4 yr	5–9 yr	10–15 yr	>15 yr
Head	19	17	13	11	9
Neck	2	2	2	2	2
Trunk	13	13	13	13	13
Buttock	2.5	2.5	2.5	2.5	2.5
Upper arm	4	4	4	4	4
Lower arm	3	3	3	3	3
Hand	2.5	2.5	2.5	2.5	2.5
Thigh	5.5	6.5	8	8.5	9
Leg	5	5	5.5	6	6.5
Foot	3.5	3.5	3.5	3.5	3.5

- **>12 yr:** Rule of 9s: Head 9%, front and back of torso 18%, arms 9% each, leg 18% each
- **<12 yr:** Modified Rule of 9s, head and neck 18%, each lower extremity 15%, each upper extremity 10%, and anterior and posterior torsos each 16%
- Irregular/non-confluent burns: Rule of palms: Palmar surface of pt's hand ~1% of BSA

Resuscitation Formula
- First 24 hr (no colloid); Parkland formula now renamed the Consensus formula
  - Adults and children >20 kg; LR 2–4 mL/kg/% burn/24 hr (1st 1/2 in 1st 8 hr)
  - Child <20 kg; LR: 2–3 mL/kg/%burn/24 hr (1st 1/2 in 1st 8 hr); then D5LR
- **Second 24 hr** (all patients)
  - Crystalloid: To maintain UOP; if silver nitrate used, need isotonic fluid 2/2 Na leeching. If other topical, free H_2O requirement significant; follow serum Na; begin enteral feeds if appropriate
  - Colloid: (5% albumin in LR): 0–30% burn: None, 30–50% burn: 0.3 mL/kg/%burn/24 hr, 50–70% burn: 0.4 mL/kg/%burn/24 hr, 70–100% burn: 0.5 mL/kg/%burn/24 hr

Management of Burns
- **Stabilization:**
  - **Airway:** Intubate if evidence of inhalation; avoid use of succinylcholine
  - **Breathing:** Humidified 100% O_2 to clear CO (can have nml O_2 sat even w/ ↑[CO])
  - **Circulation:** Fluid resusc: Infant w/ >10% burn, child w/ >15% burns and child w/ inhalation injury
  - **Pain relief:** First consideration in stable patients: Use morphine SC or IV
- **Survey:** Eval for other injuries (e.g., skeletal trauma from fall, injuries w/ electrical burns)
- **Eval:** CBC, T&C, carboxyHgb, coags, CMP, ABG, EKG, CXR (signs may be delayed)
- **GI:** NPO, NG tube, stress ulcer prophylaxis with H_2 blockers and antacids
- **GU:** Place Foley to monitor urine output, keep UOP = 0.5–2 cc/kg/hr
- **Eye:** Careful exam with fluorescein (refer to ophtho if suspected injury)
- Tetanus prophylaxis
- Cooling if w/i 30 min of injury to ↓ damage
  - If burn <10% BSA, apply clean towels soaked in sterile cold water
  - If >10% BSA, apply clean dry towels to avoid hypothermia
- Chemical burns → wash w/ copious amts of sterile water for 20 min
- Analgesia → consider morphine

Triage and Treatment
- **Outpatient management:**
  - Burn <10% of infant BSA or <15% of child's BSA
  - No concern for airway compromise; good outpatient support and follow-up
  - No prophylactic oral antibiotics indicated
  - Pt's providers understand dressing changes and burn care
  - **Rx:** Debride only open blisters (closed blister is best bandage), topical antimicrobial agent QD (silver sulfadiazine, combination antibiotics, and chlorhexidine. No high-quality data comparing agents, choice can be made based on cost, availability, and provider familiarity. Silver sulfadiazine with cerium or alone, and povidone-iodine are contraindicated in newborns, pregnancy, and lactation)(preferred over

Silvadene [sulfadiazine], which is toxic if ingested, risk of skin rxn), Gauze, r/o infection. F/u next day w/ PCP
- **Inpatient management:** Referred to nearest pediatric burn center
  - Burns of larger BSA than above, electrical or chemical burns, burns of face, hands, feet, perineum or joints, full-thickness burns, circumferential burns; suspicion of abuse/neglect; burns in a child w/ underlying illness; evidence of smoke inhalation; **CO poisoning or burns assoc w/ life-threatening injuries**

CARBON MONOXIDE INHALATION

Definition (Pediatr Rev 2005;26:150; N Engl J Med 2009;360:1217)
- Inhalation of carbon monoxide (colorless, odorless, tasteless), binds to Hgb w/ 250× the affinity of O_2 forming carboxyhemoglobin, which blocks O_2 disassociation from Hgb
- Damage occurs 2/2 hypoxia as well as direct CO toxic effects
- Higher metabolic activity (inc O_2 demand), increased vulnerability (e.g., infants)
- Source of CO include motor exhaust, smoke inhalation, poorly functioning heaters; lethal levels achieved w/i 10 min w/ running engine in closed garage or blocked exhaust

Clinical Manifestations (Pediatr Rev 2005;26:150)
- P/w sx of asphyxia in pt w/ nml O_2 sat, pink & well perfused or can look cyanotic and pale
- Can p/w HA, N/V, fatigue, dizziness, dyspnea, syncope, lethargy; similar to viral URI
- Severity of sx can but does not always closely correlate w/ degree of exposure
- Can see ↑ HR & ↑ RR (2/2 tissue hypoxia), may p/w chest pain, pulm edema &/or szrs
- Can see delayed neuropsychiatric syndrome in 10–30% from 3–240 d after exposure

Diagnostic Studies (Pediatr Rev 2005;26:150)
- Check serum carboxyhemoglobin level, ABG (metab acidosis w/ nml PaO_2), oximetry falsely ↑. Check for rhabdomyolysis w/ serum CK and U/A for myoglobinuria
- Serum carboxyhemoglobin levels 1–3% in nonsmokers, up to 10–15% in smokers
- Administer **C**arbon **M**onoxide **N**europsychological **S**creening **B**attery (J Clin Psychol 1991;47:675)
- Consider cyanide (CN) toxicity if smoke exposure w/ metabolic acidosis & normal carboxyHgb and MetHgb levels
- Non-invasive CO tests not shown to correlate well w/ serum levels, especially in kids

Management (Pediatr Rev 2005;26:150; N Engl J Med 2009;360:1217)
- Provide 100% O_2 until carboxyhemoglobin level <5%
  - Elim $t^{1}/_2$ of CO in 100% O_2 = 1 hr, 21% O_2 = 4–5 hr, 2–3 atm hyperbaric O_2 < 30 min
- Indications for hyperbaric rx (carboxyhemoglobin level >40% (at MGH/MEEI ≥20, >15% if pregnant), coma, any unconsciousness, abnormal CMNSB score, cardiac ischemia, continued symptoms w/ conventional rx × 4–6 hr or recurrent sx up to 3 wk); controversial

TRAUMA OVERVIEW

Primary Survey (Emerg Med Clin N Am 2007;25:803)
Airway and C-spine control: Protect C-spine. Need for patency, chin lift/jaw thrust/oral airways/LMA/ETT as needed. Surgical cricothyroidotomy rare in pediatrics,↑ risk tracheal stenosis in pts < 9–12 yo as cricothryoid membrane immature
- Intubate if (1) unable to ventilate w/ bag-mask, (2) GCS ≤ 8, (3) respiratory failure from hypoxemia or hypoventilation, (4) decompensated shock resistant to fluid (5) loss of laryngeal protective reflexes. See PICU section for ETT size chart

- **Breathing:** Seriously injured patients receive 100% NRB mask. Early monitoring w/ pulse oximetry. Assess inspiratory effort/mechanical fxn. Assess for tension/ hemo/pneumothorax, flail chest. Pulmonary contusions common, particularly in younger pts
- **Circulation:** Eval extremities/cap refill/central pulses; HoTN usually late finding; volume resusc as need; bolus LR or NS 20 cc/kg × 3 (warm fluids for significant trauma) followed by pRBC xfusion 10 mL/kg. Control external bleeding. Pressors as needed. Consider internal bleeding, if not stable → FAST exam → potentially w/ evaluation w/ ex lap
- **Disability:** Evaluate GCS (See Head Trauma) or AVPU:
  A = **A**lert, **V** = Responds to **V**erbal stim, **P** = Responds to **P**ainful stim,
  U = **U**nresponsive
- Rule out hypoglycemia in any patient with altered mental status
- **Exposure:** Fully undress patient to assess for hidden injury. Maintain temperature with warm lights, warm blankets, warm fluids and warm inspired air

Secondary Survey (Emerg Med Clin N Am 2007;25:803)
- 2° survey performed after initial resuscitation to include:
  - AMPLE history – **A**llergies, **M**eds, **P**MH, **L**ast meal, **E**vents related to injury
  - Age-appropriate motor and sensory examination
  - Detailed head-to-toe inspection for unsuspected injury
    - Head exam includes pupillary size/reactivity, fundoscopic exam, palpation of skull
    - Assess chest for wounds and crepitus, auscultation
    - Back and buttocks exposed by rolling pt while maintaining cervical spine alignment. Rectal exam to assess sphincter tone, and bleeding (guaiac)
    - Lacerations, abrasions, ecchymosis, deformities, or tenderness should be noted
- **Labs:** CBC, CMP, coags, type and cross ± serum/urine tox, urine β-HCG
- **Diagnostic testing**
  - **Plain films:** AP chest, lateral C-spine, pelvis, & selected extremities of blunt trauma (consider trauma series during primary survey)
    - Can obtain cross-table lat views for free air, AP/odontoid views to eval C-spine
  - **FAST scan:** Consists of U/S scanning of 4 areas: (Am J Emerg Med 2000;18:244)
    - Subxiphoid: To visualize the heart (assess for pericardial effusion)
    - RUQ: To visualize Morison pouch and paracolic gutter; can see lung base (PTX)
    - LUQ: To visualize the splenorenal recess and paracolic gutter; can see lung base
    - Suprapubic: To visualize Douglas pouch
    - Limited data in peds: Sens 75%; spec 97%; PPV 90%; NPV 92% in a small study
    - Cannot detect injury to bowel, diaphragm, or retroperitoneal organs
  - **Head CT:** To evaluate for acute intracranial bleed
  - **Abd/Pelv CT:** Test of choice to assess intra-abdominal injury. Only for hemodynamically stable patients. Does not rule out duodenal hematoma

HEAD TRAUMA

(Lancet 2009;374:1160; Pediatrics 2011;127:1067)

Minor Head Injury
- Normal mental status at initial exam, no abnormal or focal findings on neurologic (including funduscopic) exam. No physical evidence of skull fracture

Clinical Presentation
- Variable; nml or w/ vomiting, poor feeding, lethargy, seizure, respiratory distress, apnea, and lifelessness
  - **Pertinent history:** When did it happen?, mechanism of injury, when did pt return to nml MS and activity (beware "temporary lucid interval" in epidural hemorrhage)
  - Concerning history findings: Loss of consciousness (LOC), assess how long, Δ mental status, any seizure, vomiting, HA (postconcussive syndrome, also sign o ↑ ICP [rare]) abn gait, weakness, visual changes (sign of cerebral injury), amnesia
- **Exam:** Detailed general exam, eval for fractures, check mental status, cranial nerve muscle strength, coordination, and gait

Modified Pediatric Glasgow Coma Scale		
Eyes opening	Spontaneous	4
	To speech	3
	To pain	2
	None	1
Verbal	Oriented (coos, babbles)	5
	Confused (irritable)	4
	Inappropriate words (cries to pain)	3
	Nonspecific sounds (moans to pain)	2
	None	1
Motor	Follows commands (spontaneous movements)	6
	Localizes pain (withdraws to touch)	5
	Withdraws to pain	4
	Abnormal flexion	3
	Abnormal extension	2
	None	1

- GCS score has limited ability to predict outcome in children. For GCS <14, risk of traumatic brain injury on CT >20%

Diagnostic Studies

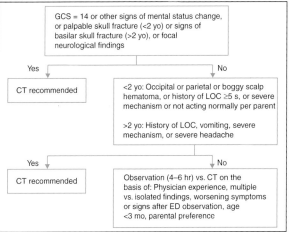

- **Labs:** Consider CBC, w/ platelet count, PT/PTT to evaluate for coagulation disorders, blood bank sample
- **Imaging:**
  - Noncontrast head CT: Obtain immediately as guided above
  - Rapid Sequence T2-weighted MR: If available, consider MR as an alternative to CT given risk of radiation w/ CT. MR can demonstrate structural changes (midline shift, mass effect), hematomas, & volume Δ's. (Arch Phys Med Rehabil 2010;91:1661)
  - Skull films: Not sensitive for brain injury; if +fracture, CT is indicated

Management

Stabilize patient following ABC rules, call trauma team or neurosurgery if needed
Look for signs suggestive of ↑ ICP and manage if necessary (see later discussion)
Observation: All children w/ minor head injury obs 4–6 hr in ED. Patients who are observed before making the decision for CT scan have significantly lower rates of CT use and similar rate of clinically important TBI
Admission criteria
- Δ in mental status, neurologic deficits, seizures, persistent HA, persistent vomiting status
- CSF otorrhea/rhinorrhea (requires antibiotics) or hemotympanum
- Linear skull fracture crossing middle meningeal artery groove, venous sinus, foramen magnum

- Depressed skull fracture, skull base fracture
- Suspected child abuse or bleeding disorder
- **Discharge instructions:** F/u w/i 24 hr, at least by phone, should be arranged for all children who are discharged following a head injury
  - **Immediate medical attention** required if the following conditions are noted:
    - Inability to awaken the child as instructed. Persistent or worsening headache
    - Continued vomiting or vomiting that begins/continues 4–6 hr after injury
    - Change in mental status or behavior. Unsteady gait or clumsiness/incoordination
    - Seizure

Concussion (Pediatrics 2010;126:597)

- Caused by direct or transmitted blow to head/neck. Results in a set of graded clinical sx that may or may not involve LOC. Nml neuroimaging. May result in neuropathologic Δ's
- Estimated 3.8 million recreation and sports-related concussions annually
- F > M in similar sports. Football highest for boys, soccer for girls
- When seen in the ED, athlete should not return to play the same day

Stepwise Return to Play (AAP Guidelines; Pediatrics 2010;126:597)

- Each stage in concussion rehabilitation should last no less than 24 hr with a minimum of 5 d required to consider a full return to competition. If symptoms recur during the rehabilitation program, the athlete should stop immediately. Once asymptomatic after at least another 24 hr, the athlete should resume at the previous asymptomatic level and try to progress again. Athletes should contact their healthcare provider if symptoms recur. Any athlete with multiple concussions or prolonged symptoms may require a longer concussion-rehabilitation program, which is ideally created by a physician who is experienced in concussion management

Rehabilitation Stage	Functional Exercise
1. No activity	Complete physical and cognitive rest
2. Light aerobic activity	Walking, swimming, stationary cycling at 70% maximum heart rate; no resistance exercises
3. Sport-specific exercise	Specific sports-related drills but no head impact
4. Noncontact training drills	More complex drills, may start light resistance training
5. Full-contact practice	After medical clearance, participate in normal training
6. Return to play	Normal game play

FOREIGN BODIES ASPIRATION AND INGESTION

(Curr Gastroenerol Rep 2005 7:212; Pediatr Rev 2009;30:295)

Aspiration

- **Classic Hx:** Acute choking episode followed by coughing/wheezing/stridor
  - Unless seen, history unreliable; should be on differential w/ Hx of chronic cough
- **Exam:** Cough (most common sx), localized wheeze, & localized ↓ breath sounds
- **Location:** Can be either side as children have approx symmetric bronchial angles
- **Evaluation:** Start w/ AP/lateral inspiratory/expiratory films
  - If unable to cooperate, consider left and right lateral decubitus inspiratory films
  - ↓ inflation on affected side. CXR can be nml. Freq w/ localized air trapping or atelectasis
  - Clinical symptoms and radiologic findings before bronchoscopy have low diagnostic value. Usually foreign bodies are nuts/vegetables ~80%, both radiolucent
- **Management:** If concern for aspiration or partial obstruction, rigid bronchoscopy under general anesthesia
  - Postbronchoscopy will require observation, pulmonary toilet, and possible antibiotics
  - Complete airway obstruction requires back slaps and chest thrusts in head down position for infants or abdominal thrusts for older children
  - Asymptomatic patients who have normal exam and normal radiography can be observed at home

Ingestion

- Common foreign bodies ingested are coins (most common), toys, sharp objects, batteries, magnets, bones, & food
- 80–90% of foreign bodies that come to medical attention pass uneventfully, 10–20% require endoscopic removal & <1% require surgery
- **Location:** 5–10% in oropharynx, 20% in esophagus, 60% in stomach, and 10% distal to the stomach, usually in intestine (Eur J Emerg Med 1995;2:83)
- **Symptoms:** Drooling, choking, poor feeding, odynophagia, dysphagia, and chest pain. Fever suggests deep ulceration or perforation

- **Evaluation:** H&P, x-ray of neck, chest, and abdomen. Include lateral view of esophagus
  - Metal detectors sensitive and specific for localizing coins
  - For battery ingestions, call National Battery Ingestion Hotline at 202–625–3333
- **Management** of foreign body dependent on object, location, and patient's age/size
  - **Esophagus:** Early intervention 2/2 risk resp distress, esophageal erosions or fistulas
    - No evidence for the use of motility agents such as glucagon
    - Disc batteries are of great concern and need immediate removal
    - If object is close to LES, could wait and repeat x-ray if passes into stomach
    - Multiple magnets in esophagus or stomach should be removed endoscopically to prevent fistulization or perforation
  - **Stomach:** Objects continue to pass uneventfully in GI tract. Prokinetics not helpful
    - Endoscopy deferred unless pt is still symptomatic until 4–6 wk after ingestion
    - Some FBs will not pass pylorus. FB >10 cm cannot pass in adults. Unclear in children
    - Have greater concern for sharp objects, such as pins/needles
    - Disc batteries often pass w/o issue; some cause ulcers & may need endoscopy
  - **Intestine:** Safety pins in duodenum need removal because they can become lodged
    - Coins/disc batteries eventually pass
    - Rarely obstruct unless w/ anatomical abn (Meckel diverticulum or in appendix)
    - Magnets – if multiple and beyond reach of endoscope, need careful follow-up or surgical intervention
- **Outpatient management:** Not necessary to sieve feces to find object
  - Follow-up x-ray in 1–2 wk for passage
  - If witnessed ingest of radiolucent FB, may need f/u endoscopy or contrast x-ray eval

THE CRYING INFANT

Definition (Emerg Med Clin North Am 2007;25:1137)
- In outpatient setting, <5% of infants with complaint of crying have organic disease
  - In ER, may be as high as 60%
  - Use H&P (completely undress pt and complete exam; ears, nares, genitals, anus, fingers and toes) to guide w/u
  - Focused Ddx: IT CRIES
  - **Infection** (sepsis, meningitis, encephalitis, UTI, PNA, osteomyelitis, septic arthritis, cellulitis, gastro, Kawasaki, dermatitis, OM, herpes stomatitis/herpangina, thrush)
  - **Trauma** (accidental and non-accidental), **testicular torsion**
  - **Cardiac** (CHF, MI, SVT), **colic**
  - **Reflux, reactions to meds/formulas**
  - **Immunizations, insect bites**
  - **Eye** (corneal abrasion, foreign body, glaucoma)
  - **Surgical** (volvulus, intussusception, hernias), **strangulation** (hair/fiber tourniquet)
- Review of 237 cases w/ 5% w/ serious illness, UTI most prevalent (3/12) w/ H&P alone leading to dx in 66.3% (Pediatrics 2009;123:841)

Child with a Limp
- Limp 2/2 pain, weakness, or deformity; may be 2/2 lower extremity, spine, or abdomen
- Always examine 1 joint above and below the joint initially suspected

Common Causes By Age (Am Fam Physician 2000;61:1011; Pediatr Emerg Care 1985;1:7)	
AGE	DDX
All ages	Cellulitis, fracture, septic arthritis, osteomyelitis Less common: Neoplasm (including leukemia), neuromuscular disease
0–3 yr	Septic hip, leg-length discrepancy, developmental dysplasia of the hip Occult fractures, Toddler's fractures
4–10 yr	Legg-Calve–Perthes dz, transient synovitis, juvenile rheumatoid arthritis
11–16 yr	Slipped capital femoral epiphysis, avascular necrosis of the femoral head Overuse syndromes (i.e., Osgood–Schlatter), tarsal coalitions, gonococcal septic arthritis
Requiring urgent care	Osteomyelitis, septic joint, paraspinal abscess, cord tumor, Guillain–Barré Intracranial: Cerebral abscess, meningitis, encephalitis Appendicitis

Transient Synovitis versus Septic Arthritis in a Child with a Limp
Transient synovitis: Pain & limited motion of joint that resolves with conservative management; inflammation of synovium; classic picture is afebrile, nontoxic child w/ a limp. Ages 3–10

- **Septic arthritis:** More likely to have fever (>101.3°F), ↑CRP (>2 mg/dL), ↑ESR (40 mm/hr), and ↑WBC (>12 × 10⁹/L) w/ inability to bear weight. If all the five factors present, then 98% probability of septic arthritis. Elevated CRP is an independent risk factor. Diagnosed by >50,000 WBC in joint aspirate (J Bone Joint Surg Am 2006;88:1251)

Salter–Harris Classification (SALTR)
- **Type I (S**traight**):** Fracture through physis. Nml x-ray w/ pain over site (open growth plate)
- **Type II (A**bove**):** Fracture extends into metaphysis
- **Type III (L**ower**):** Fracture extends into epiphysis
- **Type IV (T**hrough**):** Fracture extends through both metaphysis and epiphysis
- **Type V (R**uined/need **ER):** Physis is crushed or compressed axially
- Severity of injury & assoc morbidity ↑ing SALTR class; type V most severe

Fractures Requiring Immediate, Same-day, Attention
- **Supracondylar fracture of the humerus**
  - Supracondylar fx can compromise (1) brachial artery, (2) median, & (3) radial nerve
  - Test the median nerve sensory pathway on the ventral index finger and the motor pathway by asking to make an OK sign with the thumb and forefinger
  - Test the radial nerve sensor pathway in the dorsal web-spaces and the motor pathway by asking the patient to hold up their hand indicating "stop"
- **Open fractures**
- **Slipped capital femoral epiphysis** (Am Fam Physician 1998;57:2135)
  - Can lead to osteonecrosis of femoral head
  - Usually obese, early puberty, p/w pain and altered gait (several wk) 25–40% bilateral

Ottawa Ankle Rules
- Prediction rules designed to eliminate unnecessary x-rays of ankle in **adults**
- **ADULTS** do not require an x-ray if they are
  - ANKLE: (1) Able to walk immediately following an injury or can take 4 steps in the ER and (2) have no tenderness over the posterior malleoli or
  - MIDFOOT: (1) Able to walk immediately following an injury or can take 4 steps in the ER and (2) have no tenderness over the navicular, or the proximal 5th metatarsal
  - Sensitivity of 1 (i.e., there is zero likelihood of having a fracture if these criteria are not met) (JAMA 1993;269:1127)
- In **children,** these rules likely apply after growth is completed
  - Will miss 14 fractures per 1,000 children w/ a neg exam by the Ottawa ankle rules (Arch Dis Child 2005;90:1309)

Fractures Suggestive of Non-accidental Trauma
- Fracture Type: Fractures in various stages of healing; metaphyseal–epiphyseal fractures; distal humerus transphyseal fracture; femur fracture in child before walking; humerus diaphyseal fracture <3 yo; rib fractures, especially posterior; scapular fractures; vertebral fractures; complex skull fractures; digital fractures before walking; multiple fractures especially bilateral (Emerg Med Clin North Am 2010;28:85; Clin Orthop Relat Res 2011;469:790)

TOXICOLOGY

Recognizable Tox-syndromes		
Toxidrome	**Signs and Symptoms**	**Sources**
Anticholinergic	Dry skin, hyperthermia, thirst, dysphagia, mydriasis, ↑HR, urinary retention, delirium, hallucinations	Belladonna, Jimson weed, antihistamines, TCAs
Cholinergic: Muscarinic	Dec HR, salivation, lacrimation, urination, defecation, emesis, bronchial secretions	Acetylcholine, pilocarpine, organophosphates
Cholinergic: Nicotinic	Tachycardia, HTN, muscle fasciculations, paralysis	Insecticides, tobacco, black widow venom
Opiates	Sedation, hypoventilation, HoTN, miosis	Narcotics
Sympatho-mimetics	Agitation, seizures, HTN, tachycardia, cool moist skin	Theophylline, caffeine, LSD, PCP, amphetamines, cocaine, PPA
SSRIs	Stupor, confusion, flushing, tachycardia, trembling, hyperreflexia	SSRI overdose
α-adrenergic	Stupor, hypotension, bradycardia	Clonidine

- Consider complete workup if the above syndrome suspected or in the setting of altered mental status
- Stabilize airway, breathing, and circulation
- Patients may be hyper-alert/agitated or have reduced alertness
- Perform a complete neurologic evaluation
- Consider infection, particularly if fever is present
- Check electrolytes (esp glucose)
- Assess for trauma
- Perform toxicology screen & call local poison control center if + or high suspicion

Decontamination
- **Activated charcoal:** 1 g/kg PO/NG (max 50–60 g) (see below for sorbitol)
  - Contraindicated in ileus/obstruction, hydrocarbons, caustics, lithium, Fe, boric acid, electrolyte solution, obtunded patient
  - Substances poorly absorbed by charcoal: Electrolytes, iron, mineral acids/bases, alcohols, cyanide, most solvents, most water-insoluble compounds per recommendation of Poison Control, as standard for administration changes
- **Orogastric lavage:** Intubate prior to procedure if airway cannot be protected; lavage can be used if ingestion <1 hr PTA
  - Contraindicated with caustic or hydrocarbon ingestions, co-ingestion of sharp objects
  - Method: Pt on left w/ head lower than body. Place OG tube (18–20°F in children, 36–40°F in adults). Lavage w/ NS 15 mL/kg/cycle (up to 200 mL) until gastric contents are clear
- **Cathartics:** May be used in conjunction with 1st dose of activated charcoal
- Sorbitol 2 cc/kg if >2 yr (not for children <2 yr), or Mg citrate 4–8 cc/kg – max 300 cc
- Contraindications: Caustic ingestions, no bowel sounds, recent bowel surgery. Avoid magnesium with poor renal function
- **Whole bowel irrigation:**
  - Polyethylene glycol solution via cont NG infusion may be useful for toxic iron, lithium, or sustained release prep, ingestion of vials or whole packets of illicits or lead chips
  - Contraindications: GI bleed or obstruction, ileus, unintubated obtunded/comatose pt
  - Children: Polyethylene glycol (e.g., GoLYTELY) @ 500 mL/hr for 4–6 hr or till stools clear. Adults: 1–2 L/hr for 4–6 hr
- **Urine alkalinization:**
  - For elimination of weak acids (i.e., salicylates, barbiturates, and MTX)
  - Bolus $NaHCO_3$ 1–2 mEq/kg, then D_5W w/ $NaHCO_3$ 132 mEq/L at 1.5–2× maint
- **Hemodialysis:**
  - For low–molecular-weight drugs; aspirin, theophylline, lithium, phenobarb, & alcohols

Acetaminophen Overdose (Pediatrics 2001;108:1020)
- Metabolites are hepatotoxic. Reactive intermediates can cause liver necrosis
- 5–10% of acetaminophen metabolized to NAPQI (toxic), detoxed by glutathione
- **Four phases** of intoxication
  - First: P/w nausea, vomiting, anorexia, malaise, diaphoresis; nonspecific
  - Second: Above sx resolve & develop RUQ pain, hepatomegaly & in some oliguria
    - Inc LFTs and bilirubin levels, prolonged PT
  - Third: 3–5 d into course return of N/V, anorexia w/ evidence of hepatic failure (jaundice, encephalopathy, coagulopathy, hypoglycemia). Can see renal and cardiac failure too
  - Fourth: Recovery or death from liver failure
- **Risk factors** assoc w/ hepatotoxicity; multi-ingestion, <10 yo w/ inapprop dosing, delay initiation NAC, use sustained release form or co-admin w/ OTC drugs w/ acetaminophen
  - Rectal admin w/ peak drug levels, which can vary up to 9-fold, often fail to reach therapeutic levels and have longer dosing intervals (q6–8h vs. q4h)
  - **History:** Timing critical. Initial nonspecific symptoms NOT predictive of outcome
  - **Dose of ingestion:** 120–150 mg/kg or >7.5 g is considered toxic
  - **PE:** As above; in the -1st 24 hr nonspecific. Evidence of hepatotoxicity in 24–36 hr
  - **Labs:** Plasma acetaminophen level at 4 hr predictive (use Rumack–Matthew nomogram) (Pediatrics 1975;55:871) or available online at www.utoronto.ca/kids/aceta. htm. Check baseline Chem 7, LFTs, coags
  - Serum transaminases peak by 3–4 d after ingestion. Serum and urine toxicology
  - **Treatment**
  - Activated charcoal given if <8 hr since ingestion or if co-ingestion suspected
  - Mucomyst: N-acetylcysteine: 20% NAC diluted 1:4 in carbonated beverage PO/PNG
    - Loading: 140 mg/kg then 70 mg/kg/dose q4h × 17 doses. IV dosing below

Specific Agents and Their Antidotes (POISINDEX®)

Ingested Agent	Antidote
Acetaminophen	N-acetylcysteine (e.g., Mucomyst) 140 mg/kg PO × 1 then 70 mg/kg q4h × 17 doses or 150 mg/kg IV infused over 1 hr, followed by a 4-hr infusion of 50 mg/kg IV, followed by a 16-hr infusion of 100 mg/kg IV
Anticholinergics	**Physostigmine:** Adult 2 mg IV, child 0.2 mg/kg up to 0.5 mg IV—repeat q15min until desired effect, then q2–3h PRN; if wide QRS: NaHCO$_3$ 1–2 mEq/kg IV (pH 7.45–7.55) **Lidocaine:** Load 1 mg/kg, then infuse 20–50 mcg/min
Anticholinesterase	**Atropine:** Adults 2–5 mg IM/IV rpt q30min, child 0.02 mg/kg IM/IV, rpt q2–5min until effect; min dose 0.1 mg
Organophosphates	**Pralidoxime:** Adults 1–2 g, child 25–50 mg/kg IV. Rpt q1h PRN then q10–12h for 24–48 hr
Carbamates	**Atropine:** As above, **pralidoxime** if severe
Benzodiazepines	**Flumazenil:** 0.01 mg/kg IV × 1 followed 5 mcg/kg/min infusion
Beta blockers	**Atropine:** 0.02 mg/kg IV q5min (min 0.1 mg/max 0.5 mg); **Glucagon:** 50–150 mcg/kg IV, infuse 50–100 mcg/kg/h; **Insulin/Dextrose:** 1 unit/kg 25–50 mL D$_{50}$W, then 1 unit/kg/hr and titrate dextrose; NS for HoTN, pressors if needed
Calcium channel blockers	**CaCl:** 10%: Adult 10 cc, child 0.2 cc/kg IV; **CaGluc:** 10%: Adult 30 cc, child 0.6 cc/kg IV; **Glucagon:** 50 mcg/kg IV
Carbon monoxide	**100% O$_2$** — consider hyperbaric if severe case
Clonidine/α-adrenergic	**Narcan:** Infants, children <20 kg: 0.01 mg/kg/dose IM/IV/SC/ETT >20 kg or >5 yo: 2 mg/dose may repeat PRN q2–3min
Cyanide	**Adult:** Amyl nitrite inhalation (inhale 15–30 sec q60sec) until given **NaNitrite** 300 mg (10 mL of 3%) IV over 2–4 min. Follow w/ 12.5 g (50 mL) 25% **NaThiosulfate** IV. **Child:** Dose depends on Hgb to avoid methemoglobinemia (call poison control), 0.15–0.33 mL/kg of 3% **NaNitrite,** follow w/ 1.65 mL/kg of 25% **NaThiolsulfate**
Digitalis	**Digibind** (Fab antibodies): Dose based on amt ingested
Ethylene glycol	*See methanol*
Fluoride	**Milk** to bind fluoride; if Ca abn; **CaGluc** 10%: 0.6 cc/kg IV slowly until sx resolve and serum calcium normalizes, repeat PRN
Heavy metals	*Usual chelators*
Arsenic	**Dimercaprol (BAL)** 2.5–3 mg/kg IM q4–12h; **Penicillamine:** 100 mg/kg/d up to 1 g divided q6h; **DMSA** 10 mg/kg q8h for 5 d → q12h for 14 d.
Lead	**Dimercaprol (BAL):** 2.5–3 mg/kg q4h for 2 d → q4–6h for 2 d → q4–12h for 7 d, **EDTA** 50–75 mg/kg/d divided q3–6doses; **Penicillamine:** 15–20 mg/kg/d divided q6h; **DMSA** 10 mg/kg q8h for 5 d → q12h for 14 d.
Mercury	**DMSA:** 10 mg/kg q8h for 5 d → 10 mg/kg q12h for 14 d; **Penicillamine:** 25–100 mg/kg/d divided in 2–4 doses; **BAL:** 3–5 mg/kg/q4h for 3 d → 2.5–3 mg/kg q6h for 2 d → 2.5–3 mg/kg q15h for 7 d
Iron	**Deferoxamine:** 15–35 mg/kg/hr IV—use higher end dose for severe symptoms
Isoniazid	**Pyridoxine: 5–10%:** 1 g/1 g INH ingested (5 mg if dose unknown)—IV over 30–60 min
Methanol and ethylene glycol	**Ethanol to achieve blood level of 100 mg/dL.** Adults 0.6 mg/kg/7–10 g infused over 1 hr. Child 0.6 mg/kg over 1 hr. Maintenance: 110 mg/kg/hr in adults; 66 mg/kg/hr in children; if levels of methanol or ethylene glycol exceed 20 mg/dL or if high anion gap acidosis give **Fomepizole:** 15 mg/kg × 1 → 10 mg/kg doses q12h × 4 → 15 mg/kg q12h until leaves <20 mg/dL. Consider hemodialysis if severe. Also give folate (if methanol) or thiamine/pyridoxine (if ethylene glycol).

Methemoglobinemic agents	**Methylene blue**1%: 1–2 mg/kg IV slowly over 5–10 min if cyanosis with metHgb level >40%
Opioids	**Narcan:** Infants, children <20 kg: 0.1 mg/kg/dose IM/IV/SC/ETT >20 kg or >5 yo: 2 mg/dose, may repeat PRN q2–3min
Phenothiazines	**Diphenhydramine:** 1.25 mg/kg IV/IM; **Benztropine:** 1–2 mg IM/IV
SSRI	Benzos: **Diazepam:** 0.2–0.5 mg/kg q5min; **Lorazepam:** 0.05–0.1 mg/kg; **Cyproheptadine:** (Periactin) 60 mcg/kg q6h max:12 mg/d
Sulfonylureas	**Dextrose:** 0.5–1 g/kg (2–4 cc/kg of D25); **Octreotide:** adult 50–100 mcg SC q6–12h
TCA	**NaHCO$_3$** 1–2 mEq/kg IV (serum pH 7.45–7.55); **MgSulfate** 50 mg/kg IV
Warfarin	**Vitamin K** Child: 1–5 mg; Adult 5–10 mg

FACIAL TRAUMA

Eye Trauma (Emerg Med Clin North Am 2008;26:199; Int J Clin Pract 2008;62:1776; Philos Trans R Soc Lond B Biol Sci 2011;366:251, CD004166)

- **Corneal abrasion**
  - Traumatic defect in corneal epithelium
  - Symptoms of pain, photophobia, tearing, foreign body sensation
  - Topical anesthetic (proparacaine) can facilitate exam. Conjunctival injection (common), visual acuity usually normal. Very important to evert upper/lower lids
  - Diagnosis made with topical fluorescein staining
  - Treated with antibiotic ointment and +/− oral analgesics. Contact lens wearers need to have contact lens removed, pseudomonas coverage, and referral to ophthalmology. Eye patching is not recommended
- **Traumatic hyphema**
  - Layering of blood in the anterior chamber
  - Caused by blunt trauma directly to eye. May be associated with head trauma or fall
  - Symptoms of pain, photophobia, visual loss, nausea and vomiting
  - Remember ABCs and trauma evaluation. Often trauma can be seen with pen-light exam. Microhyphema requires slit lamp exam
  - Apply eye shield immediately. Do not patch. Place on bed rest with head of bed elevated 30–45 degrees. Emergent ophthalmology exam
- **Open globe injuries**
  - Full-thickness wound of eye wall
  - Caused by sharp objects, BB guns, ball sports, MVAs
  - Males 10–30 years old at greatest risk
  - Symptoms of pain, diplopia, decreased visual acuity
  - Do not touch the eye. Usually presents with sub-conjunctival hemorrhage, hyphema and teardrop pupil (narrow segment points toward rupture)
  - Apply eye shield immediately. Can use bottom of Styrofoam cup as shield. Immediate referral to ophthalmology
- **Pinna hematoma**
  - Often due to athletic injury, fall, blow to head. May cause disruption of perichondrial blood vessels causing cartilage necrosis
  - Emergent evacuation to avoid cauliflower ear complication
- **CSF otorrhea**
  - May be secondary to temporal bone fracture
  - Do not use otoscope or other instruments. Place on bed rest and elevate head of bed
  - Neurosurgical referral and head imaging

Nasal Trauma (Pediatr Clin North Am 2006;53:195; Pediatr Rev 1998;19:142; Int J Pediatr Otorhinolaryngol 2011;75:186)

- **Epistaxis**
  - 90% due to anterior bleeding and usually arises from Kiesselbach's plexus. Anterior bleeding is slow, persistent oozing
  - Commonly due to trauma, nose picking, URI, allergic rhinitis, foreign body
  - Management includes internal/external exam, then direct nasal pressure for 5–10 min while patient is sitting upright

- Posterior bleeds originate from sphenopalatine artery and bleed more profusely. May be associated with hemoptysis, hematemesis, blood in posterior pharynx, and failure to identify an anterior source of bleeding. Higher risk for airway compromise, aspiration of blood and hemorrhage. Requires ENT referral

- **Nasal fractures and septal hematoma**
  - Children have more soft cartilage which can cause more soft tissue swelling with trauma. Septal hematoma develops when there is disruption of septal cartilage from perichondrium, which can develop pressure-induced avascular necrosis
  - Require internal/external exam which may be difficult due to edema. Septal hematoma has septal asymmetry and swelling of nasal mucosa with obstruction of nasal passage. Size of mass does not change with topical vasoconstrictor
    - Radiographs are not helpful
    - If not septal hematoma, intracranial or ocular injury, should follow-up in 3–4 d when swelling has subsided
    - Management of septal hematoma includes prompt surgical evacuation and antimicrobial therapy if nasal septal abscess is suspected.
    - Improperly treated septal hematoma can lead to saddle nose deformity

- **Clear rhinorrhea**
  - Differential is broad but think of CSF leak caused by skull base fracture
  - Allow rhinorrhea to drip onto piece of paper and classic pattern is central area of blood with halo of clear CSF. Not a sensitive test
  - If CSF rhinorrhea is suspected, place patient on bed rest and elevate head of bed 30 degrees. Consult neurosurgery and otolaryngology

Oropharyngeal Injuries (Pediatr Clin North Am 2006:53:195; Pediatrics 2010;126:e1578)

- **Dental injuries**
  - Patients with a fracture, luxation, tooth pain, or discoloration should undergo dental radiography
  - Uncomplicated fractures affect the outer enamel or dentin only. Patient can be seen by dentist in 48 hr
  - Complicated fractures involve enamel, dentin, and pulp. Symptoms include tooth pain with pressure, temperature sensitivity, bleeding from core of tooth, and malocclusion. Requires immediate dental referral
    - Avulsion refers to complete displacement of tooth from socket. If primary tooth, do not reimplant. Permanent teeth begin to erupt at age 6. If permanent tooth, handle by crown, rinse with water or normal saline and attempt reimplantation. If unable to reimplant, place in milk or other commercial product. Patients require immediate dental referral. Tooth survival outside oral cavity at 1 hr is near 0

- **Tongue and frenulum injuries**
  - Careful examination of teeth, oropharyngeal foreign bodies, bite for malocclusion (mandibular fracture) and TMJ (condylar fracture)
  - Most frenulum injuries heal spontaneously and do not require repair
  - Tongue lacerations <1 cm and non-gaping usually do not require repair
  - Tongue lacerations >1 cm, into muscle or lateral tongue, large flaps, or do not achieve hemostasis usually require repair

- **Palate injuries**
  - Superficial and puncture wounds to the central palate that are <2 cm usually do not need repair after careful exam for foreign body
  - Injury to lateral aspect of palate, posterior pharyngeal wall, >2 cm, or with unknown depth or foreign body will likely need repair. These injuries carry a small risk of injury to the carotid arteries and jugular veins. Consider further imaging and close observation for neurologic deterioration. Obtain otolaryngology consult

FOOD ALLERGY

NIAID-Sponsored Food Allergy Guidelines (J Allergy Clin Immunol 2010;126:S1)
www.niaid.nih.gov/topics/foodAllergy/clinical/Documents/FAGuidelinesExecSummary.pdf

Definition (Pediatrics 2011;128:955)
- **Food allergy (FA):** Adverse health effect arising from a specific response that occurs reproducibly on exposure to a given food
- **Anaphylaxis:** A serious immunologic reaction that is rapid in onset and may cause death (see ED chapter for more on anaphylaxis)

Classification (Pediatr Clin N Am 2011;58:315)
- **IgE mediated:** Urticaria/angioedema, rhinoconjunctivitis/asthma, anaphylaxis, pollen-food allergy syndrome (PFAS) (aka oral allergy syndrome (OAS))
- **Mixed IgE and cell mediated:** Atopic dermatitis (AD), eosinophilic gastrointestinal disorders (EGIDs)
- **Cell mediated:** Dietary protein-induced proctitis/proctocolitis, food protein-induced enterocolitis syndrome (FPIES), Celiac disease, Heiner syndrome

Pathophysiology (Annu Rev Med 2009;60:261)
- IgE mediated: Dendritic cells interact w/ dietary antigens → T-helper-2 response → B-cell IgE production → IgE binds on the surface of mast cells
- PFAS: Cross-reactivity btw proteins in pollen & proteins in certain fruits/veg
- FPIES: May relate to increased TNF-α, decreased TGF-β

Epidemiology (Pediatr Clin N Am 2011;58:327)
- Self-reported FA is 10 times higher than what can be confirmed with testing
- FA is more common in early childhood and decreases with age
- Self-reported FA ranges from 3–35%; confirmed FA ranges from 1–10.8%
- Most common allergens (kids): Cow's milk, egg, wheat, soy, peanut/tree nut, fish/shellfish

Clinical Manifestations (Pediatr Clin N Am 2011;58:315)
- **IgE-mediated:** Onset of sx min to 2 hr after ingestion (urticaria, angioedema, rhino-conjunctivitis, asthma, GI sx, anaphylaxis) vs. **Cell Mediated:** Delayed rxn
- **OAS:** Pruritis, tingling, mild swelling of lips, tongue, palate, and throat; 10% have systemic findings; 1–2% develop anaphylaxis
- **Eosinophilic esophagitis:** Presentation varies w/ age: Feeding difficulty + FTT in young kids, vomiting + abd pain in older kids, dysphagia + food impaction in teens
- **Eosinophilic gastroenteritis:** Abd pain, nausea, diarrhea, weight loss 2/2 malabsorption
- **Dietary protein-induced proctitis/proctocolitis:** Typically breastfed infants age 2–8 wk, mucus + blood in stools but otherwise well-appearing, removing allergenic food from mother's diet leads to rapid improvement
- **FPIES:** Peak incidence 1 wk–3 mo, usually formula fed; severe GI symptoms: Vomiting, diarrhea, FTT, anemia, hypotension and lethargy 2/2 dehydration

Evaluation (J Allergy Clin Immunol 2010;126:S1, Ann Allergy Asthma Immunol 2006;96:S1, J Allergy Clin Immunol 2004;114:213)
- History is key: Identify culprit foods, time course of rxn, quantity ingested, ancillary factors, Hx of similar sx, and FHx and personal hx of atopy
- IgE mediated: Skin prick testing (SPT) and specific serum IgE (sIgE) measurements can be helpful but not diagnostic; to avoid false+, pts should be tested only to suspect foods and when there is high pretest probability
- Skin prick tests (for IgE-mediated disorders): A wheal ≥3 mm is considered positive
  - SPT: Sensitivity >90%; specificity approx 50%
- CAP-FEIA (formerly RAST): Measures food-specific serum IgE
  - ImmunoCAP is the preferred CAP-FEIA
- Double-blind, placebo-controlled food challenge gold std for dx; only in controlled setting; should be done if dx of FA unclear or to confirm suspected resolution of FA
- EGIDs: SPT, atopy patch testing may be helpful but mucosal bx needed for dx
- Dietary protein-induced proctitis/proctocolitis/FPIES: Dx based on history, sx resolution with causative food elimination, and sx recurrence with food challenge

Management and Prevention (Pediatrics 2011;128:955, Pediatr Clin N Am 2011;58:481, J Allergy Clin Immunol 2011;127:654)
- Key to mgmt is avoidance of allergen (www.foodallergy.org has practical tips)
- Tx: Antihistamines for OAS and nonsevere rxns, epi for all pts w/ systemic rxns
- Current research for tx of FA includes immunotherapy and anti-IgE antibodies

- Oral immunotherapy has been shown to induce desensitization and enable patients to ingest a greater amount of allergenic food protein
- Restricting mother's diet in pregnancy or lactation to prevent FA not recommended
- No evidence that delayed intro of solid food >4 mo prevents FA and some evidence that delayed intro of solids may promote allergy
- Vaccines containing egg include influenza, MMR, yellow fever, rabies
  - MMR vaccine is not contraindicated for children with egg allergy
  - Flu vaccine: If mild rxn to egg (hives only) → safe to give vaccine in office with precautions (resuscitative equipment available and observe pt for 30 min); if severe rxn (CV, resp, GI sx) → allergy consultation for evaluation of egg allergy and vaccine administration (Pediatrics 2011;128:813–825)

ATOPIC DERMATITIS (AD)

Definition (J Allergy Clin Immunol 2006;118:152)
- Chronic, immune-mediated, inflammatory, pruritic skin dz occurring in pts w/ atopic diathesis, w/ variable clinical pattern depending on age

Pathophysiology (J Invest Dermatol 2012;132:949)
- Impaired epidermal barrier: Stratum corneum defects → ↓ epidermal water content
  - Mutations in the filaggrin gene predispose to AD (filaggrin is a protein in the stratum corneum that helps maintain hydration and has anti-staph properties)
  - Dry skin → pruritis and scratching → trauma and inflammation
  - Water loss → changes in epidermal lipids → cracks in the stratum corneum
- Antigenic and irritant agents penetrate the skin and activate immune cells
- Immune dysfunction w/ exaggerated T_h2 response: IgE prod, eosinophilia, and proinflammatory cytokines → hyperactive immune response → extravasation of inflammatory cells, cellular signaling at injury site
- Pruritus mechanism not just 2/2 histamine
- Triggers: Stress-induced immunomodulation, food + inhalant allergens, chemical irritants, skin infection, hot/humid or cold/dry weather, viral infections esp w/ fever

Epidemiology (N Engl J Med 2008;358:1483, N Engl J Med 2005;352:2314)
- Affects 15–30% of children and 2–10% of adults
- Age of onset: 45% in 1st 6 mo of life, 60% before age 1; 85% before age 5
- 70% of children have spontaneous remission before adolescence
- 77% concordance rate for monozygotic twins; 15% for dizygotic
- Asthma develops in approx 30% and allergic rhinitis in 35% of children with AD

Clinical Manifestations (J Allergy Clin Immunol 2006;118:152)
- *Infantile stage* (infancy–2 yo)
  - Location: Cheeks, forehead, scalp, may spread to trunk
  - Intensely pruritic, erythematous, scaly lesions, may have vesicles or serous exudate in severe cases
- *Childhood stage* (2 yo–puberty)
  - Location: Flexural surfaces, wrists, ankles, hands, feet, neck, dorsum of extremities
  - Less exudation; more lichenified papules and plaques
- *Adult stage* (puberty+)
  - Location: Flexural surfaces, face, neck, upper arms, back, hands, feet
  - Dry, scaly erythematous papules & plaques; lichenified plaques in areas of chronicity
- W/ severe cases, any area involved, but axillary, groin, & gluteal areas usually spared
- Complications: Bacterial or viral superinfxn of eczematous sites (e.g., eczema herpeticum)

Diagnostic Studies (N Engl J Med 2005;352:2314)
- Clinical criteria: Evidence of *itchy skin* + 3 of the following:
  - H/o involvement of skin creases
  - H/o generally dry skin in the past year
  - H/o asthma or hay fever (or FHx atopy in 1st-degree relative for pts <4 yo)
  - Onset of sx at <2 yo (criterion not used if child <4 yo)
  - Dermatitis of flex surfaces (or cheeks/forehead/outer aspects of ext for pts <4 yo)
- Specific allergy testing not routinely recommended, depends on dz severity
- Ddx: Psoriasis, contact dermatitis, seborrheic dermatitis, scabies, vit def, drug rxns

Management (Pediatrics 2008;122:812, Am Fam Physician 2007;75:523)
- *Eliminate exacerbating factors:* Soap, hot water, abrasive materials (synthetics, wool), physiologic/emotional stress, individual-specific allergens and irritants
- *Skin hydration* w/ emollients even when asymptomatic: Avoid lotions (worsen xerosis via water evap); use thick creams/ointments (hydrolated petrolatum, petroleum jelly) are most effective; apply immediately after bathing
- *Topical steroids:* Limit to bid; only low potency on face, genital, intertriginous areas
  - 1–2.5% hydrocortisone (low potency) for mild AD
  - 0.1% triamcinolone (medium potency) for more severe AD
- *Topical calcineurin inhibitors* (1% pimecrolimus & 0.03% tacrolimus): Approved as 2nd-line Rx in kids >2 yo who respond poorly or are intolerant to topical steroids
  - Adverse effects: Burning sensation of skin and irritation; should use sun protection
  - Benefits: Not assoc w/ skin atrophy, safe for use on face
  - FDA "black box warning" safety not clear w/ long-term/continuous use & in pts <2 yo
- *Systemic tx* used in severe cases: UV light, systemic immunosuppressants
- *Adjunctive tx:* Sedating antihistamines for pruritis – due to sedative effect (non-sedating antihistamines *not* effective for itch), wet dressings, bleach baths to ↓ local skin infections

DRUG ALLERGY

Definition (Ann Allergy Asthma Immunol. 2010;105:259)
- Immunologically mediated response to pharmacologic agent
- Differs from pseudoallergic rxn (e.g., contrast): Non–IgE-mediated release of mediators from mast cells and basophils → classic end organ effects
- **Hypersensitivity:** (Gell PGH, Coombs RRA. Clin Aspects Immunol 1975;761)
  - **Type I:** IgE mediated: urticaria, laryngoedema, bronchospasm, cardiovascular collapse immediately after drug admin; commonly with antibiotics
  - **Type II:** Cytotoxic (e.g., acquired hemolytic anemia from large doses of PCN)
  - **Type III:** Immune complex: Fevers, arthralgias, lymphadenopathy, and urticarial rash 1–3 wk after initial drug exposure; w/ PCN, sulfonamides, phenytoin
  - **Type IV:** Cell mediated (e.g., contact dermatitis w/ topical med use)
- Can categorize drug rxn by tissue/organ involved (e.g., systemic, cutaneous, visceral)

Penicillins (JAMA 2001;285:2498)
- Most common BUT 80–90% pts reporting PCN allergy not truly allergic by skin test
- Incidence of skin rxns: 5.1% w/ amox, 4.5% w/ amp, 1.6% with PCN; rates of PCN-induced anaphylaxis: 0.015–0.04% of pts receiving PCN
- Hx (age, rxn, timing, route, other meds, response to d/c, Hx of taking similar Abx)
- Immediate rxn (<1 hr): Type I/IgE mediated. Usually in pts 20–49 yo. Risk not ↑ w/ atopy but if occurs, may be more severe rxn
  - Skin testing most reliable for IgE-mediated allergy (NOT SJS/TEN or Types II–IV). CAP-FEIA not as reliable; neg predictive value of PCN skin testing almost 100%
- Late rxn (>72 hr): Types II–IV. None involve IgE, so skin testing useless
- Idiopathic: Commonly maculopapular (MP)/morbilliform rash. Unclear mech. 1–4%
  - ↑ w/ EBV, CMV, or leukemia. Also infectious causes of MP rash
  - If rash strictly MP (nonpruritic, nonurticarial), no signs Type I; safe to readmin

Cephalosporins (Pediatrics 2005;115:1048)
- Causes allergic rxn in 1–3% w/ or w/o hx PCN allergy, but anaphylaxis is rare
- Rates cephalosporin allergy in pt w/ PCN allergy Hx or skin testing differs w/ gen
  - Risk ↑ 'd by 0.5% with 1st generation, likely not most 2nd, 3rd, or 4th
- Risk 2/2 to side chains; PCN similar to cefoxitin, cephalothin, cephaloridine; amoxicillin/ampicillin similar to cephalexin, cephradine, cefatrizine, cefaclor, cefprozil

Other Beta-lactams
- **Carbapenems** (imipenem): Are cross-reactive; use w/ caution in PCN allergic
- **Monobactams** (aztreonam): Not considered cross reactive

Vancomycin
- Red man syndrome = pseudoallergic (non–IgE-mediated histamine release)
  - Affects >50% of pts; prevent by slowing infusion rate + premed w/ antihistamines
- Rarely causes IgE-mediated reactions

URTICARIA

(Allergy 2003;58:1224, Immunol Allergy Clin North Am 2005;25:353)

- **Definition:** Rapid appearance of wheals (pruritic, central swellings of variable size, almost always surrounded by reflex erythema that blanches w/ pressure); histamine release is the primary mediator; affects the superficial dermis
- **Clinical sx:** Pruritic, at times burning; transient (1–24 hr); +/– angioedema
- **Epidemiology** (Immunol Allergy Clin N Am 2005;25:353)
  - Incidence 15–25%. Affects 6–7% of preschoolers, 17% of kids w/ AD
  - 50% w/ urticaria and angioedema, 40% w/ just urticaria, 10% w/ angioedema alone

Angioedema (Am J Med 2008;121:282)

- **Definition:** Pronounced asymmetric, nonpitting swelling that occurs in nondependent areas caused by leakage of plasma into deep dermis and subcutaneous tissues
- **Clinical sx:** Sudden onset. Can be painful rather than itching (few mast cells in deep skin layers). Commonly affects mucosa. Slower resolution (up to 72 hr)
- **Epidemiology:** 15% of general population

Etiologies: Urticaria +/– Angioedema

- **Spontaneous urticaria:** Spont appearance of wheals, ↑ in atopic individuals
  - Acute <6 wk: Mostly viral infxns (also consider parasitic and bacterial), drug and transfusion rxns, foods (in young kids: Egg, milk, peanut, soy, wheat; older kids: Fish, seafood, nuts, peanuts; food less common cause in adults)
  - Chronic >6 wk: Less common in kids; cause is rarely identified; etiologies include infectious (H. pylori, parasites, Hep A and B), autoimmune (anti-IgE receptor Abs, thyroid Abs), FA, pseudoallergy (non–IgE-mediated histamine release), chronic inflammatory process (SLE, neoplasia)
- **Physical urticaria:** Urticarial reaction to specific physical stimuli
  - Dermographic urticaria: Rapidly appears 2/2 shearing force on skin, usually resolve in 1–2 hr without treatment; most common
  - Delayed pressure urticaria: Deep, painful swelling 4–8 hr after static pressure
  - Cold urticaria; heat urticaria (rare); solar urticaria (mostly from UV light)
- **Special types of urticaria:**
  - Cholinergic urticaria: 2/2 brief ↑ in body core temp (physical exercise, warm bath); w/ small transient wheals, may include angioedema, wheezing, syncope
  - Adrenergic urticaria: Rare, elicited by stress; red wheals w/ white halo
  - Contact urticaria: Wheals at site of substance contact; can have generalized sx
  - Aquagenic urticaria: $H_2O \rightarrow H_2O$-soluble allergen → diffuses into dermis → wheal
- **Other diseases in differential diagnosis:**
  - Urticarial vasculitis (UV) & erythema multiforme (EM): Suspect if lesions >24 hr old
    - EM w/ targetoid lesions from med or infxn (e.g., HSV)
    - UV w/ palpable purpura and bruising when disappears
  - Mastocytoma: Hyperpigmented macule/papule → wheal when mech irritated
  - Mastocytosis: Excess mast cells in skin, BM, GI tract, liver, spleen, LNs, are usually sporadic. Flares w/ pruritus, flushing, palps, ↑ HR, syncope, GI sx
- **Angioedema:** (Amer J Med 2008;121:282, Immunol Allergy Clin North Am 2005;25:353)
  - Hereditary angioedema: 1% of all angioedema (see later discussion)
  - Acquired angioedema: Type 1 (lymphoprolif dz [malign cells consume C1 inhib prot]); Type 2 (autoAb to C1 inhib prot); Meds: ACE-I 0.1–2.2%, less w/ ARBs

Diagnostic Studies (Allergy 2003;58:1224)

- Hx most important (duration, pruritus, blanching, when, where, viral illness, drugs, skin contact, fever, joint pain, sx thyroid dz) (Immunol Allergy Clin North Am 2005;25:353)
- Acute urticaria: No routine diagnostic tests
- Chronic urticaria: CBC w/ diff, ESR/CRP (indicates systemic dz), stop drugs (e.g., NSAIDs)
  - Consider: Eval H. pylori, ANA, gastroscopy, stool for O and P, skin tests, specific IgE, thyroid fxn, and autoAbs, food elimination diet for 3 wk
- Physical urticaria: Elicit rxn from various physical stim, consider CBC w/ diff and ESR
- Cholinergic urticaria: Exercise or hot bath according to patient history

Management (Allergy 2003;58:1224)

- Avoid or eliminate eliciting stimulus (e.g., d/c drugs, rarely IgE FA)
- Therapy of target tissues of mast cell mediators: H1-antihistamines—mainstay of Rx
- Inhibit mast cell mediator release: Systemic steroids (avoid long-term use), cyclosporine A (for resistant chronic urticaria, expensive), PUVA (psoralen plus UV light) → ↓ # mast cells

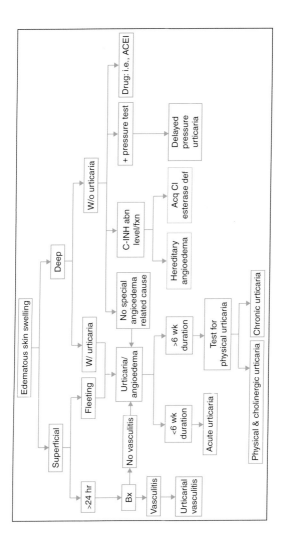

IMMUNE DEFICIENCIES

(J Allergy Clin Immunol 2010;125:S182)

Overview (N Engl J Med 2000;343:37, N Engl J Med 2000;343:108)
- **1° immunity:** Occurs on 1st encounter with antigen; slower response
- **2° immunity:** Preformed Ab by memory B cell; quicker response on 2nd exposure
- **Passive:** Transplacental transfer of IgG: Provides protective effect for 1st 6–12 mo; breast milk contains IgA and IgG; large amt of IgA in colostrum

Immune Deficiencies
- Can be 1° (usually inherited and present during early childhood) or 2° (due to underlying disorder or immunosuppressive treatment) (Ann Allergy Asthma Immunol 2005;94:S1)
- Normal to have up to 11 respiratory infections per yr in infancy, 8 episodes per yr at pre-school age, 4 episodes per yr at school age (Pediatr Allergy Immunol 2008;19:505)
- **When to suspect primary immunodeficiency (PID)** (Clin Exp Immunol 2008;152:389 Pediatrics 2011;127:810)
  - ≥8 new infections in 1 yr; ≥2 serious sinus infections or episodes of PNA in 1 yr
  - ≥2 mo on abx with little effect; need for IV abx to clear infections
  - Recurrent deep skin or organ abscesses; persistent superficial candidiasis after 1 yr
  - Opportunistic infections; ≥2 invasive infections; complications after live vaccines
  - Unexplained autoimmune disease; failure to thrive; + FHx of PID
  - Strongest identifiers of PID: Family hx of PID, use of IV abx for sepsis, failure to thrive

Evaluating for PID (Ann Allergy Asthma Immunol 2005;94:S1)
- History + physical exam; consider possibility of secondary immunodeficiency; CBC w/ diff, lytes, glucose, BUN/Cr, albumin, urinalysis, immunoglobulin levels
  - Lymphopenia = <2500 cells/uL if <5 yo; <1500 cell/uL if >5 yo;
- Most PIDs are caused by B cell or combined B + T cell dysfunction; these diseases should be considered initially unless clinical presentation suggests otherwise
- **Evaluation of humoral immunity:** Suspect with sinopulmonary bacterial infections
  - Screening: Immunoglobulins (IgG, IgA, IgM), antibodies to protein antigens (diphtheria or tetanus vaccines) + polysaccharide antigens (pneumococcal vaccine)
  - Further testing: IgG subclasses, B-cell subset analysis by flow cytometry, antibody response to booster immunization, in vitro assessment of B-cell function
- **Evaluation of cell-mediated immunity:** Suspect with atypical mycobacteria, disseminated infection, opportunistic infection
  - Screening: T-cell subset analysis by flow cytometry, delayed-type hypersensitivity skin testing: PPD, Candida, and mumps antigens applied → most immunocompetent individuals will develop induration to at least 1 antigen
  - Further testing: In vitro assessment of T-cell function
- **Evaluation of phagocytic cells:** Suspect with abscesses and/or fungal infection
  - Screening: Neutrophil staining and morphology
  - Further testing: Oxidase function (dihydrorhodamine assay), assessment of phagocytosis, chemotaxis, bactericidal activity
- **Evaluation of complement:** Suspect with Neisserial infection
  - Screening: CH50 (total hemolytic complement activity) + AH50 (alternative pathway hemolytic activity): Normal levels exclude most hereditary complement deficiencies
  - Further testing: Assessment of individual complement components

B-CELL DEFICIENCY (HUMORAL IMMUNITY)

X-linked Agammaglobulinemia (XLA) a.k.a. Bruton
Agammaglobulinemia (J Allergy Clin Immunol 2002;109:581)
- **Definition:** Disorder in which pts are unable to generate mature B cells → absence or severe deficiency of serum immunoglobulins → freq infections beginning at 6–9 mo
- **Pathophysiology:**
  - Mutation in Bruton tyrosine kinase (Btk) gene located on the midportion of X chromo
  - Absence of Btk → block in B-cell maturation → low Ig in all classes
  - % of T cells generally increased and T-cell function is normal
- **Epidemiology:** X-linked, 1 in 100,000 males
  - Accounts for 85% of pts w/ early onset hypogammaglobulinemia and no B cells

- **Clinical manifestations:**
  - At 6–9 mo, begin w/ ↑ frequency of upper and lower resp tract infxns, cellulitis, chronic conjunctivitis, gastroenteritis, arthritis, meningitis/encephalitis
  - Common pathogens: *H. influenza, S. pneumoniae* (encapsulated pyogenic organisms)
  - Often nml response to viruses (T cells intact), except hepatitis, polio, enterovirus
  - Lymphoid tissue often ↓ in size; look for hypoplastic adenoids, tonsils, spleen
- **Diagnostic studies:** (X-linked Agammaglobulinemia in *GeneReviews* PMID 20301626)
  - Serum IgG, IgA, IgM, more than 2 SD below normal for age
  - Less than 2% CD19 + B cells
  - Abn antibody response to vaccines
  - Mutation in BTK gene or absent Btk protein
  - Differentiate from transient hypogammaglobulinemia (prolongation of infant hypogammaglobulinemia >6 mo, self-resolves, usually vaccine Abs nml)
- **Management:** (X-linked Agammaglobulinemia in *GeneReviews* 1997–2011)
  - Mainstay of treatment is IVIG; some centers use chronic prophylactic antibiotics
  - With acute infections tx course should be 2× as long as in healthy pts
  - Live viral vaccines (esp oral polio) should be avoided
- **Complications:**
  - Unclear if same predisposition for malignancy as other immune deficiencies
  - Chronic meningoencephalitis from coxsackie or enterovirus
  - Higher incidence of aseptic polyarthritis, JIA, dermatomyositis

Common Variable Immunodef (CVID) (J Allergy Clin Immunol 2002;109:581)

- **Definition:** Hypogammaglobulinemia with onset later in life; often associated with T-cell dysfunction, autoimmunity, malignancy
- **Pathophysiology:** No single molecular dx; catch-all for several immunodefs
  - Drug induced: Phenytoin, gold, or sulfasalazine may be trigger
  - B cells usually nml in # but do not differentiate into Ig producing cells
- **Epidemiology:** Average age of onset is 25 yo w/ even sex distribution
- **Clinical manifestations:**
  - Similar to XLA; encapsulated organisms, sinopulm infxns (see previous discussion) often leading to bronchiectasis if continued pulmonary infections
  - Exam: Lymphoid hyperplasia (in contrast to X-linked): Large tonsils, nodes, spleen
  - GI tract affected in about ½ of pts: Lymphoid proliferation of gut, chronic diarrhea, malabsorption, lactose intolerance, infection with Campylobacter, Yersinia, Giardia
  - Approx 22% of pts have autoimmune disorders: RA, hemolytic anemia, pernicious anemia, autoimmune endocrinopathies
  - Increased incidence of malignancy (esp involving GI tract + lymphoid tissues)
- **Diagnostic studies:**
  - Total Ig is markedly decreased, but generally not as depressed as in XLA
  - Any or all classes of Ig can be affected; degree of hypogammaglobulinemia is variable
  - T-cell function is variable (can be affected in about 50% of patients)
  - Abn Ab response to vaccines
- **Management:** Same as above for XLA; monitoring pulmonary function

IgA Deficiency (J Clin Immunol 2010;30:10)

- **Definition:** IgA antibody deficiency with normal levels of other Ig isotypes in pts >4 yo
- **Pathophysiology:**
  - B cells fail to differentiate into plasma cells expressing/secreting IgA
  - No well-defined genetic susceptibility; likely heterogeneous group of genetic defects
- **Epidemiology:** Most common in Middle East, Africa, and Caucasian populations
  - Incidence 1:223 to 1:3000 in US, most common primary immunodeficiency
- **Clinical manifestations:** Asymp in 85–90% of pts
  - If symptomatic: Recurrent sinopulmonary infections (*S. pneumoniae, H. influenzae*), GI infections and disorders (lactose intolerance, celiac, UC)
  - Predisposition to allergic and autoimmune disorders
- **Diagnostic studies:** Send total Ig and Ig isotypes and subclasses
  - IgA <7 mg/dL, normal IgG and IgM, normal T cells
- **Management:** If asymptomatic → no tx; if recurrent infections → prophylactic abx; if concurrent IgG subclass deficiency → IVIG
  - **Complications:** Risk of anaphylaxis with transfusions as may develop anti-IgA Ab: Blood products should be from IgA deficient individual or saline washed RBCs

T-CELL DEFICIENCIES (CELLULAR IMMUNITY)

DiGeorge Syndrome (DGS)/Thymic Aplasia (N Engl J Med 2000;343:1313)

- **Definition** (J Pediatr 2001;139:715)
  - Thymic and parathyroid aplasia/hypoplasia w/ ↓ T cells and frequent opportunistic infections as well as hypocalcemia, presents neonatally
  - Divided into partial and complete types: 1% of pts have complete DGS (a form of SCID) w/ severe immunodeficiency; pts w/ partial DGS have milder immunodeficiency
- **Pathophysiology:** Embryologically 3rd and 4th pharyngeal pouches form incorrectly
  - Microdeletion of 22q11.2 is the most common defect, generally de novo mutation
- **Epidemiology:** 1:4000 to 1:6000 prevalence
- **Clinical manifestations:** P/w tetany/szrs 2/2 hypocalcemia in 1st few days of life
  - All T-cell def generally present within 1st 1–3 mo of age w/ opportunistic infections, viral infections, fungal infections (PCP), intracellular bacteria
  - Can have similar facies to fetal alcohol syndrome: Short filtrum, low set ears
- **Diagnostic studies:** Absolute lymphocyte count ↓, B-cell count ↑, Ig nml
  - ↓ mitogen stimulation response, can have delayed hypersensitivity skin testing
- **Management:** Bone marrow transplant w/ HLA match
  - Thymic transplant in neonatal period (N Engl J Med 1999;341:1180)
- **Complications:** Can have other structural anomalies; conotruncal cardiac anomalies, right-sided aortic arch, esophageal atresia, bifid uvula, congenital heart disease, hypertelorism, mandibular hypoplasia, low set ears
  - GVHD to nonirradiated blood products or to BMT with T cells

COMBINED IMMUNE DEFICIENCIES

Severe Combined Immunodeficiency (SCID)

- **Definition:** (N Engl J Med 2000;343:1313)
  - Most severe 1° immunodef, lymphopenia, no thymocytes, incompatible w/ life
  - Mostly T-cell deficiency, but can also involve B cells and NK cells (combined)
- **Pathophysiology:** (J Allergy Clin Immunol 2009;124:1161)
  - Multiple gene loci including: **T-B+ SCID:** *IL2RG* encoding γ-chains of interleukins (most common), *Jak3, IL7RA, CD3, CD45*; **T-B− SCID:** RAG1/RAG2, ADA deficiency, Omenn syndrome, Artemis mutation
  - Inheritance autosomal recessive and X-linked (for *IL2RG*)
  - Generally small thymus, w/ poor thymocyte production (no T cells)
- **Epidemiology:** Affects 1 in 100,000 (Pediatrics 2010;125:e1226)
  - For X-linked all are male, but overall SCID has small female predominance
- **Clinical manifestations:** (J Pediatr 1997;130:378)
  - Infant p/w FTT, chronic diarrhea, PNA, OM, sepsis, opportunistic infxns, cutaneous *Candida*, thrush, recurrent RSV, frequent HSV outbreaks
  - *Candida albicans*, PCP, varicella, measles, Paraflu3, CMV, EBV, Adeno
- **Diagnostic studies:** At birth, WBC <2,000/mm^3, abs lymphocytes very ↓, ↓/absent T cells (<20% of total lymphocytes are T cells)
  - Can have absent B cells as well and absent NK cells depending on genotype
  - Absent mitogen stim response, can have delayed hypersensitivity skin testing
  - Serum immunoglobulins ↓, no antibodies after vaccination
- **Newborn screening** (Curr Opin Allergy Clin Immunol 2010;10:521)
  - Detection of T-cell receptor excision circles (TRECs) = marker of # of naïve T cells
  - Low TRECs → repeat analysis of TRECs and β-actin (to ensure integrity of DNA) → TRECs still low → flow cytometry
- **Management: Pediatric emergency** (Eur J Pediatr 2011;170:561)
  - Hematopoietic stem cell transplant (success rate ≈90% in best circumstances)
  - For ADA deficiency: Enzyme replacement is an alternative tx
  - New innovations: Gene Rx (for ADA and IL2RG)
- **Complications:** GVHD to nonirradiated blood products or to BMT w/ T cells
  - Severe sepsis, severe viral infections because of immunocompromised state

Ataxia-Telangiectasia
- **Definition:** (Pediatr Allergy Immunol 2005;16:615)
  - Progressive disorder w/ cerebellar ataxia, oculocutaneous telangiectasias and combined immunodeficiency (T and sometimes B)
- **Pathophysiology**
  - Mutation in *AT* on long arm chromo 11q22–23 (encodes DNA-dependent protein kinase involved in DNA repair, cell cycle signaling and meiotic control)
  - ↓ CD3 & CD4 counts, ↓ response to T- & B-cell mitogens, helper T-cell & B-cell defects
- **Epidemiology:** Equal male and female incidence, 1 in 40,000–100,000 births
  - Autosomal recessive, so consanguinity increases risk of disease
- **Clinical manifestations:** (J Pediatr 2004;144:505)
  - Early deterioration of gait beginning 1–4 yo with ataxia (wheelchair by 10–12 yo)
  - Extrapyramidal deterioration, oculomotor apraxia, nystagmus, poor articulation
  - Telangiectasia in conjunctiva and skin appear by age 3–6 yr after neurologic signs
  - Concurrent sinopulmonary infections (70%) severe PNA
- **Diagnostic studies**
  - Selective absence of IgA (50–80%), IgG and IgE generally ↓, often T-cell deficiency (60–75%), and more rarely B cells ↓ as well
  - Elevated AFP, abnormal ATM kinase activity (if lab can obtain test)
  - MRI w/ degeneration of granular and Purkinje cells (Neuroradiology 2003;45:315)
- **Management:** Prophylactic antibiotics if indicated; IVIG for hypogammaglobulinemia or specific antibody defect; supportive measures
- **Complications:** ↑ incidence (200×) malignancies; lymphoma, leukemia, and adeno Ca
  - Extreme sensitivity to radiation

Wiskott–Aldrich
- **Definition:** (N Engl J Med 2006;355:1759, Curr Opin Hematol 2008;15:30)
  - X-linked d/o w/ AD, thrombocytopenic purpura, dysfunction of platelets leading to bleeding and predisposition to infection
- **Pathophysiology** (Curr Opin Hematol 2005;12:284)
  - WASP (Wiskott–Aldrich syndrome protein) mutated (Xp11.22–11.23) >160 muts
  - WASP, normally expressed in lymphocytes and megakaryocytes, controls actin assembly for microvesicles involved with tyrosine kinase and protein kinase c signaling affecting B, T, and NK cells
  - T cells cannot interact w/ APC, B-cell adhesion inhibited by poor cytoskeleton reorganization and poor cell motility
- **Epidemiology:** X-linked recessive syndrome, generally only affects males
- **Clinical manifestations:** (N Engl J Med 1995;333:431)
  - Bloody diarrhea, bruising, bleeding after circ, thrombocytopenia neonatally
  - Frequent OM, PNA, sinusitis, and opportunistic infections; severe eczema
- **Diagnostic studies:** Serum IgM decreased, IgA and IgE often increased, total Ig normal
  - T cells low w/ poor mitogen response, B cells can be increased
  - Thrombocytopenia <50,000/μL and small volume platelets seen
- **Management:** (J Allergy Clin Immunol 2006;117:725, Curr Opin Hematol 2008;15:30)
  - Hematopoietic stem cell transplantation (HSCT) is the mainstay of treatment (5 yr survival rate of 87% if HLA match)
  - If HSCT not possible: IVIG q3–4wk, consider antibiotic prophylaxis (amoxicillin 20 mg/kg qd), Splenectomy: Increased platelets but also increased risk of sepsis
  - Gene Rx w/ WASP shown to be feasible & effective (N Engl J Med 2010;363:1918)
- **Complications:** Autoimmune disease in as high as 40% of affected pts; ITP, hemolytic anemia, vasculitis, IBD, nephritis
  - Lymphoma and other malignancies (13%) (J Allergy Clin Immunol 2007;120:795)

COMPLEMENT DEFICIENCIES

Overview (N Engl J Med 2001;344:1058, N Engl J Med 2001;344:1140)
- Divided into 3 pathways: Classical, mannose-binding lectin, and alternative
- Functions of complement: Defense against infection (opsonization, chemotaxis, lysis), interface between innate and adaptive immunity, clearance of waste
- Complement works as predetermined cascade pattern, all pathways activate C3

Hereditary Angioneurotic Edema (Pediatrics 2011;128:1173, J Allergy Clin Immunol 2008;121:S398)
- **Definition:** Recurrent self-limited episodes of tissue swelling affecting the skin, upper respiratory and GI tracts

- Type 1 (85%) w/ ↓ amount and activity of C1-inhibitor (C1-INH) in serum
- Type 2 (15%) w/ normal amount, but functional impairment of C1-INH
- Type 3 w/ normal level and fxn of C1-INH; associated w/ mutation in coagulation factor XII protease
- **Pathophysiology:** Autosomal dominant, >200 mutations of C1-INH gene identified
- C1 activates classical complement pathway; C1-INH prevents spont activation
- **Epidemiology:** Usually presents in 1st or 2nd decade of life; 1:10,000 to 1:150,000
- 25% of pts have no family history and are presumed new mutations
- **Clinical manifestations:**
  - 50% have attacks ≤5 times/yr; 30% have attacks >12 times/yr
  - Patients generally feel prodrome 1–2 hr before onset
  - Recurrent edema lasting up to 1 wk after stress or traumatic events
  - Edema tends to be nonpainful, nonpitting; subcutis (face, trunk, genitals, extremities) and submucosal (intestines, larynx), laryngeal swelling can be life-threatening
  - Intestinal swelling → significant abdominal pain, vomiting, diarrhea; sx can be similar to appendicitis/other causes of acute abdomen
- **Diagnostic studies:**
  - ↓ C1-INH and ↓ levels of C4 (↑ C1 levels result in↑ cleavage of C4 from pathway)
  - Nml complement levels and C1 inhib levels reached from 2–3 yo, infant eval uncertain
- **Management:**
  - Not a histamine release so typical agents (anti-histamines, epi, steroids) will not help
  - Acute attacks: Hydration, pain relief, plasma derived C1-INH or ecallantide (kallikrein inhibitor) or icatibant (bradykinin B2 receptor antagonist); 2nd-line agents: FFP and solvent detergent-treated plasma
  - Short-term ppx (before high-risk procedure): C1-INH (off-label); or danazol (androgen) +/- C1-INH, icatibant, or ecallantide; or FFP
  - Long-term ppx: (If attacks >1/mo); danazol or antifibrinolytic agent (tranexamic acid)
  - New therapies: Nano-filtered C1-INH concentrate (FDA approved for long-term prophy), recombinant human C1-INH (under FDA review for acute attacks)
- **Complications:** Critical airway management
  - ACE inhibitors, OCP (estrogen), dental work can bring on an episode
  - Higher incidence of autoimmune disease, no higher incidence of atopy

Other Complement Deficiencies (Mol Immunol 2011;48:1643)
- C1q def; sepsis, meningitis, pneumonia; *S. pneumoniae, N. meningitidis*; SLE-like syndrome
- C2 def; sepsis, meningitis, pneumonia; *S. pneumoniae, N. meningitidis, S. aureus*; rheumatic disease, CV disease
- C5, C6, C7, C8, C9 def; meningococcal meningitis
- CD59, CD55 def: Thrombosis, hematopoietic cytopenia

PHAGOCYTIC DISORDERS

Overview (N Engl J Med 2000;343:1703)
- Include congenital neutropenias (cyclic neutropenia, severe congenital neutropenia, Shwachman–Diamond), adhesion defects (leukocyte adhesion deficiency), abnormal chemotaxis (Hyper IgE syndrome), intracellular killing defects (CGD), defects in formation/fxn of neutrophil granules (Chediak–Higashi)
- Consider phagocytic disorder if pt continues having severe or unusual bacterial or fungal infxns and all other workup for B- and T-cell deficiencies negative

Chronic Granulomatous Disease (CGD) (N Engl J Med 2000;343:1703)
- **Definition:** Defect in NADPH oxidase resulting in impaired ability to kill bacteria + fungi
- **Pathophysiology:**
  - Normally, NADPH oxidase → hydrogen peroxide formation → hypochlorous acid (bleach) formation → respiratory burst
  - In CGD, 5 known gene mutations affect assembly and activation of NADPH oxidase → failure to activate neutrophil resp burst → failure to kill catalase positive bacteria
  - Most common mutation (gp91phox) is X-linked, accounts for 70%
- **Epidemiology:** Quite rare, 4–5/million, 2/3 are male; can be X-linked or AR
- **Clinical manifestations:** (J Allergy Clin Immunol 2011;127:1319)
  - Most infxns 2/2 *S. aureus, S. marcescens, Burkholderia cepacia, nocardia, & Aspergillus*
  - Commonly develop PNA, lymphadenitis, liver abscess, osteo, skin + soft tissue infxn
  - Noncaseating granulomas in brain, lung, liver, spleen, GI tract; autoimmune dz
  - X-linked: Earlier diagnosis, higher mortality rate

- **Diagnostic studies:** (Clin Rev Allergy Immunol 2010;38:3)
  - See "Evaluating for PID" above: Abnormal neutrophil oxidase function suggests CGD
  - NBT testing replaced by dihydrorhodamine oxidation (DHR) testing
- **Management:** (J Allergy Clin Immunol 2011;127:1319)
  - Hematopoietic transplant is only curative Rx, 90–95% survival over previous 10 yr
  - Antibacterial (TMP-SMX) and antifungal (itraconazole) prophylaxis +/–
    immunomodulatory therapy (IFN-gamma)
  - Steroids used to decrease granulomas, low-dose prednisone
- **Complications:** Gastric outlet or ureteral obstruction from granulomas

Chediak–Higashi Syndrome (N Engl J Med 2000;343:1703)
- **Definition:** Rare defect in chemotaxis w/ ↑ susceptibility to bacterial infections,
  neuropathy, platelet dysfxn, oculocutaneous albinism
- **Pathophysiology:** AR disorder w/ abn degranulation of lysosomal granules
  - Mutation in *LYST* cytoplasmic protein involved in vesicle transport affecting all cells
    including melanocytes, which results in poor delivery pigment to skin and hair
- **Epidemiology:** Rare; 1 in 1 million, AR, dx early childhood, fatal by early adulthood
- **Clinical manifestations:**
  - Oculocutaneous albinism, progressive periph neuropathy, mild MR, periodontal dz
  - Infections: Sinopulmonary, skin, susceptible to *S. aureus*, and β-*hemolytic-strep*
  - Defective platelets: Easy bruising, mucosal bleeding
- **Diagnostic studies:** # of neutrophils slightly ↓ and smear w/ giant cytoplasmic granules
- **Management:** Prophylactic antibiotics
  - BMT (does not correct/prevent central and peripheral neuro defects) (Bone Marrow
    Transplant 2007;39:411)
- **Complications:** (J Clin Oncol 2006;24:3505)
  - Accelerated dz in 85% of pts: Lymphoma-like syndrome (nonmalignant cells) w/
    pancytopenia, fever, lymphocyte infiltration of liver, spleen, nodes that may be related
    to EBV infection, often becomes uncontrolled and leads to death
  - If pt survives, can lead to severe neuro manifestations by 20s and wheelchair bound

EKG INTERPRETATION

Approach to the EKG

- Indication for EKG: W/u for chest pain, syncope, cyanotic episodes, drug ingestion, CHD eval, palpitations, pericarditis, Kawasaki dz, myocarditis, rheumatic heart fever, FHx sudden death, and electrolyte abn (Emerg Med Clin North Am 2006;24:195)
- Basic EKG: 12 leads w/ 6 precordial leads and 3 limb leads (BMJ 2002;324:1382)
  - Paper speed usually 25 mm/sec so each small box 0.04 sec, 5 boxes 0.20 sec
  - Standard voltage is 10 mm/mV; 1 mm = 0.1 mV; can be modified on request
  - Leads: R and L arm, R and L leg give rise to I, II, III, aVL, aVR, aVF
  - Dipolar: I, II, III; represent differential from one lead to another
    - In **I,** positive deflection of wave is signal traveling from RA to L**A**
    - In **II,** positive deflection of wave is signal traveling from RA to L**L**
    - In **III,** positive deflection of wave is signal traveling from L**A** to L**L**
  - Unipolar: + deflect = center out to limb; aVR (RA), aVL (LA), aVF (LL)
  - Pericardial leads: Views cardiac activity in the horizontal plain

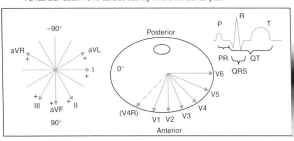

- Initial EKG read: Always take a systematic approach; check paper speed and voltage
  - Rhythm: Regular or irregular; then if sinus (every P followed by QRS, unique P wave morphology, constant PR)
  - Rate: # of large (5 mm) boxes btw R waves; 1 = 300 bpm, 2 = 150, 3 = 100; pattern is 300, 150, 100, 75, 60, 50; can also use 1500/# small boxes
  - Axis: If R + in limb lead, vector goes toward that lead; nml axis based on age
    - R waves +I and + aVF = 0 to –90° (noted as normal axis; but can be abn for age)
    - R waves +I and = 0 to –90° (left axis deviation) actually –30 to –90°
    - R waves –I and +aVF = 90–180° (right axis deviation)
    - R waves –I and –aVF = –90° to –180° (extreme right/NW deviation)
    - Neonates w/ transitioning from R-sided dominance; initially w/ R axis as nml
    - P wave axis; if sinus then +I, +aVF, if not consider ectopic atrial pacer (EAP)
  - P waves: Should have same morphology in a given lead, otherwise multi-pacemakers
    - 2.5 mm wide in II and/or biphasic in V1 = p mitrale; left atrial enlargement
    - 2.5 mm high in II = p pulmonale; right atrial enlargement
  - Q wave: Can be nml (II, III, aVF, V5, V6), max amp at 3–5 yrs (0.6–0.8 mV nml)
  - QRS complex: R:S ratio initially >1 in V1 and V2, and <1 in V5 and V6; at about 3 yo R:S ratio becomes <1 in V1 and V2, and >1 in V5 and V6; some pts w/ juvenile pattern until 8–12 yr (Heart 2005;91:1626)
    - EKG assessment of LVH very poor in pediatrics; sens 19.4%, spec 85%
  - T wave: Progressive changes through childhood, very different from adult pattern
    - 1st 2–3 DOL upright T wave in V1–V3 normal, then inverts in 1st wk of life
    - T wave becomes upright during childhood, starting w/ V3, then V2, then V1
    - 50% nml 3–5 yo have inverted T in V2, only 5–10% nml 8–12 yo w/ inverted T
    - T wave in V5 and V6 should be upright in all ages (Heart 2005;91:1626)
  - RVH criteria: Pure R wave in V1 >10 mm, upright T wave in V1, RSR' pattern in V1, where R' >15 mm (<1 yo) or R' >10 mm (>1 yo) (Ped ECG Interpretation 2004)
  - Intervals: Interpretation varies based on age group (Heart 2005;91:1626)
    - PR: ↑ w/ ↑ vagal tone, heart block, endocarditis w/ abscess, hyperK, digoxin, tox, short w/ pre-excitation (WPW), EAP, glycogen storage dz
    - QRS: >0.08 msec if <8 yo or >0.10 msec if >8 yo = bundle branch block, junctional or ventricular rhythm (not via His-Purkinje) (Emerg Med Clin North Am 2006;24:195)
    - QT: Start of Q to end of T; correct for HR w/ Bazett formula QT/√RR
    - Both old and recent reviews place upper limit nml QTc at 450 msec

- Nml limits prev from Davignon et al. (2,141 Caucasian pts), more recent by Rijnbeek et al. w/ higher sampling rate w/ sign diff in nml limits (Euro Heart J 2001;22:702)

	HR	PR Interval	QRS Axis	QRS Interval	QTc Limit
0–1 wk	90–160	0.08–0.15	60–180°	0.03–0.08	<0.49
1 wk–2 mo	100–180	0.08–0.15	45–160°	0.03–0.08	<0.49
2–6 mo	105–185	0.08–0.15	0–135°	0.03–0.08	<0.49
6 mo–1 yr	110–170	0.07–0.16	0–135°	0.03–0.08	<0.45
1–8 yr	90–165 (1–2 yr) 65–140 (>2 yr)	0.09–0.17	0–110°	0.04–0.08	<0.45
8–16 yr	60–130	0.09–0.17	–15–110°	0.04–0.09	<0.45
>16 yr	50–120	0.12–0.20	–15–110°	0.05–0.10	<0.45

HEART MURMURS

Definition
- Result of turbulent blood flow; can be 2/2 ↑ blood flow (fever, anemia), abn cardiac structures (abn valve, cardiac defect), or combination
- 50–70% seen annual exam, sports physicals, etc. w/ murmur on exam but only 0.8–1% of pop w/ structural congenital heart disease (Pediatr Rev 2007;28:e19)

Cardiac Examination (Pediatr Rev 2007;28:e19)
- Observation for syndromic appearance, central cyanosis, breathing, JVP
- Palpation for thrills and point of max impulse for displacement, hyperdynamic flow
  - Pulse exam: Bounding (inc pulse pressure; PDA, AR, hyperthyroid, AVF), pulsus parvus (weak)/tardus (late) in AS, unequal in all 4 ext (aortic coarc)
  - Abdominal exam: Hepatosplenomegaly (CHF), pulsatile liver (TR)
- Auscultation characterizing S_1 (AV valves) and S_2 (aortic and pulmonic often split)
  - S_3 (rapid filling of ventric) often normal in children; sounds like slosh-ing-**in**
  - S_4 (atrial contraction against stiff ventricle) always pathologic; sounds like **a**-thick-wall
  - Heart sound order; S_4 --- S_1 ----S_2----S_3; S_2 nml split to A_2--P_2; can mistake for S_3

       -----slosh-ing---**in**

       a------thick-wall----

  - Murmurs: Define timing (systolic vs. diastolic; early, mid, late), intensity, location, quality, configuration (crescendo, decrescendo, etc.), duration
    - Systolic: Holosystolic (involves S_1, cont to S_2 at same intensity) and heard w/ AV valve regurg or VSDs; ejection murmurs (begin after S_1 w/ cres-decres) and related to flow in great vessels (Pediatr Clin North Am 2004;51:1515)
    - Diastolic: Almost always pathologic (aside from venous hum)
    - Continuous: Flow through vessel/communication distal to aortic/pulm valves
      - Pathologic (PDA, continuous machinery murmur) or benign (venous hum)

Innocent Murmurs of Childhood (Circulation 2005;111:e20; Pediatr Clin North Am 2004;51:1515)
- **Stills murmur:** Most common innocent murmur in children; 1st described in 1909
  - Typically heard in patients aged 2–6 yo, but can be heard in infants and adolescents
  - Vibratory systolic murmur, low pitched, best at LLSB radiating to apex, no thrill
  - 2/2 turbulence in LV outflow tract; change w/ position and dec w/ Valsalva
- **Pulmonary flow murmur:** Cres-decres, early to mid-peaking systolic at LUSB
  - Rough & dissonant, best heard in supine position; inc w/ expiration, dec upright
  - Can be difficult to distinguish from ASD murmur but w/ ASD have fixed split S_2
  - Pulm stenosis distinguished by possible presence of thrill, ejection click, soft S_2
- **Peripheral pulmonary artery stenosis:** Common <1yo, usually gone by 6 mo
  - Low/mod-pitched ejection murmur in early/mid systole best at axilla or back
  - In utero pulm outflow tract well developed, pulm arterial branches comparatively underdeveloped and arise at sharp angles, which resolves w/ growth
  - May be difficult to distinguish btw this and pathologic periph pulm artery stenosis w/ Williams or rubella syndrome; murmur may persist beyond S_2 w/ these
- **Supraclavicular flow murmurs:** Cres-decres harsh, high-pitched 2/2 nml bld flow in aorta and head/neck vessels; hear best above the clavicles (e.g., over carotids)
  - Same sitting or supine; diminished w/ shoulder girdle hyperextension (arms back)
  - **Aortic systolic flow murmur:** Systolic ejection in aortic area 2/2 increased, cardiac output; anxiety, anemia, hyperthyroidism, fever, extreme fitness
  - If murmur inc w/ dec preload (Valsalva, squat to stand) → HOCM

- **Venous hum:** Most common type of continuous murmur and benign
  - Best at infraclavicular region while sitting or standing; usually > on R side
  - Diminished w/ supine position or pressure over jugular vein

Pathologic Murmurs (Circulation 2005;111:e20)
- Systolic—usually longer and louder than innocent counterparts
  - Pansystolic: Involves/obscures S_1; if constant; VSD, MR, TR; if crescendo, then PDA
  - Ejection (AS, PS): Signs of pathology are presence of ejection click, abn S_2 split
    - Assess pulses, presence of cardiac failure (JVD, etc.), diastolic murmur as well
- Diastolic: W/ exception of venous hum, all diastolic murmurs are pathologic
  - Often need to reposition patient to best auscultate (sitting up leaning forward for aortic sounds and left lateral decubitus to best hear mitral sounds)
  - Early: Usually decres; assoc w/ aortic or pulmonic regurgitation
  - Mid: Cres-decres 2/2 inc flow across nml MV/TV or 2/2 MS/TS
  - Late: Cres and also assoc w/ mitral or tricuspid stenosis (MS/TS)
- Continuous: Harsh machine-like murmur classic for PDA

Further Evaluation (Circulation 2005;111:e20)
- Depends on clinical assessment of patient; if asymptomatic, exam is usually sufficient
- Echo is gold standard to assess cardiac structure; ancillary testing w/ EKG or CXR may be helpful; some suggest referral to pediatric cardiology before imaging

SYNCOPE

Definition (Pediatr Rev 2000;21:384; Pediatr Rev 2000;21:201)
- Sudden, often brief loss of consciousness and postural tone 2/2 ↓ cerebral blood flow
- Presyncope is the feeling one is about to pass out

Etiology
- Breath-holding spells: Incidence of 4.6% and primarily 1–5 yr of age, strong FHx
  - Provoked by pain, anger, or frustration; normal physical and neuro exam
  - Cyanotic type (80%): Peaks at 2 yo and resolves by 5 yo
    - Characterized by a prodromal period of crying then forced expiration and apnea
    - Involuntary Valsalva → ↑ intrathoracic pressure → ↓ cardiac output → ↓ cerebral blood flow, LOC, and loss of muscle tone
    - May be assoc w/ generalized clonic jerks, opisthotonos, and bradycardia
  - Pallid type (20%): Preceded by frustration, pain, sudden startle, or minor trauma
    - Initial quieting and breath holding → pallor → LOC and loss of muscle tone
    - Abnormal slowing of HR w/ ocular compression seen in >50%
    - Ocular compression test w/ at least 3 sec of asystole, followed by pallid syncope, and no epileptiform discharges on EEG confirms dx
- Neurocardiogenic (vasovagal): ~75% syncope in kids. 2/2 autonomic dysfxn; often +FHx
  - Usually in adolescents after prolonged standing in a crowded, warm environment
  - Characteristically preceded by nausea, diaphoresis, light-headedness, or yawning
- Cardiac syncope
  - Arrhythmogenic: Prolonged QT, WPW, heart block, sick sinus syndrome, SVT
    - Recent study of QTc in children presenting to ED; 1/3 w/ QTc ≥440 ms (borderline prolonged); of these 31% w/ f/u and 62.5% w/ significant normalization of QTc in follow-up (Pediatrics 2011;128: e1395)
  - Structural: HOCM, severe aortic/pulmonic stenosis, pHTN, anom L coronary
  - POTS (postural orthostatic tachycardia syndrome)
  - Myxomas
- Neuropsychiatric
  - Seizures/drop attacks
  - Hyperventilation syndrome/panic attacks
  - Hypoglycemia: Gradual onset w/ weakness, hunger, sweating, agitation, confusion
  - Migraines assoc w/ vertebrobasilar vascular spasm: HA persists after awakening
  - Benign paroxysmal vertigo: Sudden falling attacks w/ dizziness in pts <6 yo
- Cough syncope: Most common in children w/ asthma
  - Recovery w/i seconds, and consciousness restored w/i minutes

Clinical Manifestations
- Hx most important in selecting dx studies and guiding Rx
- Should include the time of day, time of last meal, and details of preceding activities
  - Syncope at rest/recumbent suggests sz or arrhythmias
  - Syncope w/ exercise suggests HOCM

- Syncope while standing suggests vasovagal
- Syncope w/o warning suggests primary cardiac
- Medication Hx including prescribed, OTC, and illicit drugs
- FHx: Sudden unexplained death, deafness, arrhythmias, congenital heart disease, sz, metabolic diseases, or MI at young age

Physical Exam
- Cardiac exam: Pulse, BP, orthostatics, murmurs, clicks; detailed neuro exam

Diagnostic Studies: Guided by History and Physical Exam
- Measurement of serum glucose & lytes rarely of value unless an acute episode
- EKG: Assess rhythm, conduction, premature beats, delta waves, chamber enlargement, PR, QRS, and QTc; further testing w/ exercise tests or 24-hr Holter if needed
- Toxicology screen
- Echocardiography w/ Doppler studies
- Tilt-table testing for positional syncope
- EEG: In pt w/ prolonged LOC, suspected sz; postictal, drowsiness or confusion
- Cardiology c/s indicated for pathologic heart murmur, CP preceding syncope, arrhythmia, ↑QTc, Q waves, RV strain (suggestive of pHTN), or LVH on EKG, or w/ FHx of cardiomyopathy or sudden death

Treatment
- Breath-holding spells: Reassurance and explanation of pathophysiology most important
  - Iron therapy has been shown to decrease incidence in cyanotic type
  - Consider anticholinergics in pallid type if they become severe or frequent
- Neurocardiogenic: (H&P negative for other causes and EKG nml; trial of fluid therapy w/ 1 8 oz glass liquid q2–4h and 2 8 oz glasses prior to athletic participation. 90% will respond w/o need for further referral. Non-responders referred to Cardiology, may need PO salt suppl +/– fludrocortisone (Pediatr Rev 2003;24:269)
- Cardiac: Include drug therapy, radiofrequency ablation, or pacemaker placement
  - Pts w/ long QT should not receive macrolides or cisapride
- Seizures: Appropriate anticonvulsants

CHEST PAIN

Definition (Pediatr Clin North Am 2004;51:1553; Pediatr Rev 2010;31:e1)

Chest pain (CP) in the pediatric population is overwhelmingly benign, but can have significant impact on patients; ½ miss school, 69% self-limit activity
Source can be 2/2 musculoskeletal, respiratory, cardiac, GI, or nervous system
Incidence of chest pain 2/2 cardiac etiology 2–5%

Epidemiology (Pediatr Rev 1986;8:56; Pediatr Rev 2010;31:e1)

Primary complaint in 0.3–0.6% of pediatric patients in ED or outpt care
May be chronic lasting up to 6 mo in 15–36% of patients, 1 yr in 8%
Mean age of presentation is 12–14 yr

Clinical Manifestations

Detailed Hx: Describe **p**ain (location and duration) **q**uality, **r**adiation, **s**everity, **t**emporal assoc (w/ breathing, eating, activity), exacerb or alleviating factors
In younger patients, assess history of occult toxic ingestion
Chest pain assoc w/ exertion, syncope, light-headedness, or palpitations is concerning
FHx of sudden death, HOCM, MVP, Marfan's or personal Hx of Kawasaki concerning

Etiologies (Pediatr Rev 2010;31:e1; Pediatr Clin North Am 2004;51:1553)

Cardiac: Rare; responsible for <5–6% of pediatric chest pain
- **Mitral valve prolapse:** 18% pts w/ MVP have chest pain, though pain not 2/2 valve prolapse, unclear if neuroendocrine or autonomic dysfunction
  - Check flat, sitting, and standing for midsystolic click and late systolic murmur
  - Association with anxiety exists; echo diagnosis
- **Pericarditis:** Sharp and stabbing, often pleuritic and positional; improved w/ leaning forward; may have recent URI sx, fever. Viral cause most common
  - Can be infectious, inflammatory (w/ CTDs), neoplastic, or 2/2 XRT
  - Exam w/ pericardial rub; EKG w/ PR depressions and diffuse ST elevations across all leads. PR elevation in aVR is the most specific finding
  - Myocarditis can also p/w chest pain but usually 2/2 assoc pericarditis
- **Coronary vasospasm:** P/w crushing, diffuse chest pain w/ assoc SOB, diaphoresis, radiation to L arm, neck, or jaw; light-headedness/syncope

- Exam may have gallop (S_3 and S_4), +/– signs of poor cardiac function
- Consider cocaine induced, check tox screen, and if suspected use combined α- and β-antagonist (pure β-antagonist → unopposed α activity and periph vasospasm)
- Can also see vaso-occlusive dz w/ some types of systemic dz; e.g., sickle cell
- **Anomalous coronary artery:** Rare; coronary arteries arise from opposite sinus of Valsalva, increases risk for ischemia and sudden death
  - Usually p/w sudden death but 5/27 in 1 study w/ CP in prior 2 yr
  - Chest pain associated w/ exertion; often nml physical exam
  - EKG and stress test have not shown to be helpful in identifying at-risk pts
- **Aortic dissection:** Pts w/ Marfan, Turner, type IV Ehlers–Danlos, or homocystinuria; p/w severe tearing chest pain radiating to back
- **Kawasaki dz:** If c/b coronaryartery aneurysm, can see stenosis or aneurismal thrombus; if Hx prior Kawasaki w/ aneurysm & p/w CP, ischemia until proven not
  - **LV outflow obstruction:** Hypertrophic obstructive cardiomyopathy (HOCM) most common though rarely p/w chest pain; exam w/ systolic murmur at aortic region that amplifies w/ standing or Valsalva
  - **Pulm HTN:** Unclear mech; may be 2/2 pulm art stretch or RV ischemia (Am Fam Physician 2001;63:1789)
  - **Tachyarrhythmias:** Abrupt onset and cessation, w/ or w/o activity, often w/ N/V
- **Idiopathic: 21% cases,** no cause identified in prospective study (Pediatrics 1988;82:319)
  - Avg pt w/ wks to mos intermittent CP, sharp, w/ or w/o exertion, short duration, no assoc sx, recurrence common, PE nml, and pain not reproducible
- **Musculoskeletal: 15–31% cases** in prospective study (Pediatrics 1988;82:319)
  - Strain or costochondritis from overuse or trauma. Reproducible on exam
  - Hx of exertion/activity, pain usually sharp and radiating, can be pleuritic
  - Costochondritis w/ tenderness on palpation of site of rib attachment to sternum
  - Tietze syndrome—localized nonsuppurative inflammation of costochondral, costosternal, or sternoclavicular joints in adolescents; usually only a single joint
  - Precordial catch syndrome—sharp, well-localized twinge of pain, acute onset at rest and lasts sec to min; not reproducible on palpation
  - Slipping rib syndrome: 8th, 9th, 10th ribs slip over one another (Pediatrics 1985;76:810)
    - Pop or click → dull chest wall/abd pain, reproduced by lifting rib anteriorly
- **Psychosomatic/anxiety: 9–20% cases;** often chronic and usually adol females
- 1/3 w/ Hx of sign sleep disturbance, ½ w/ +FHx of chest pain
- **Respiratory—2–11% cases**
  - Specific etiologies include asthma (most common) and exercise-induced asthma (check for wheeze, +FHx; trial of albuterol), PNA (fever, cough), PE
  - Pneumothorax p/w sharp chest pain; steady, pleuritic, tachycardic and w/ dec breath sounds (not always appreciable). Inc risk w/ CF, asthma, and Marfan
- **GI: 8% cases;** GERD (burning pain, assoc w/ meals, worse when supine; trial of PPI) also consider peptic ulcer disease, esophageal spasm or inflammation, & cholecystitis
  - Foreign body ingestion or caustic substance ingestion can p/w chest pain
- Other: Important to assess for breast masses in both M and F; usually in puberty
  - Pleurodynia (devil's grip) paroxysms of sharp pain 2/2 coxsackie virus infection

Evaluation

- Examine chest for evidence of trauma, symmetry, and palpation for reproducibility
- Focused cardiovascular exam to assess pulses, BP, JVP, PMI, murmurs, and extra heart sounds, peripheral perfusion. Hx will guide further focused evaluation
- EKG rarely useful outside of suspected congenital or structural heart disease or dysrhythmia, f/u with echo and consult cardiology if these are suspected
  - In prospective study EKG in 47% cases; only 4/191 EKGs w/ abn related to final dx. Echo in 34% cases; only 17/139 abn (12/17 w/ MVP) (Pediatrics 1988;82:319)

CYANOTIC CHILD

Pathophysiology
- Blue to dusky hue in the newborn; 5 g/dL of deoxyhemoglobin produces cyanosis
- Dependent on absolute concentration of reduced hemoglobin
- 2/2 hypoventilation, R to L shunt/intrapulmonary shunting, V–Q mismatch, diffusion impairment

Etiology (Pediatr Clin North Am 2004;51:999)

Pulmonary	Miscellaneous
Parenchymal	Methemoglobinemia
Transient tachypnea of newborn (TTN)	Hemoglobin M
Hyaline membrane disease (HMD)	Metabolic acidosis
Aspiration—meconium, blood, mucus, or milk	Sulfhemoglobinemia
Pneumonia, pulmonary hemorrhage	Hypoglycemia
Pulmonary edema	Sepsis
Pulmonary hypoplasia	Polycythemia
Pulmonary lymphangiectasia	Associated w/ feeding: GER
Nonparenchymal	Central nervous system (CNS)
Tracheoesophageal fistula (TEF)	Cerebral edema
Congenital diaphragmatic hernia (CDH)	Hemorrhage
Congenital cystic adenomatoid malformation (CCAM)	Infection
Pulmonary sequestration	Hypoventilation
Pneumothorax, pneumomediastinum	Vocal cord paralysis or paresis
Pleural effusion	
Choanal atresia	
Laryngeal web	
Lobar emphysema	
Persistent pulmonary hypertension of newborn (PPHN)	

Cardiac
  The 5 Ts (transposition of great arteries [TGA], tetralogy of Fallot [TOF], total anomalous pulm venous drainage [TAPVD], truncus arteriosus, tricuspid atresia)
  Critical pulmonary stenosis/atresia, Ebstein anomaly, L to R shunt w/ pulmonary edema, single ventricle physiology, low cardiac output states

Clinical Manifestations
- Central cyanosis: Decreased arterial oxygen content
- Periph cyanosis: Nml PaO_2; w/ cold exposure, Raynauds, polycythemia, early shock
- Differential cyanosis: Pink upper body, cyanotic lower part (R to L shunt from PDA)
- Reverse diff cyanosis: Upper part of body cyanotic, lower part pink (Transposition w/ pHTN, interrupted aortic arch, critical aortic coarctation)
- Harlequin condition: 1 quadrant or ½ of body cyanotic (vasomotor instability)

Diagnostic Studies

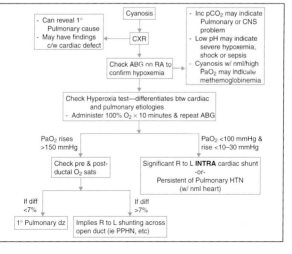

- Management and prognosis depends on the dx, severity, and the time of presentation
- Requires initial stabilization, assuring hemodyn stability w/ IVFs, oxygen administration, and possible referral to a NICU, **use Prostaglandin E if failed hyperoxia test**

CONGENITAL HEART DISEASE

Tetralogy of Fallot	**Transposition of the Great Arteries**
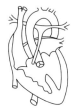	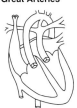
1. VSD 3. RVOT obstruction 2. Overriding aorta 4. RVH	1. Aorta from RV, pulmonary artery from LV 2. Intact ventricular septum 3. PDA
Truncus Arteriosus	**Tricuspid Atresia**
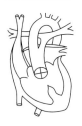	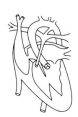
1. Common aterial trunk (Aorta+PA) 2. VSD	1. Tricuspid atresia 3. Pulmonary stenosis 2. VSD 4. Hypoplastic RV

Elena Grant 2012

Cyanotic Lesions (Pediatr Rev 2007;28:123; N Engl J Med 2000;342:334)
- **Tetralogy of Fallot:** Most common cyanotic CHD after infancy; anterior malalignment of conal septum leading to VSD, overriding aorta, RV outflow tract obstruction, and RVH
  - Exam: SEM at LUSB, loud single S_2; EKG w/ RAD, RVH
  - CXR: **"Boot-shaped"** heart, nml heart size, decreased PVMs, +/– right arch
  - Degree of cyanosis related to degree of pulmonary outflow obstruction, which ca vary. Can present as severe cyanosis DOL#1 or later (pink Tet)
    - Hypercyanotic **spells:** W/ tachypnea, hyperpnea, worsening cyanosis 2/2 ↑ in RVOT obstruction
    - Treat hypercyanotic spells acutely with volume, oxygen, agent to increase SVR, squatting position, morphine
    - Murmur disappears during spells 2/2 ↑ RV outflow tract obstruction
  - Tetralogy is ductal dependent if PS is severe (use prostaglandin)
  - Treatment is surgical with repair of RV outflow tract obstruction and closure of VSD
- **Transposition of Great Arteries (D-TGA):** Aorta arises from the right ventricle an pulmonary artery arises from the left ventricle. Need communication between systemic and pulmonary circulations
  - Nonspecific; single loud S_2; no murmur w/o other defect, **worst cyanosis ever!**

- EKG: RAD, RVH
- CXR: **"Egg on string"**; increased PVMs
- Ductal dependent (prostaglandin, balloon atrial septostomy & surgical arterial switch)
- **Total Anomalous Pulmonary Venous Return:** Total or partial abnormal return of pulm veins to R side circ
  - 3 main types: Supracardiac (left cardinal vein), infracardiac (ductus venosus), or intracardiac (coronary sinus). May be complicated by obstruction of venous return with earlier presentation
  - Exam: ↑ RV impulse; fixed, split S_2; SEM at LUSB; mid-diastolic rumble LLSB
  - EKG: RAD, RVH, ± RAE
  - CXR w/ cardiomegaly, nml to ↑ peripheral vascular markings (PVM); if obstructed venous flow—**"snowman in a storm,"** edema, congestion
  - Treatment is surgical repair
- **Tricuspid atresia:** Failure of tricuspid valve to form leading to incomplete development of right ventricle (hypoplastic RV) and pulmonary artery
  - Exam: PDA murmur; ± single S_2; ± VSD murmur
  - EKG: LAD or superior axis; RAE, LVH
  - CXR: Normal; mild cardiomegaly; usually decreased PVMs
  - Degree of cyanosis and hypoxemia depend on patency of duct and size of VSD and overall obstruct to RV outflow; can present later if VSD large and minimal PS
  - Ductal dependent. Treatment is surgical repair
- **Ebstein anomaly:** Inferior displacement of tricuspid valve with atrialization of right ventricle. Often with tricuspid regurgitation. Variable severity
  - Exam: Widely split S_1 and S_2, S_3 and S_4 often present, systolic M at LLSB
  - EKG: Tall and broad P waves, RBBB; **20% assoc with WPW**
  - CXR: **Biggest heart you will ever see;** narrow mediastinum; decreased PVMs
  - ↑ rate of intrauterine mortality, neonate p/w severe cyanosis, older kid usually p/w murmur, adol/adults usually p/w supravent arrhythmia. Rx w/ PGE acutely
- **Hypoplastic left heart syndrome (HLHS):** Spectrum of defects characterized by underdevelopment of the LV outflow tract resulting in varying degrees of hypoplasia of left-sided structures including the mitral valve, LV, and aorta. The right ventricle provides systemic and pulmonary blood flow
  - Exam: Increased RV impulse; single loud S_2; +/– soft HSM at LLSB, HM
  - EKG: Nml to increased PVMs, cardiomegaly
  - Ductal dependent. Symptoms depend on ductal patency. With closure of ductus get cardiogenic shock and circulatory collapse. Need to keep PVR high and SVR low. Needs staged surgical palliation (Norwood, Glenn, Fontan)
- **Pulmonary atresia:** Atresia of pulmonary valve, can be with or without VSD. Pulmonary atresia with VSD is managed as a severe form of TOF. Pulmonary atresia with intact ventricular septum usually associated with hypoplastic RV and anomalous connections between the RV and coronary arteries (sinusoids)
  - Exam: Murmur of PDA; EKG: Mild LAD, RAE; CXR: Decreased PVMs
  - Severe cyanosis, day 1 with closing PDA. Decreased PaO_2
  - Ductal dependent. Treatment is surgical repair
- **Truncus arteriosus:** Failure of conotruncal septum to separate the aorta and pulmonary artery resulting in a single great vessel (truncal artery) arising from the heart which gives rise to the aorta and pulmonary arteries. VSD present. Variable origin of branch PAs from truncal artery. Commonly have truncal valve abnormalities
  - Exam: Active. Single S_2; ± SEM, click; ± regurg murmur; inc pulse press, bounding pulses; EKG: Bi-ventricular hypertrophy (BVH)
  - CXR: Cardiomegaly, increased PVMs; ± right arch
  - Presents with cyanosis and signs/symptoms of heart failure due to pulmonary overcirculation from L to R shunt
  - Not a ductal dependent lesion. Treatment is surgical repair

Acyanotic Lesions (N Engl J Med 2000;342:256)
- **Atrial septal defects:** (1) Ostium secundum defect; (2) ostium primum defect (actually form of atrioventricular septal or AV canal defect); (3) sinus venosus ASD at the base of atrial septum; sinus venosus ASD; (associated with partial anomalous pulmonary venous return); (4) unroofed coronary sinus
  - Exam: Wide fixed split S_2; SEM at LUSB
  - EKG: Normal to RAD; incomplete RBBB, RV volume overload
  - CXR: Increased pulm vascular markings and a peripheral vascular pattern
  - Magnitude and direction of shunt determined by size of defect and compliance of ventricles. Can be asymp or lead to CHF (due to L to R shunt), poor feeding, recurrent pulm infections
  - Rx includes surgical patch or cath device. Ostium secundum can spont close

- **Ventricular septal defects:** Most common congenital cardiac defect. Types include (1) inlet (beneath AV valves), (2) outlet (gives rise to great vessels), (3) perimembranous (junction between inlet and outlet, 70% cases), and (4) muscular (between LV and RV, 20% cases). Causes L to R shunt
  - Exam: Dynamic and laterally displaced LV; HSM at LLSB; ± apical diastolic rumble (only if a large VSD is present)
  - EKG: Small defects – nml; large – LAE/LVH to BVH
  - CXR: Small – nml; large – cardiomegaly, increased PVMs
  - Presentation, depends on size of defect and resistance in pulm and systemic vasc. Large → LV failure or pHTN w/ RV failure. Muscular VSDs usually spontaneously close by 12 mo. Inlet and malalignment VSDs never close
- **AV canal:** Endocardial cushion defect. Spectrum of lesions. Complete AV canal: Includes primum ASD, inlet VSD, and common AV valve. Results in L to R shunting. Often associated with Trisomy 21
  - Exam: Murmurs of ASD, VSD; active. ± gallop
  - EKG: Superior QRS axis; Q in I, aVL; ± RVH, LVH
  - CXR: Cardiomegaly, increased PVMs
  - If complete, presents like large VSD. Treat like ASD or VSD
- **Patent ductus arteriosus:** Persistence of fetal circulation w/ connection btw pulmonary artery & aorta. 10% of CHD; ↑ incidence in preemies, infants born at high altitudes, and pregnancies c/b perinatal hypoxemia or maternal rubella infxn
  - Direction of shunt determined by relative resistance of systemic & pulmonary circ
  - Exam: **Continuous machinery murmur at LUSB,** bounding pulses, widened pulse pressure due to aortic diastolic runoff
  - EKG: Small – nml; large – LAE/LVH to BVH
  - CXR: Nml to inc PVMs, prox pulm a. dilation, prominent ascending aorta
  - Usually presents with murmur, ± CHF later. Can close PDAs with ibuprofen, indomethacin, cath coil, or surgical ligation
- **Pulmonary stenosis:** Valvular (assoc w/ **Noonan** syndrome), supravalvular (narrowing of pulm trunk, its bifurcation, or its branches), or subvalvular (narrowing of RV infundibulum)
  - Exam: Cres–decres systolic @ LUSB; wide split S_2 that moves w/ respiration
  - EKG: Normal to RAD, RVH to RVH with strain
  - CXR: Poststenotic dilatation of main pulm a., decreased PVMs
  - Symptoms determined by severity of stenosis, RV fxn, and competence of tricuspid valve; ductal dependent if there is critical stenosis
  - Rx is percutaneous balloon valvuloplasty or surgical valve replacement or resection
- **Aortic stenosis:** Valvular, subvalvular (subaortic) or supravalvular (assoc w/ **Williams** syndrome). Valvular AS assoc w/ other cardiac anom (PDA or coarct). Subvalvular may be fixed or dynamic (hypertrophic cardiomyopathy) at RUSB, can radiate to the neck
  - EKG: Normal to LVH ± strain; CXR: Normal to cardiomegaly w/ LV dilatation
  - Valvular AS can present <1 yo w/ CHF even shock; or >1 yo w/ murmur. Subvalvular AS usually presents w/ murmur
  - Ductal dependent if there is critical stenosis
- **Aortic coarctation:** Narrowing of aorta usually distal to L subclav artery origin opposite ductus arteriosus; M > F, assoc w/ Turner, bicusp AV, and aneurysms of circ of Willis
  - Exam: SEM at LUSB to back; ↑ SBP and widened pulse press in arms, femoral pulses are weak and delayed
  - EKG: LVH in older children
  - CXR: Rib notching in older children; indentation of aorta (reverse E or 3 sign)
  - 3 presentations: Infant in CHF, child w/ HTN in upper ext, or child w/ murmur
  - Tx: ↑ incidence of subsequent aortic aneurysm or recurrent coarctation w/ percutaneous balloon dilatation vs. surgical repair

ESSENTIAL HYPERTENSION

Definition
- Essential HTN is BP >95th percentile (sex, age, and height specific) in the absence of other etiologies (Pediatr Rev 2007;28:283) Per published BP charts. (Pediatrics 2004;114:555)
  - Pre-HTN: Avg SBP and/or DBP ≥90th but <95th percentile or adol ≥120/80
  - Stage I HTN: Avg SBP and/or DBP ≥95th percentile
  - Stage II HTN: Avg SBP and/or DBP 5 mm Hg >95th percentile
  - HTN urgency/emergency: Avg SBP and/or DBP 5 mm Hg >95th percentile w/ clinical signs or sx (chest pain, HA, epistaxis, lethargy, seizure, encephalopathy, diplopia)

- ~2–5% of children have essential hypertension but only 23% carry the dx (even w/ elevated BPs × 3 documented by PCP) (JAMA 2007;298:874)
- BP should be checked at R arm w/ cuff width ~40% or arm circ at midpoint humerus
  - Measured after seated for 5 min in controlled environment w/ R arm at heart level
  - Cuff too large underestimates BP, cuff too small overestimates BP

Epidemiology (Am Fam Physician 2006;73:1558)
- Familial patterns of essential HTN well established; heritability estimated at 50%
- BMI has been demonstrated to be a strong risk factor for development of HTN
- Insuff data to define role of ethnicity; some studies show AA > Caucasian children
- Obesity: Defined as >95 percentile for age and sex; 3–5× inc risk of HTN
  - 30% of obese pediatric patients have hypertension (Pediatrics 2004;114:555)
- Essential HTN linked w/ risk factors of metabolic syndrome (low HDL, inc trigs, abd obesity, insulin resistance/hyperinsulinemia); prevalence 4.2–8.4% in adolescents

Etiology (Pediatr Rev 2007;28:283)
- Most childhood HTN due to 2° causes (60–70% renal dz, rarely essential HTN <10 yo); adolesc HTN 85–90% essential HTN
- Initial eval should assess 2° causes but more strongly suggested in younger children, those w/ stage II HTN and w/ other systemic symptoms (Pediatrics 2004;114:555)
  - Renal: Renal artery stenosis (abd bruit), polycystic kidney dz, parenchymal dz, Wilms tumor, neuroblastoma
  - Obstructive sleep apnea (OSA): Affects 1–3% of children, assoc w/ inc DBP
  - Drugs—albuterol, amphetamines, antidepressants, antipsychotics, caffeine, cocaine, EtOH, NSAIDs, OCPs, OTC allergy/cold meds, and steroids
  - Endocrine: Pheochromocytoma (w/ flushing and diaphoresis), Cushing (moon facies, hirsutism, acne, obesity), hyperthyroidism (thyromegaly, tachy, weight loss), hyperaldosteronism (muscle weakness)
  - Neonatal Hx: Umbilical artery catheter, asphyxia, BDP, maternal substance use, unequal peripheral pulses (aortic coarctation)
  - Systemic lupus erythematosus and other CTD (joint pain, malar rash)

Evaluation (Pediatr Rev 2007;28:283; Pediatrics 2004;114:555)
- BP checks start at 3 yo at regular checkups (Pediatrics 2004;114:555)
- Initial focused history for FHx, medication Hx, and possible 2° causes as above
- Exam w/ BMI, 4 ext BPs, retinal exam for chronicity (presence of copper wiring and AV knicking), cardiovascular exam for extra heart sounds, murmurs, and bruits
  - Moon facies, truncal obesity, violaceous striae in Cushing syndrome
  - Webbed neck and wide-spaced nipples in Turner syndrome
  - Abd mass/palpable kidney in Wilms tumor, neuroblastoma, pheochromocytoma, polycystic kidney disease, hydronephrosis
  - Malar rash, friction rub, & joint swelling & pains in SLE or other CTD
- Lab testing and imaging to assess end organs and identify possible etiologies
  - CBC w/ diff (anemia 2/2 CKD), electrolytes w/ BUN/Cr and Ca++, Phos, Mg++ (assess renal dz, calculi dz), U/A (assess for infection, hematuria, proteinuria), 24-hr urine protein and creatinine (to calculate CrCl)
  - Imaging: Renal U/S w/ Doppler (assess renal scarring, cong anom, unequal size), may need further imaging assess renovasc dz (CTA, MRA, arteriography)
  - Studies assessing end organs; echo (presence of LVH), retinal exam, and renal U/S
  - Hormonal studies: Plasma rennin (mineralocorticoid dz), thyroid, adrenal, urine, and plasma catecholamines (pheo)
  - ↑ serum uric acid assoc w/ HTN; >5.5 mg/dL in 89% pts w/ essent HTN; 30% w/ 2° HTN

Treatment (Pediatrics 2004;114:555)
- Lifestyle modification 1st line for all pts w/ HTN (weight reduction if overweight, regular physical act, dietary mod, all more successful when family based)
  - Indication for drugs; inadeq resp to lifestyle mod or 2° HTN (goal to ↓BP <95th %ile)
  - First-line therapy ACE-I, ARBs, BB, CCBs, and diuretics
  - Can tailor Rx to underlying dz (i.e., ACE-I or ARB w/ DM or proteinuria)
  - Regular monitoring for drug toxicity and for end organ BP damage necessary
- Patient's HTN emergency must be managed w/ IV antihypertensives w/ goal to dec BP by <25% in the 1st 8 hr and normalized BP over next 24–48 hr

Approach to Dysrhythmia (Pediatr Clin North Am 2006;53:85)

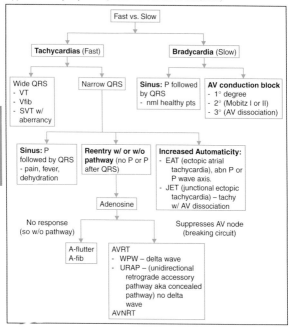

Sinus Tachycardia (50% of arrhythmias)
- Generally benign, defined by age (roughly >140 in children, >160 in infants)
- Narrow QRS and P wave before every QRS
- For every 1°C inc body temp can expect 9.6 bpm increase in HR
- Ddx: Fever, pain, hypoxia, hypovol, anemia, shock, MI, PE, hyperthyroid, hypoCa, illicit, meds
- Treat the underlying disorder

Supraventricular Tachycardia (13% of arrhythmias)
- Most common symptomatic dysrhythmia (roughly >180 in children, >220 in infants)
- Narrow regular complex tachycardia, w/o P waves or w/ retrograde P waves w/ abnormal axis, abrupt onset
- **Two types:**
  - Reentry tachycardias (w/ pathway as below, or w/o as w/ Afib or Aflutter)
    - **AV reentrant** (most common): 2/2 accessory pathway that is an anatomically separate bypass tract; (e.g., WPW-short PR, wide QRS, delta wave in sinus)
    - **AV nodal/junctional:** Dual AV node pathways
  - Increase automaticity (foci other than SA node is driving tachycardia)
    - **Ectopic atrial tachycardia** (different P waves; MAT)
    - **Junctional ectopic tachycardia** (foci w/i or adjacent to AV junction)
      - Only AV dissociation in which ventricular rate is faster than the sinus rate
      - Very rarely w/ 1:1 association w/ retrograde p waves
      - Classically seen postoperatively from cardiac surgery (6–72 hr)
- **Etiologies:** Most idiopathic; also w/ drugs, myocarditis/CM, Ebstein, transposition
  - In infants <4 mo, 50% idiopathic, 24% fever or drug related, 23% CHD (commonly Ebstein, single ventricle, or L-transposition), 10–20% WPW
- Infants may present w/ irritability, poor feeding, diaphoresis

- Younger children (<12 yo) more commonly AVRT (i.e., WPW)
- Older children (>12 yo) AVNRT more common
- **Treatment:**
  - **Stable SVT:** Attempt vagal maneuver: Valsalva, ice bag to face, etc.
    - Adenosine IV rapid push w/ rapid saline flush in vein close to heart (i.e., antecub)
  - **Unstable SVT:** See PALS card
    - Immediate synchronized cardioversion (0.5 J/Kg, may repeat 1 J/kg)
    - Consult cardiology: May give digoxin, BB for longer term (ONLY in conjunction with cardiology)

Atrial Flutter: Hallmark pattern is "saw-toothed" flutter waves
- Avg atrial rate ~300 bpm (240–450) w/ 2:1, 3:1, or 4:1 AV block
- **Etiologies:** Often seen in healthy newborns with structurally normal hearts
  - Structural heart disease (dilated atria, myocarditis, or acute infection)
  - Postop complications (ASD repairs, Mustard procedure, or Fontan)
  - Occasionally seen in Duchenne muscular dystrophy or CNS injury
- **Treatment**
  - Unstable: Electrical cardioversion +/– heparinization
  - Stable: Medications (digoxin, propranolol)
  - Recurrences may be prevented w/ quinidine

Atrial Fibrillation (4.6% of arrhythmias)
- "Irregularly irregular," generally seen in settings of RAE or LAE
- Disorganized rapid atrial activity w/ rates ranging from 350 to 600 bpm
- **Etiologies:** Often seen in adolescents w/ healthy hearts after drinking binges
  - Structural heart disease (underlying mitral valve disease w/ hyperthyroidism)
  - Intra-atrial operative procedures
  - Familial atrial fibrillation syndrome (structurally normal but w/ channelopathy)
- **Treatment**
  - **Unstable:** Immediate synchronized cardioversion
  - **Stable:** Rate control w/ BB (Lopressor) or w/ CCB (diltiazem), can use digoxin (if not improved in 24 hr, consider adding propranolol or procainamide)

Ventricular Tachycardia
- Three or more consecutive PVCs; wide QRS complexes (0.06–0.14 sec)
- AV dissociation, sometimes with ventricular rate > atrial rate
  - Monomorphic: Uniform contour w/ absent or retrograde P waves
  - Polymorphic: Ex torsades de pointes
- **Etiologies:** Electrolyte abn (hyperK, hypoK, hypocalcemia, hypomagnesemia), metabolic abnormalities (acidosis), congenital heart disorders, myocarditis or acquired heart disease, drug toxicity, idiopathic, prolonged QT, cardiac tumors
- **Treatment**
  - **Pulseless:** Treat as Vfib
  - **Pulse**
    - Unstable: Synchronized cardioversion (0.5–1 J/kg)
    - Stable: Medications (amiodarone, procainamide, or lidocaine)

Ventricular Fibrillation
- Chaotic, irregular ventricular contractions w/o effective circulation to the body
- Bizarre QRS complexes w/ varying sizes and rapid, irregular rate
- **Etiologies:** Postop complications, severe hypoxemia, hyperK, meds, myocarditis, and MI
- **Treatment**
  - Immediate CPR
  - Defibrillation as soon as possible: 2 J/kg → 2–4 J/kg → 4 J/kg

Bradycardias (6% of arrhythmias)
- No need to treat bradycardia w/o symptoms or hemodynamic compromise
- **Sinus bradycardia:** (<80 bpm in infants or <60 bpm in children)
  - Usually benign but ensure not assoc w/ inc ICP (Cushing triad: Bradycardia, HTN, and irreg RR), resp distress or HoTN
  - Assess for inc K, inc Ca, hypoxia, hypothermia, hypothyroidism, meds
  - Treatment = treat cause (but ensure P waves present and not a junctional rhythm)
- **1° AV block:** Prolonged PR interval (>200 msec) but no dropped QRSs
  - Seen commonly in healthy children w/ infections (sometimes just in healthy kids)
  - Also in rheumatic fever & Lyme dz, cardiomyopathy & CHD (ASD & Ebstein)
- **2° AV block, Mobitz I:** (Wenckebach) Progressive ↑ PR w/ eventual dropped QRS
  - Benign or assoc w/ myocarditis, MI, cardiomyopathy, CHD, dig tox, or postop
  - Because of increased refractory period at the level of the AV node
- **2° AV block, Mobitz II:** Regular PR interval w/ intermittently dropped QRS

- Failure of conduction at the level of the bundle of His
- More concerning as it can progress to complete heart block
- Prophylactic pacemaker may be warranted
- Cannot distinguish btwn Mobitz type I vs. Mobitz type II when there is 2:1 block
- **3° AV block:** Complete AV dissociation
  - Congenital (assoc w/ L TGA), maternal CTD (SLE w/ anti-Ro, anti-La), underlying rhythm is often a junctional escape
  - Assoc w/ myocarditis, Lyme, rheumatic fever, diphtheria, Kawasaki dz, and SLE
  - Older children may present w/ syncopal attacks (Stokes–Adams attacks)
  - Sx include fatigue, dizziness, impaired exercise tol, syncope, or sudden death
  - Rx is pacemaker placement (atropine, isoproterenol, or temp wire in interim)

PERICARDITIS AND PERICARDIAL EFFUSION

Definition (Pediatr Infect Dis J 2006;25:165)
- Pericardium w/ 2 layers, outer (parietal) and inner (visceral) w/ small amount of fluid
- Pericarditis is inflammation of these layers; can be inflammation alone, inflammation w/ purulent, serosanguineous or hemorrhagic effusion +/– tamponade, and fibrosis +/– constriction

Pathophysiology (Pediatr Infect Dis J 2006;25:165)
- Inflammation of the pericardium results in pain and can result in fluid accumulation
- With purulent pericarditis, effusion can accumulate quickly resulting in right heart failure or tamponade; if develops slowly, greater amt of accum can be tolerated
- Tamponade = accumulated pericardial fluid compresses heart, prevents nml venous return on insp (↓ SBP and cardiac output w/ insp 2/2 ventricular interdependence w/ bowing of interventricular septum into LV impairing filling); **"pulsus paradoxus"**

Etiology: Multi-etiologies possible for pediatric pericarditis (Pediatr Infect Dis J 2006;25:165)
- Bacterial: *Staph, Strep, Haemophilus, Neisseria, Tularemia, TB, Bartonella, Actinomyces, Nocardia, Salmonella, Coxiella*
- Viral: Enteroviruses (coxsackie B), adenovirus, CMV, VZV, EBV, flu, HIV
- Parasites: *E. histolytica* and *Echinococcus*
- Fungi: *Candida* and *Aspergillus*
- Other infections: Spirochetes, *Mycoplasma, Chlamydia,* rickettsiae
- Noninfectious: Postsurgical, CTD, autoimmune, toxin mediated, Kawasaki
- Genetic/metabolic: Glycogen storage disease, hypothyroidism, FMF, uremia
- Cancer associated: Leukemia, metastatic or solid tumor, 2/2 chemo or XRT
- Trauma: Blunt or penetrating or iatrogenic/surgical
- Contemporary studies of mod to large pericardial effusions in ages 1 d–17.8 yr w/ neoplastic dz (39%), idiopathic (37%), collagen vascular dz (9%), renal dz (8%), bacterial infection (3%), HIV (2%) (Pediatr Cardiol 2007;29:90)

Diagnosis (Pediatr Infect Dis J 2006;25:165)
- EKG w/ diffuse ST elevation in all vascular distributions and PR depression in all but aVR, PR elevation in aVR most sens (QRSs +/– low voltage, electrical alternans, if effusion
- Eval of etiology includes CBC w/ diff, electrolytes w/ BUN/Cr, cardiac enzymes, viral assays, blood cx, & possibly evaluation for CTD, autoimmunity, or malignancy
- CXR +/– "globular" cardiac enlargement on PA film; huge heart but nml pulm vasc
- Echo is gold std for eval; cannot determine kind of fluid (hemorrhagic, infectious, etc.)
- Constrictive pericarditis: Assessment by echo limited, usually dx made by cath
- CT and MRI can both evaluate pericardium but echo is sufficiently sens and spec
- Pericardiocentesis if tamponade or suspected bact infxn; diagnostic in pts w/ unknown etiology (cell count, diff, cx, along w/ AFB, fungal & viral cx, viral PCR, cytology)
  - **Acute mgmt of tamponade is VOLUME resuscitation while arranging pericardiocentesis**
- Assessment of tamponade via pulsus paradoxus; measure diff btw SBP at which Korotkoff sounds 1st audible (at 1st audible only w/ expiration) & pressure at which audible throughout full resp cycle; >10 mm Hg is a +pulsus (JAMA 2007;297:1810)

Treatment (Eur Heart J 2004;25:587)
- Management depends on type and underlying etiology of pericarditis
- Pain management and treatment of inflammation with NSAIDs, theoretical risk of hemorrhagic conversion exists but not established
- Colchicine demonstrated to be effective in adult trials, not approved in peds

- Acutely, steroids only for pts recalcitrant to NSAIDs or pts w/ acute pericarditis 2/2 connective tissue disease, autoimmune pericarditis or uremic pericarditis
  - Purulent pericarditis w/ severe inflam resp may benefit from 1–2 wk steroids, as may TB pericarditis both acutely & chronically (Pediatr Infect Dis J 2006;25:165)
- Pericardiocentesis indicated in tamponade physiology, or if purulent, tuberculous, or malignant effusion suspected

Complications
- Fibrosis and constrictive pericarditis can occur 2/2 purulent pericarditis resulting in heart failure w/ a small rather than large globular appearing heart

CARDIOMYOPATHIES (CM)

Dilated Cardiomyopathy (DCM)
- **Epidemiology:** Annual incidence is 0.57 per 100,000 kids (JAMA 2006;296:1867)
  - Most common cardiomyopathy and cause of cardiac transplantation in children
  - More common M > F, African-Americans > Whites, and infants (<1 yo) > children
- **Etiologies:** Idiopathic most common; also 2/2 myocarditis, doxorubicin, neuromuscular dz (Duchenne, Becker), inborn errors of metab, malformation synd, & familial
- **Clinical manifestations** (Circulation 2006;114:2671)
  - Severe sx are found in majority of pts presenting to early medical attention
  - Presenting sx CHF (89.7%), sudden death (4.9%), exercise intolerance or arrhythmias (2.2%), or on routine screening (3.3%) in one study
- **Treatment:** Etiology dependent, diuretics, digoxin, ACEI, BB, or aldosterone antag in CHF, anticoagulation
  - Immune modulators (cyclosporine, steroids, γ-globulin) used in some pts w/ myocarditis
- **Prognosis** (JAMA 2006;296:1867; Circulation 2006;114:2671)
  - Risk factors for death or transplantation include older age at dx (>6 yo), those w/ idiopathic disease, and CHF at time of dx
  - Mortality or transplantation more common to occur w/i 2 yr of presentation
  - 1- and 5-yr rate of death or transplantation found to be 31% and 46% in 1 study

Hypertrophic Cardiomyopathy (JAMA 2002;287:1308)
- **Definition:** Complex, relatively common genetic dz; presents at any age
  - AD inheritance 2/2 mutations in any 1 of 10 genes (most commonly β-myosin heavy chain, cardiac troponin T, or myosin-binding protein C)
- **Epidemiology:** Most common genetic CV dz; most common cause sudden death in kids
  - A prevalence of 1:500 in the general population
- **Clinical manifestations**
  - Most HCM pts w/ nonobstructive dz (75% w/o sizable resting outflow tract obst)
  - May p/w sudden death, CP, syncope, heart murmur, + FHx, or abn EKG
- **Diagnostic studies:** EKG abn in 75–95% of pts
  - Echo w/ hypertrophied nondilated LV in the absence of other cardiac or systemic dz
  - MRI may show asymmetric LVH undetectable on echo
- **Prognosis:** Overall annual mortality rate is 1%
  - Risk factors for sudden death: Prior Hx of cardiac arrest, spontaneous VT, FHx of sudden death, syncope, hypotension during exercise, and extreme LVH
- **Treatment**
  - Genotype w/o Phenotype
  - Genotype + Phenotype—exercise restriction, control arrhythmias, pacemaker therapy
  - Consider automated ICDefib
  - Genotpy + Phenotype + Heart failure—drug therapy, pacemaker, consider myotomy/ myomectomy/EtOH septal ablation
  - End-stage systolic dysfxn—heart transplant

Restrictive Cardiomyopathy—
- **Definition:** Diastolic dysfxn w/ preserved systolic fxn w/o ventricular hypertrophy or dilation
  - Impaired ventricular filling w/ nml or ↓ diastolic volume 2/2 heart muscle dz
- **Epidemiology** (Heart 2005;91:1199; N Engl J Med 1997;336:267)
  - Rare in children (only 2–5% of pt w/ pediatric cardiomyopathy)
  - Etiologies: Idiopathic, familial, infiltrative dz (Gaucher, Hurler, amyloid), storage dz (Fabry, glycogen storage, hemochromatosis), hemosiderosis, drugs, XRT
- **Clinical manifestations**
  - Etiology dependent; dyspnea, tachypnea, fatigue, PND, orthopnea, periph edema

- Cardiac conduction abnormalities are also common
- Elevated JVP, S_3, w/ tachycardia and low pulse volume can be found on exam
- **Diagnostic evaluation**
  - CXR usually w/ normal cardiac size but pulmonary congestion often seen
  - EKG often w/ nonspec ST and T wave abn, but BBB, LVH, and conduct abn as well
  - Doppler echo w/ ↑ early diastolic filling velocity, ↓ atrial filling velocity, ↑ ratio of early diastolic filling to atrial filling ratio, and ↓ relaxation time
- **Treatment:** Specific Rx varies w/ etiology
  - Symptomatic therapy includes diuretic for venous congestion, antiarrhythmics or pacemaker for conduction abnormalities, and warfarin for thrombus formation
- **Prognosis:** Worse than in adults w/ a median survival of 1.4 yr in 1 study
  - Pts presenting w/ pulmonary venous congestion have worse outcomes

CONGESTIVE HEART FAILURE

Definition
- Acquired or inborn state in which the heart cannot meet metabolic demands of the body at nml physiologic venous pressures
- Accounts for ~10% of pediatric heart transplant, w/ DCM as most common cause

Pathophysiology
- Preload = loading force on the heart (amt of venous blood return) that stretches myocardial fibers, which (to a point) results in ↑ contraction strength and thus ↑ cardiac output (represented by Frank–Starling law) (Pediatr Rev 1980;1:180)
- As filling pressures ↑ beyond point of maximal contractile response, myocardial contraction becomes increasingly inefficient, resulting in ↓ cardiac output
- As tissue perfusion impaired 2/2 ↓ cardiac output, renin–angiotensin sys activated resulting in ↑ renal Na & H_2O retention → ↑ extracellular volume & cardiac preload
- Response, while initially adaptive, is maladaptive in the long run → ↑ afterload against which the heart must work and results in volume overload

Etiology (Pediatr Rev 1980;1:321; Heart 2002;88:198)
- **Increased demand for cardiac output** (high-output cardiac failure)
  - Hypermetabolic states: Hyperthyroidism, anemia, sepsis
  - Valvular insufficiency: Can be inherited or acquired
  - Fluid overload: Renal disease or iatrogenic
  - Left- to right-sided shunting: PDA, VSD, ASD, etc.
- **Increased afterload**
  - Aortic or pulmonic valvular stenosis
  - Coarctation of the aorta, pulmonary artery stenosis
  - Systemic or pulmonary hypertension
- **Impaired myocardial function/contractility**
  - Myocarditis: Lymphocytic myocarditis accounts for 10% of recent onset CM
    - Viruses, most common causes in dev countries; coxsackie B and adenovirus
    - Chagas disease is the most common cause in C. and S. America
  - Dilated cardiomyopathies: 1° indication for xplant aside from CHD in infancy
    - Prognosis for DCM is 60% at 5 yr from presentation
    - DCM genetic etiology at present a "molecular maze"; mutations assoc w/ cytoskeleton, troponin T, and other sarcomere protein genes
  - Coronary artery disease, rare aside from anomalous cardiac vasculature or high-risk patients (ESRD, familial hyperlipidemia, DM, etc.)
  - Metabolic abnormalities (Pompe disease)
  - Nutritional or toxic insults (thiamine deficiencies, chemotherapeutics)
  - Electrolyte disturbances
  - Dysrhythmias

History and Physical Exam
- Hx poor feeding, poor weight gain, sweating w/ feeds, poor exercise tolerance, cyanosis, chest pain, nocturnal cough, orthopnea, paroxysmal nocturnal dyspnea
- Physical exam may reveal tachycardia or tachypnea
  - Edema not common; in infants, assess eyelids & sacrum (most dependent areas)
  - Heart may be enlarged w/ displaced point of max impulse
  - Heart murmur may be present, as may extra heart sounds (S_3, S_4, etc.)
  - Crackles on pulmonary exam indicate pulmonary edema with left-sided failure
  - Elevated jugular venous pulsations or enlarged liver seen with right-sided failure

Evaluation (Heart 2002;88:198)
- EKG rarely nml but very nonspecific, CXR may have cardiac enlargement, pulm edema
- BNP (normal values vary with age)
- Echocardiography can assess cardiac function and for anomalous coronary anatomy
- Myocarditis: Viral PCR (coxsackie, adenovirus, echo, influenza, parainfluenza, VZV, RSV, rubella, CMV, EBV, HIV, parvovirus, *Mycoplasma,* and other endemic infections such as Chagas, dengue, diphtheria, *Coxiella*), troponin, CBC (for lymphocytosis), and myocardial bx for histology and PCR, toxicology (cocaine)
- Autoimmune: Anti-Ro and La, ANA, RF, ESR, dsDNA, and other autoantibodies
- Mitochondrial: Carnitine, acylcarnitine, lactate, glucose, CBC (for neutropenia), urine AA for methylglutaconic aciduria, muscle bx, molecular genetics (Barth syndrome)

Treatment (Heart 2002;88:198)
- Pharmacokinetics in pediatrics not as clear for the core CHF drugs
- ACE inhibitors: 1 retrospective study demonstrating reduced mortality in children w/ DCM compared to standard Rx with digoxin and diuretics. (Pediatr Cardiol 1993;14:9)
- BB: In children, 2 RCTs have shown improvement of LV fx, inc exercise tolerance and dec need for heart xplant in idiopathic, drug-induced, or inherited DCM. (Heart 1998;79:337; J Heart Lung Transplant 1999;18:269)
- Diuretics: Clear clinical benefit but little published in the last 30 yr
  - Chlorothiazide, ethacrynic acid, and furosemide are all used
  - Spironolactone; small RCT in peds showed safety and efficacy; no mortality impact
    - Use derived from benefit seen in larger RALES study in adults
- Digoxin: Long-standing corner stone of pediatric CHF management
  - Only studies published that evaluate efficacy of digoxin in children show modest benefits in small nonrandomized or unblinded trials (all were in infants w/ large VSDs) (Am J Cardiol 1999;83:1408; Am J Cardiol 1991;68:1377)
  - Increased contractility does not consistently correlate with clinical improvement
- Oldest core of CHF therapy is digoxin and diuretics, now w/ data supporting use of ACE-Is and BB as well as spironolactone

DIABETES MELLITUS

Definition (Pediatr Diabetes 2009;10(Suppl. 12):3)
- Fasting glucose ≥126 mg/dL, 2 hr oral glucose tolerance test (ODTT) glucose ≥200 mg/dL, or random glucose ≥200 mg/dL in the presence of symptoms. In the absence of symptoms, level needs to be repeated on diff day

Classification
- **Type 1 diabetes:** Autoimmune disorder w/ T cell–mediated destruction of pancreatic islet cells, causing insulin deficiency. +pancreatic autoantibodies. Rx w/ insulin
- **Type 2 diabetes:** Peripheral resistance to insulin action and variably dysregulated/diminished insulin secretion. Rx w/ oral hypoglycemic agents and/or insulin
- Others:
  - **Monogenic diabetes** (formerly maturity-onset diabetes of the young [MODY]): Heterogeneous group of genetic disorders caused by mutations in beta-cell genes
    - AD inheritance, mild to moderate hyperglycemia, absence of autoantibodies
    - ~1–5% of diabetes Rx w/ oral hypoglycemic agents and/or insulin
  - **Mitochondrial diabetes:** May be assoc w/ sensorineural deafness; characterized by progressive non-autoimmune beta-cell failure
    - Maternal transmission of mutated mito DNA = maternally inherited diabetes
  - **Secondary diabetes:**
    - CF-related DM: ↓ insulin secretion 2/2 pancreatic damage & amyloid deposition
    - Drug induced: 2/2 meds (steroids, growth hormone, β-agonists, diazoxide, atypical antipsychotics, cyclosporine A, L-asparaginase (reversible DM)
    - Hemosiderosis/hemochromatosis: Fe overload (chronic transfusion) ↓ secrete and ↑ resistance insulin
    - 2/2 genetic syndrome: Down,* Turner*, Klinefelter*, Wolfram syndrome (a.k.a. DIDMOAD, diabetes insipidus, diabetes mellitus, optic atrophy, deafness), Prader–Willi, Bardet–Biedl, etc. (*Often autoimmune)
  - Gestational diabetes

DIABETES MELLITUS TYPE 1

(Pediatr Diabetes 2009;10(Suppl 12):1; ISPAD Clinical Practice Consensus Guidelines 2009 Compendium)

Epidemiology
- Western countries: T1DM >90% of childhood/adolescent DM; incidence greatest in Finland > Sardinia > Canada > Sweden > UK > USA
- Onset bimodal (1st peak at 4–6 yo & 2nd at early puberty) & ↑ in winter
- No recognizable pattern of inheritance though familial aggregation ~10%; 2–3× more common in offspring of diabetic men than women
- Concordance rates for monozygotic twins 30–50%; genetic factors: HLA DR 3, 4—and as yet unknown environmental triggers

Clinical Manifestations
- Asymptomatic incidental hyperglycemia/glycosuria or
- **Classic symptoms:** Polyuria and polydipsia (70%), weight loss (34%) often w/ inc in appetite (polyphagia), lethargy (16%), and nocturnal enuresis
- Diabetic ketoacidosis (DKA): Classic sx +/– vomiting and abdominal pain, fruity breath (acetone), Kussmaul respirations, obtundation, coma
  - If identified thru antibody screening and f/u (DPT1 trial) approx 70% asymptomatic but DKA initial presentation 15–70% in Europe and NA
  - DKA is freq in very young children, in families w/o FHx of diabetes, and lower socioeconomic status
- Dehydration: Mild to severe, because of osmotic diuresis
- Visual changes: 2/2 osmotic shifts in lens or cataracts if prolonged hyperglycemia
- Candidal infections (more common in younger children)

Epidemiology (Pediatrics 2004;113:e133)
- DKA as 1st presentation of DM1 more often in pts <4 yo, w/o a 1st-degree relative w/ DM1, and of lower socioeconomic status
- 25% of new onset diabetes in children presents as DKA
- Incidence of 1–10% per patient per yr in established DM1

- Risk factors for recurrent DKA: Poor control, previous episodes of DKA, peripubertal or adolescent, psychiatric disorders, lower SES, insulin not administered by responsible adult, pump failure, inadequate insulin during intercurrent illness

- Hemoglobin A1c: Glycated Hgb; good marker of serum glucose over 2–3 mo (nml RBC lifespan 100–120 d)
  - Accuracy affected by hemolysis, RBC turnover, and hemoglobinopathies (if hemoglobinopathy, measure total glycated Hgb, not HbA1C)
- Anti-islet cell Ab (ICA), anti-insulin Ab (IAA; check before admin insulin), anti-IA2 (islet antigen 2, aka ICA512) Ab, anti-GAD (glutamic acid decarboxylase, aka GAD65) Ab
- **Consider eval for other autoimmune conditions** (ISPAD)
  - Autoimmune thyroid dz (antithyroid peroxidase Ab, antithyroglobulin Ab), in up to 18% of newly dx'd DMI pts. Check TSH/free T4
  - Celiac sprue (anti-TTG Ab), + up to 5% of newly dx'd DMI
  - Also consider adrenal insufficiency, vitiligo, & autoimmune poly-endocrinopathies

- Blood glucose checked before meals and at bedtime. Consider testing at MN, at 2–4 AM, and after meals shortly after dx or when altering regimens
- HgbA1c every 3 mo (see age specific goals, below)
- Dilated retinal exam every year after 10 yr
- Fasting lipid panel at diagnosis and then q5yr if normal or yearly after 10 yr
- TSH, free T4 yearly; anti-TPO antibodies, antithyroglobulin antibodies initially
- Celiac screening every 2 yr
- Urine microalbumin: Creatinine ratio yearly after 10 yr

- Insulin regimen requires estimation of total daily dose (TDD) of insulin
- Start dose btw 0.3 and 0.6 U/kg/d; prepubertal pts may need less (0.25–0.5 U/kg/d); pubertal pts and those who present in DKA may require more (0.5–1 U/kg/d)
- Onset and action of insulins

Type	Onset (hr)	Peak (hr)	Duration (hr)	Comments
Rapid Acting				
Lispro insulin (Humalog)	0.25	1	2–3	
Insulin aspart (NovoLog)	0.25	1	2–3	
Glulisine (Apidra)	0.25	1	2–3	
Short Acting				
Regular human insulin	0.5–1	2–4	4–6	Longer action if larger dose (mass action effect) Can be used intravenously
Intermediate Acting				
NPH human	0.5–1	4–6	8–16	Peak and duration quite variable
Long Acting				
Insulin glargine (Lantus)	0.5–1	None	23–26	Basal insulin: Minimal or no peak. Cannot mix w/ other insulins
Insulin detemir (Levemir)	0.5–1	None	5.7 (low dose)–26 (high dose)	Basal insulin: Minimal or no peak Cannot mix w/ other insulins

- **Conventional insulin Rx** (2–3 injections per d)
  - NPH at least bid (before breakfast w/ 2nd dose either before dinner or bedtime), w/ rapid-acting or short-acting ("regular") insulin 2–3×/d
  - Requires fixed schedule of eating & insulin dosing and fixed amt of carbs at meals
- **Basal-bolus** (4+ injections/d) (Diabet Med 2006;23:285)
  - Assoc w/ improved HgbA1c, dec gluc fluctuations, and dec hypoglycemia
  - Long-acting 1–2×/d plus rapid-acting insulin w/ meals
    - 50% of TDD is long acting
    - 50% of TDD rapid acting—dose based on blood sugar and carb content
    - Estimate of correction factor (CF): 1500/TDD gives amt by which serum glucose expected to dec, in mg/dL
    - Estimating insulin: Carb ratio (CR); 500/TDD gives # of grams of carbs that are covered by 1 unit of rapid-acting insulin (~1/3 CF)

- Insulin pump: Use rapid-acting insulin for basal infusion and bolus corrections
  - Assoc w/ less hypoglycemia, improved HgbA1c compared with NPH-based regimens, and improvements in quality of life scales (Diabetes Care 2008;31:S140)
- Education regarding symptoms of hypoglycemia is very important (<70 mg/dL)

Treatment Goals (ADA): (Diabetes Care 2005;28:186)
- <6 yo; plasma glucose before meals 100–189; bedtime/overnight 110–200; A1c < 8.5% but >7.5%; high risk and vulnerable to hypoglycemia
- 6–12 yo; before meals 90–180; bedtime/overnight 100–180; A1c < 8%; hypoglycemia risk vs. relatively low risk of complications prior to puberty
- 13–19 yo; before meals 90–130; bedtime/overnight 90–150; A1c < 7.5%; generally w/ lower risk of hypoglycemia; if no excessive hypoglycemia, can aim for <7%

Complications
- Hypoglycemia (<70 mg/dL); Rx w/ PO glucose (15 g carbs = 4 oz juice = 1 tblspn sugar, glucose tablets, or IV dextrose bolus, consider 0.5–1 mg SC/IV glucagon if unable to swallow. Smaller doses of glucagon [20–150 mcg] minibolus therapy) every 1–2 hr can be useful if unable to take PO (J Paediatr Child Health 2006;42:108)
- Microvascular complications (retinopathy, neuropathy, renal disease)
- Macrovascular complications (coronary vascular disease, peripheral vascular disease)
  - DCCT: Significant correlation btw HgbA1c and risk of both microvascular and macrovascular complications (N Engl J Med 2000;342:381)

DIABETES MELLITUS TYPE 2

Epidemiology (Lancet 2007;369:1823; Diabetes Care 2006;29:212; Pediatr Diabetes 2009;10(Suppl. 12):3)
- U/S prevalence ↑ing; most countries <10%, Japan 60–80%
- STOPP-T2D trial: ~50% middle-school students w/ ↑BMI (≥85 percentile), 40% w/fasting glucose ≥100 mg/dL, (only 0.4% >125 mg/dL, and ⅓ w/ hyperinsulinism w/fasting insulin ≥30 µU/mL) and thus prediabetes (Diabetes Care 2006;29:212)

Diagnostic Studies (Pediatrics 2003;112:e328)
- Characteristics: Polygenic, pubertal, rarely autoimmunity, acanthosis nigricans
- At dx, screen for proteinuria/microalbuminuria, dilated funduscopic exam by ophtho
  - After metabolic stabilization (1–3 mo after dx): LFTs & fasting lipids
  - Repeat all preceding annually. (AAP guidelines for at-risk groups) HgbA1c q3mo

Complications (Acute) (Lancet 2007;369:1823)
- Multi studies, 11–25% of pts p/w ketonuria (see section on DKA)
- Hyperglycemic hyperosmolar state (glucose >600 mg/dL, osmolality >330 mOsm/L, mild acidosis w/ bicarbonate >15 mmol/L and mild ketonuria ≤15 mg/dL) 2/2 nonadherence to Rx, meds, and stresses (infections, substance abuse, chronic disease)
  - In one study at tertiary care facility, 3.7% of pts w/ T2DM had this presentation; case-mortality rates are high across studies, and range from 14% to 42%. Pts are more dehydrated than clinically apparent (J Pediatr 2011;158:9)

Complications (Chronic) (Lancet 2007;369:1823)
- Microalbuminuria and risk of AMI ↑ for pts w/ DM2 dx'd at younger ages
- HTN, dyslipidemia, retinopathy, nonalcoholic fatty liver dz, and neuropathy
- Poor glycemic control (by HgbA1c) & HTN predictive of subseq complications
- Complications may progress more rapidly in young DM2 than w/ DM1

Treatment
- Lifestyle Δ, diet mod, weight mgmt, exercise are effective but adherence is difficult
- Oral hypoglycemics; metformin (FDA approved). Dose can be titrated up slowly to avoid common side effects (headache, nausea)
- Insulin usually necessary with time

DIABETIC KETOACIDOSIS

Definition
- ↓ effective circulating insulin and ↑ counterregulatory hormones (glucagon, epinephrine) → glycogenolysis, gluconeogenesis (hyperglycemia), lipolysis
- Lipolysis + glucagon → ketogenesis and metabolic acidosis

Diagnose DKA

1) Hyperglycemia: serum glucose >200–250 mg/dL 2) Acidosis: venous pH < 7.25–7.30 and/or serum bicarbonate ≤ 15 mEq/L 3) Elevated ketones in serum or urine

**NOTE **If severe DKA (pH < 7.1, bicarb < 5 mEq/L, mental status changes, severe dehydration). Please assign critical care nursing

Fluid/Electrolytes

Assess fluid deficit (Be careful as this is often overestimated in DKA, rough guide is 7–9%)

1 or 2 boluses 10 cc/kg 0.9% saline IV over 30 min (each), unless hypotensive (shock)

Once bolus fluid completed, **IMMEDIATELY** hang **AVAILABLE** fluid until IDEAL fluid is ready.
If void: NaCl 0.9% + KCl 40 mEq/L
If NO void: NaCl 0.9% (both premixed and in ED)
See below for IDEAL fluid calculations

CALCULATE RATE: Maintenance requirement + Replace Deficit over 48 hr * (see below for more detail.)
Do NOT replace urine losses. Subtract bolus fluid. A rough estimate is 1.5 × M. Rarely need more than 2 × M

IDEAL FLUID:
Potassium: Add potassium to IV fluid (after void): 20 mEq/L Kacetate + 20 mEq/L K phosphate. K is <3.5 consider increasing to 60 mEq/L, rarely need 80 mEq/L.

Na: If the corrected serum Na+ is high or normal, use 0.45% saline should be used and if it is low 0.9% saline should be administered
BUT if signs and symptoms are suggestive of cerebral edema run 0.9% NS

Dextrose: May consider changing fluid to D5 ½NS + 40 mEq/L KCl even in early tx if treatment of BG dropping quickly.
Goal ~100 mg/dL per hour especially when initial BG is quite high > 700 mg/dL.

Helpful Equations:
**Corrected Na = Measured Na + 1.6((glucose mg/dL −100)/100) Effective osmolality =
2(measured Na+ (mEq/L)) + (glucose (mg/dL)/18) Anion gap = [Na+] − (Cl− + CO2)

Insulin/Dextrose

Order Insulin drip STAT from pharmacy IMMEDIATELY Ask nurse to page pharmacy, Notify attending IV attending from pharmacy in 5–10 min.

Start Insulin drip between hour 1 and 2 after patient arrival (0.1 U/kg per hr IV of Regular Insulin).

Check with RN to make sure tubing was primed with insulin (Because insulin adsorbs to the plastic intravenous (IV) tubing, a volume (about 50 mL) of the infusion should be run through the tubing before initiating therapy)

An early insulin bolus is NOT recommended, however if the insulin drip is not available 2 hr after patient arrival consider giving a small SC injection of Novolog Insulin DOSE: 0.05–0.1 U/kg. Discuss with endocrine prior to giving SC insulin

Add IV Dextrose to the IVFs once glucose ~ 250–300 mg/dL to keep glucose 150–250 mg/dL. Can use 2 IV bag solution

2 IV bag solution: Upon transfer to the ICU, consider ordering IVF which contains D10 + the IDEAL fluid (see 1st column). As blood sugar falls to 300 divide total volume of IVF between these bags to keep blood sugar above 150 through. start 25% as dextrose and 75% as non-dextrose containing fluid and shift to 50/50% as needed to maintain blood glucose

Continue insulin infusion until acidosis corrects (approx pH > 7.30 and bicarbonate > 18 mEq/L). Urine ketones (acetoacetate) will take longer to disappear than serum measures of acidosis and do not need to clear before starting subcutaneous insulin

Stop insulin and dextrose and saline infusions 15–30 minutes after administration of SQ Novolog Insulin or restart insulin pump at basal rate and BOLUS for meal & food.
Even if it remains depleted of acid and electrolytes, correct early at this point

LABS for new-onset diabetes: Once stable, please draw HbA1C, FT4, TSH, anti-TPO, IgA, TTG IgA, anti-insulin, anti-GAD, anti-IA2

Neurologic Status/Monitoring

Assess neurologic status for signs of **cerebral edema** hourly (GCS/pupils), blood glucose hourly, electrolytes & VBG q2–4h, ECG PRN K level, follow RR, HR, BP, O2Sat closely q1h/on monitor, more frequently PRN; NOTE: Clinical warning signs, if see sustained deceleration HR (↓ 20) and/or widened pulse pressure (↑ 10), ask MD to evaluate for cerebral edema

Strongly consider cerebral edema if patient meets:
• One (1) Diagnostic Criterion (abnormal motor or verbal response to pain, decorticate or decerebrate posture, cranial nerve palsy, abnormal neurogenic respiratory pattern)
OR
• Two (2) Major Criteria (altered mentation, sustained heart rate deceleration, incontinence)
OR
• 1 Major and 2 Minor criteria (vomiting, headache, lethargy, diastolic BP > 90, age < 5 years)
• Other signs: bradycardia (sustained HR deceleration by 20 beat/min), delirium, retina/papilledema, vomiting, change in level of consciousness/ responsiveness, unequal pupils
NOTE: CE is more common in younger, sicker patients. Occurs in 1st 24 hr, bimodal peak at 3hr and 14hr

If suspect cerebral edema IMMEDIATELY:
1. Reduce fluid rate
2. Administer mannitol (0.25–1 gm/kg IV over 20 minutes). Hypertonic saline (3%; 3–10 mL/kg over 30 min), may be an alternative. Repeat PRN. NOTE: Mannitol is standard, but prelim data suggests that hypertonic saline may be as effective with fewer side effects. Hypertonic saline regimens vary, can use as maintenance fluid
3. Intubate and ventilate (if necessary). Do: not hyperventilate
DO NOT WAIT FOR IMAGING TO CONFIRM

BICARB: Bicarbonate therapy is NOT recommended. It may be necessary in a code of cardiac dysfunction due to profound acidosis (pH<6.9) or in severe hyperkalemia. DOSE: 1–2 mEq/kg, mixed and can run of NaBicarb in 1 L ½ NS. Page endo for discussion of considering and is it so emergent.

*Maintenance fluids calculated by Holliday–Segar formula based on body weight should ideally be based on baseline body weight, but can use current weight e.g., 5% deficit for a 50 kg child would be 2500 mL; if the patient got a 1 L bolus, the remaining deficit would be replaced over 48h, thus 1500 mL. This deficit should be replaced over 48 hr, thus 1500 mL should be given over the first 24 h (31 mL/hr). Maintenance for a 50 kg child would be about 90 mL/hr. Total fluid/hr would thus amount to about 120 mL/hr (90+31)

- Hyperglycemia + acidosis → osmotic diuresis, dehydration, electrolyte loss
- Severity: **Mild** w/ venous pH <7.3, bicarbonate <15 mmol/L, **moderate** w/ venous pH <7.2, bicarbonate <10, **severe** w/ venous pH <7.1, bicarbonate <5

Clinical Manifestations
- Confirm dx and determine cause (evidence of infection; insulin omission, failure to follow sick day/pump failure mgmt guidelines)
- Exam: Weight (assess dehydration), Kussmaul respirations (rapid, deep, sighing)
- Assess clinical severity of dehydration 5%: prolonged capillary refill time, abnormal skin turgor, hyperpnea; 10%: Weak pulse, hypotension, oliguria
- Level of consciousness (Glasgow coma scale)
- Headache or focal neurologic signs (suggests cerebral edema)

Diagnostic Studies and Treatment (Courtesy of Nicole Sherry, MD at MGH)
- See flow sheet in the next page

Complications (Pediatrics 2004;113:e133; Diabetes Care 2006;29:1150)
- Mortality from DKA is 0.15% in the United States
- 0.5–1% of episodes of DKA c/b cerebral edema; mortality risk of 20–25%
  - Accounts for 60–90% of DKA-related mortality
  - Risk factors for cerebral edema: Early bolus insulin, attenuated rise or drop in serum Na, severity of acidosis or hypocapnia, elevated BUN, but NOT degree of hyperglycemia
- Electrolyte abnormalities I (hypokalemia, hyperkalemia, hypophosphatemia) also occur
- Please see Neurology chapter section on treatment of cerebral edema

Prevention (Pediatrics 2004;113:e133)
- Earlier dx, pt, family and community education, responsible adults administering insulin, establishing comprehensive treatment networks

HYPOGLYCEMIA

Definition (Pediatr Rev 1989;11:117)
- ADA: <70 mg/dL for diabetics; <45 mg/dL for everyone else
- Sx: Autonomic, neurologic, behavioral changes: Perspiration, tachycardia, pallor, paresthesia, tremor, weak, N/V, irritability

Pathophysiology
- Nml fall in glucose → ↓ insulin secretion and ↑ counterregulatory hormones
- Presence of insulin inhibits adipose tissue breakdown → no ketones

Etiology
- Decreased availability (production/intake) or increased utilization
- Increased glucose use: Hyperthermia, polycythemia, sepsis, inability to produce/use other energy substrates like FFA, ketones, hyperinsulinemia
- Decreased glycogenolysis, gluconeogenesis, use of alternative fuels
  - Inborn errors in metabolism: AA and organic acid d/o (Maple syrup urine dz, etc., G6PD, FAO defects, galactosemia (very rare)
  - Liver disease: Hepatitis, Reye's syndrome, cirrhosis
  - Abnormalities in counterregulatory hormones: GHD, adrenal insufficiency
- Neonatal: Prematurity (limited stores), infant of diabetic mother, PPHN
- Hyperinsulinism
- Congenital hyperinsulinism (infants are often LGA)
  - PHHN: Persistent hyperinsulinemic hypoglycemia of newborn-genetic eval for common mutations in K channels, or in glutamate dehydrogenase (hyperinsulinism hyperammonemia syndrome)
  - Beckwith–Wiedemann
  - Drug induced: Insulin (low serum C-peptide—fragment of proinsulin released during secretory process—not found in pharma insulin), oral hypoglycemic agents
  - Infant of a diabetic mother
- Tox/drugs: Ethanol, INH, insulin, propranolol, oral hypoglycemics, rat poison (vacor)
- Factitious: Münchhausen syndrome by proxy

Clinical Manifestations
- >2 mo w/ rapid ↓ glucose <40 (often postprandial) usually w/ hunger and adrenergic surge w/ tachycardia, diaphoresis, anxiety, weakness
- Fasting hypoglycemia usually w/ neuroglycopenic symptoms; HA, confusion, fatigue, abn behavior, mental slowness, seizure → coma
- Neonates w/ nonspecific sx; tremor, jitteriness, apnea, cyanosis, hypotonia, poor feeding, tachycardia, cyanosis, seizure → coma

- Fingerstick glucose can underestimate serum glucose, check venous but treat
- **Critical sample** = labs to be drawn during hypoglycemic episode: **Insulin, cortisol, GH, lactate, pyruvate, beta-OH butyrate, FFA** (critical sample) (urine organic acids, acylcarnitine panel, NH_3: Can be drawn separately)
- Urine ketones: Absence of ketones → hyperinsulinemia, FAO defect, adrenal insufficiency
- Newborn screen: Aminoacidemias, urea cycle d/o, organic acidurias, FAO d/o
- Management w/ PO or IV glucose (1 cc/kg D25 bolus, then D10 at 1.5 maintenance); calculate GIR (glucose utiliz rate); %dextr × IVF rate/wt (kg) × 6
  Use: Diazoxide for hyperinsulinism, then octreotide consider rapid eval, surgical rx at appropriate center if med Rx unsuccessful.

THYROID FUNCTION TESTING

	TSH	T_4	T_3	Free T_4
"Sick Euthyroid"	Nml/↓	Nml/↓	↓	↑/Nml/↓
Subclinical hypothyroid	↑	Nml	Nml	Nml
Primary hypothyroid	↑	↓	Nml/↓	↓
Secondary (central) hypothyroid	Nml/↓	↓	Nml/↓	↓
Subclinical hyperthyroid	↓	Nml	Nml	Nml
Primary hyperthyroid	↓	↑	↑	↑
Secondary (central) hyperthyroid *(very rare)*	↑	↑	↑	↑

TFT 5-6

- TSH: Thyroid-stimulating hormone, released by pituitary in response to thyrotropin-releasing hormone from hypothalamus and w/ feedback inhibition from thyroid hormone (T_3/T_4)
- T_4: Thyroxine secreted by the thyroid gland and converted to active T_3 in target cells
- T_3: Tri-iodothyroxine; more potent than T_4; released by thyroid as well but $1/20^{th}$ amount of T_4. Not diagnostic in hypothyroidism
- Thyroxine-binding globulin (TBG) increases w/ hepatitis, pregnancy, OCPs, and decreases with excess androgens, glucocorticoids, phenytoin, cirrhosis
  - ↑ TBG results in ↑ total T_3 and T_4 (↓ results in ↓) but free T_3 and T_4 are normal
  - If suspicious of 2° or 3° hypothyroidism check free T_4 not T_4 or T_3

HYPERTHYROIDISM

Definition (Pediatr Rev 2006;27:155)
- Overactivity of the thyroid gland 2/2 overstimulation, inflammation, or abnormal thyroid axis function (overproduction or failure of feedback inhibition)

Etiology (JCEM 2007;92:797)
- Graves dz (increase in thyroid-stimulating immunoglobulin [TSI]) most common childhood etiology. Incidence peaks in late childhood; ♀ >> ♂
- Other etiologies; early Hashimoto (autoimmune thyroiditis), subacute thyroiditis hyperfunctioning thyroid nodule, pituitary adenoma–secreting TSH, activating mutation of TSH receptor, pituitary resistance to T_4, or exogenous thyroxine intake (ingestion or factitious)

Clinical Manifestations (JCEM 2007;92:797; Pediatr Rev 2006;27:155)
- Classically w/ tachycardia, palpitations, widened pulse pressure, tremor, brisk DTRs, fatigue, proximal muscle weakness, heat intolerance, ↑ perspiration, ↑ appetite but often w/ weight loss, diarrhea
- May present w/ behavioral disturbance; hyperactivity, emotional lability, ↓ concentration (worsening school performance), insomnia, anxiety
- Thyroid storm: Hyperthyroidism w/ acute onset, hyperthermia, tachycardia, jaundice, liver failure. Can progress to delirium, coma, and death
- W/ Graves dz may find ophthalmopathy (less common in children) w/ proptosis and or lid lag. Pretibial myxedema is a rare finding

Diagnostic Studies (JCEM 2007;92:797)
- Labs: TSH, free T_4, total T_3, TSH-R titers (TSI), thyroid autoantibodies (antithyroid peroxidase, antithyroglobulin); TBI-Ab (neonates)

- Radioactive thyroid uptake (Tc or 123I) can help distinguish btw transient hyperthyroidism (e.g., Hashimoto thyroiditis, viral thyroiditis) and persistent (e.g., Graves disease, McCune–Albright [activating mutation of TSH receptor])

Therapy (J Clin Endocrinol Metab 2007;92:797; Clin Endocrinol 2009; Feb 25 epub ahead of print; Thyroid 2011;21(6):593)

- **Thyroid storm:**
  - Propylthiouracil (PTU) and potassium iodide for short-term control (suppress release of thyroid hormone and peripheral conversion of T_4 to T_3)
  - IV β-blocker for HTN, other sx. Glucocorticoids for metabolic support if AI
- **Graves disease:**
  - Medical management w/ methimazole (MMI), surgery, or radioactive iodine (RAI). Risk of liver failure: PTU should be avoided in children (J Clin Endocrinol Metab 2010;953260–7)
  - 0.5% w/ serious complications: MMI → agranulocytosis; up to 25% develop rash, arthralgias, pruritus, transaminitis, or leukopenia
  - Titrate MMI until euthyroid; d/c when thyroid small & pt euthyroid (high recurrence rate)
  - Surgery well tolerated; Rare complications: Recurrent laryngeal nerve injury, hypoparathyroidism. Surgery preferred for: Large goiters, significant ophthalmopathy
  - RAI: Hypothyroidism usually follows w/i few months. (2nd dose required in 10% pts) → lifetime thyroid replacement becomes necessary (J Clin Endocrinol Metab 2011 Mar;96(3):580–588)

HYPOTHYROIDISM

Definition
- Deficiency of thyroid hormone production and decreased end-organ action
- Acquired (presents >6 mo) or congenital; 1° (↓ glandular production) or 2° (central)

Epidemiology and Etiology (Pediatr Rev 2009;30:251)
- **Congenital:** Most commonly absence of thyroid or ectopic thyroid tissue (lingual thyroid). Most sporadic, only 10–15% 2/2 inherited defects. Infants can have goiter w/ or w/o hypothyroidism if mother has iodine excess or def
- **Acquired:** Hashimoto's (chronic lymphocytic thyroiditis), most common in US; iodine deficiency is most common worldwide. Other causes: XRT, infiltrative dz, large hemangioendothelioma (↑ T_4 to rT3 conversion)
- Pt at increased risk: Down syndrome, T1DM, Turner, Klinefelter

Clinical Manifestations (Pediatr Rev 2009;30:251)
- **Congenital Hypothyroidism:** W/o Rx results in MR, severe growth failure (cretinism)
  - Neonates (1st 2 wk of life)
    - Post-term and LGA, hypothermia, poor feeding, large fontanelles, protuberant abdomen, edema of hands, feet, eyelids, neonatal jaundice (prolonged)
    - >1 mo: ↓ activity, lethargy, constipation, FTT, poor suck, resp distress, darkened and mottled skin (carotenemia)
    - >3 mo: As above w/ macroglossia, myxedema, hoarse cry, umbilical hernia, poor linear growth (can be earlier in severe in utero hypothyroidism)
- **Acquired hypothyroidism**
  - **Classic symptoms:** Growth delay, impaired school performance, sluggishness, cold intolerance, lethargy, constipation, dry skin, brittle hair, myalgias
  - Onset 6 mo–3 yo: Hoarse cry, umbilical hernia, coarse facies, dry skin, dec in linear growth, constipation, pseudohypertrophy (inc size of arm/leg muscles)
  - **Onset in childhood:** Classic sx rarely w/ precocious sexual development (thelarche w/o pubarche in girls or gonadarche w/o pubarche in boys)
  - **Onset in adolescence:** Classic sx but w/ delayed puberty; girls may have galactorrhea
- **Physical exam:** Evidence of above; bradycardia, HTN, slowed DTRs, +/– myxedema (thickened, nonpitting edematous Δ's in soft tissue)
  - Often w/ palpable thyroid (goiter) can be sym or asym; firm gland in thyroiditis, nodular gland raises concern for neoplasm but it is rare in pediatrics
- Severe cases can progress to myxedema coma

Diagnostic Studies (Pediatr Rev 2009;30:251)
- TSH and free T_4 diagnose majority of cases; if gland nonpalpable, consider thyroid U/S or I-123 or technetium scan to r/o absent or ectopic gland

- Infants: Newborn screens identify most babies. Most states use T_4 with f/u TSH
  - Newborn nml ranges differ from adults; vary w/ age, highest on DOL1 (see table in the next page: Esotrix normal values)
  - If low T_4 and nml TSH, retest and screen for TBG deficiency (check free T_4) which does not require treatment
  - If abnormal, can consider radionuclide scan (I-123/Tc) to look for thyroid tissue (considered optional in AAP guidelines)
- Older children, adults: Screen with TSH and free T_4. If abn, check thyroid (antithyroid peroxidase Ab, antithyroglobulin Ab)

Infant/Child Age	TSH [µU/ml]	Total T_4 [mcg/dL]	Free T_4 [ng/dL]
Premature infant (26–32 weeks)			
DOL 3–4	0.8–6.9	2.6–14	0.4–2.8
Full-term infant			
DOL 1–3		8.2–19.9	2.0–4.9
DOL 4	1.3–16		
1st week of life		6.0–15.9	
1–11 months	0.9–7.7	6.1–14.9	0.9–2.6
Prepubertal children			
12 mo–2 yr	0.6–5.5	6.8–13.5	0.8–2.2
3–9 yr	0.6–5.5	5.5–12.8	0.8–2.2
Pubertal children	0.5–4.8	4.9–13.0	0.8–2.3

Treatment (Pediatr Rev 2009;30:251–258)
- **Congenital:** Rx w/ levothyroxine; in infants w/ low T_4 and TSH > 40 mU/L treat immediately with 10–15 mcg/kg QD, do not wait for confirmatory lab results
  - Parental instruction: Crush T_4 tab and mix w/ human milk, formula, or water. AVOID soy or Fe supplements with med admin
  - 10–20% will have transient hypothyroidism but all infants should be treated until 3 yo, then one can consider 1 mo trial off T_4
  - Check TSH/FT$_4$ q1–2mo in 1st year, every 3 mo in 2nd yr, every 4 mo till 6 yr, every 6 mo until adult ht, then yearly. Goals: TSH < 5 mU/L, T_4 = 10–16 mcg/dL
- **Acquired:** Initial dose depends on etiology, age, gender, TSH, body weight. Avg starting doses: 50 mcg (younger child), 75–100 mcg (older child/adolesc & adult). Titrate to low-nml TSH

Complications (Pediatr Rev 2004;25:94)
- Hypothyroidism prenatally w/o perinatal Rx, or delayed/insufficient Rx in cong hypothyroidism results in impaired intellect
- Hypothyroidism >3 yo generally reversible w/ Rx unless symptomatic >1 yr → results in short stature; assoc w/ hyperlipidemia, anemia, SCFE, & chronic constipation w/o Rx. Treatment of longstanding hypothyroidism may not prevent adult short stature

ADRENAL INSUFFICIENCY (AI)

Definition (Pediatrics 2007;119:e484)
- **Primary AI** (Addison disease): Adrenal gland failure, resulting in and glucocorticoid (cortisol) and usually mineralocorticoid (aldosterone) deficiency
- **Secondary or tertiary AI:** ACTH def 2/2 pituitary or hypothalamic dysfxn
  - Mineralocorticoid fxn is nml since aldosterone secretion is stimulated by K^+ and renin–angiotensin system

Pathophysiology (Pediatrics 2007;119:e484)
- **Cortisol:** Counterregulatory hormone to insulin. Has mineralocorticoid effects at high/nml levels. ↑ angiotensin synthesis, ↑ vascular reactivity to vasoconstrictors and ↓ response to vasodilators, promotes conversion of norepi to epi (↑ cardiac output and hepatic glucose production)
  - ↓ cortisol → ↓urinary flow 2/2 ↓GFR and ↑ water absorption
- **Aldosterone** level mediated by renin–angiotensin axis, serum potassium, and ACTH
  - Deficiency → ↑ renin, ↑ K+, ↓ Na+, mild acidosis

Etiology (Pediatrics 2007;119:e484; N Engl J Med 2009;360:2328)
Most common 2/2 chronic steroid use c/b infxn or med d/c (CentralAI)

- **Primary AI:** ↓ glucocorticoid and freq, mineralocorticoid hormones
  - In one series pts <18 yo, 72% w/ congenital adrenal hyperplasia (CAH), 13% w/ autoimmune AI, and 15% w/ adrenoleukodystrophy, syndromes (Wollman, Zellweger); also can be 2/2 drug or infxn, infiltrative, or idiopathic etiology
- **Central AI:** Lack of corticotropin-releasing hormone (CRH) from hypothalamus and/or ACTH from pituitary → dec cortisol nml aldo
  - Abrupt glucocorticoid w/d after courses as short as 2 wk can cause deficiency
- Prolonged steroid use can suppress the HPA axis for 6–9 mo or longer
  - Pituitary insult and/or anatomic abnormality of HPA axis are other causes
- "Relative adrenal insufficiency" in ICU refers to vasopressor-resistant HoTN
  - Indications for steroids under investigation
  - Hypoproteinemia complicates interpretation of cortisol levels. Can be <18 mcg/dL in the absence of AI as cortisol is 90% protein bound (free cortisol nml)

Clinical Manifestations (Pediatrics 2007;119:e484; Clin Dermatol 2006;24:276; J Clin Endocrinol Metab 2011;96:E925; Pediatr Rev 2009;30:e49)
- Can present with nonspecific Sx, Dx often delayed
- **21-hydroxylase deficiency** (most common cause of CAH)
  - Newborn girls p/w virilized genitalia; boys at 2–3 wk w/ salt-wasting crisis
  - Newborn screening improves rate of detection; reduces morbidity/mortality
- **Acute AI:** Dehydration, other electrolyte abnormalities (HypoNa/HyperK) hypoglycemia, abdominal pain, fever, HoTN, and/or ΔMS/shock
- **Chronic AI:** Fatigue, anorexia, N/V, loss of appetite, weight loss, recurrent abdominal pain, back and joint pain, skin pigmentation, salt craving
- Hyperpigmentation (2/2 ↑ pro-opiomelanocortin and derivative melanocyte-stimulating hormone) and salt craving occur in primary but not in central AI
- Central AI may be assoc w/ other sx of pituitary failure; growth failure, delayed puberty, 2° hypothyroidism, and/or diabetes insipidus (AI can mask signs of DI because of water retention)

Diagnosis (Pediatrics 2007;119:e484; JAMA 2005;294:2481; Pediatr Rev 2009;30:e49)
- **1° AI:** High plasma ACTH (often >100 pg/mL) & low cortisol (often <10 mcg/dL)
  - Labs: Cortisol, ACTH, chem 20, bedside glucose, ABG/serum pH, aldosterone, plasma–renin activity, urine Na + K to evaluate mineralocorticoid status
  - Infants w/ suspected CAH: Additionally order 17-OHP, karyotype, pelvic U/S
  - **ACTH stim test** (250 mcg or 15 mcg/kg high dose ACTH test) w/ subnormal cortisol peak (<18 mcg/dL) drawn at 60 min after administration is diagnostic (some use low dose 1 mcg/M2 ACTH w/ cortisol peak <16 as diagnostic at 30 or 60 min)
  - ACTH stim testing inaccurate if patient treated with exogenous steroid (prednisone, cortisol interfere c cortisol assay/not dexamethasone); do not delay treatment for testing if unstable
  - Suspect aldosterone def if: Aldosterone low + renin high +/– HypoNa/HyperK
- **Central AI:** Confirmed by 8 AM cortisol <3 mcg/dL, r/o if >18 mcg/dL in >4 mo
  - Confirmation is difficult. Assays include insulin-induced hypoglycemia response (less safe), CRH stim, ACTH stim (can be false neg acutely), glucagon stim
  - Low-dose ACTH may be most sensitive used but not fully validated in children
- **Evaluation of etiology**: once diagnosis made often guided by H&P
  - Anti-adrenal Abs specific but not 100% sensitive for autoimmune dz
  - Check very long chain fatty acid levels and head CT/MRI for adrenoleukodystrophy
  - Abd CT for evaluation for adrenal hemorrhage, neoplasm, infection
  - Head CT/MRI if central AI suspected

Management (Pediatrics 2007;119:e484; Pediatr Rev 2009;30:e49)
- Treatment should NOT be withheld even if the diagnosis is not yet confirmed!
- **Hypotension:** Isotonic volume resuscitation, if in shock proceed per PALS, may require central access and pressors. **Hypoglycemia:** $D_{25}W$ (2–3 mL/kg)
- **Stress-dose glucocorticoids** (IM/SC/IV, IV faster, more reliable response)
  - **Hydrocortisone** (w/ mineralocorticoid activity) 50–75 mg/m² × 1 → 50–75 mg/m²/q6h
  - Methylprednisolone (min mineralocorticoid activity) 10–15 mg/m²
  - Dexamethasone (no mineralocorticoid activity, **allows subsequent ACTH-stim testing,** and does not interfere w/ cortisol assay) 1.5–2 mg/m²
  - Fludrocortisone (0.1–0.2 mg qd) replaces mineralocorticoid if able to take PO
  - Note: Prednisone requires hepatic conversion to Fludrocortisone to exert glucocorticoid activity; not a good choice for stress-dose glucocorticoid
- Once stabilized, **physiologic replacement** doses initiated
- Daily cortisol production is 5–6 mg/m²; decreased oral bioavailability results in starting daily hydrocortisone doses of 9–12 mg/m² divided q8h

- May give increased proportion in AM to mimic physiologic dosing
- Prednisone and dexamethasone w/ longer $t^{1/2}$ (convenient, but difficult to titrate)
- Infants may require daily sodium suppl (about 8 mEq/kg/d, or about 1–2 g/d)
- Titrate physiologic replacement to clinical status, not ACTH levels

Complications (Pediatrics 2007;119:e484)
- Life-threatening cardiovascular collapse can occur with failure to inc glucocorticoid supplementation w/ physical stress (infection, etc.)
- Life-threatening hyperkalemia requiring immediate attention

Prevention (Pediatrics 2007;119:e484)
- Patients should wear medical alert bracelets
- Routine vaccine, mild URI, exercise, & emot/psych stress need no replacement
- Moderate stress (fever >101, significant N/V/diarrhea) → triple TDD of hydrocortisone (30–50 mg/m^2/d divided q6h)
- If pt cannot take PO, give 50 mg/m^2 IM or SC (not usually rec but works unless pt is in shock) hydrocortisone Na succinate & seek immed medical attention
- For sepsis or major surgery, pts need ~48 hr of 100 mg/m^2/d IV divided q6h then taper over several days until back at maintenance dose

HYPOPITUITARISM

Definition (Lancet 2007;369:1461)
- Inadequate pituitary hormone production either 2/2 hypothalamic or pituitary def
- Can involve all pituitary axes ("panhypopituitarism") or only some
- Ant pit hormones stimulated by hypothalamic hormones, post pit (vasopressin/oxytocin) produced in hypothal travel down neurons to be stored in post pit

Pathophysiology (Lancet 2007;369:1461)
- Pituitary blood supply via branches of internal carotid, forming capillary plexus at median eminence of hypothalamus, which feeds the pituitary via long and short portal veins; pituitary stalk is fed by the middle hypophyseal artery
- Cellular damage can occur from compression 2/2 mass occupying lesion (adenoma) after XRT, vascular insufficiency 2/2 stalk injury w/ subsequent anterior lobe infarction
- Defects in multiple gene products can result in pituitary malformation and malfunction

Etiology (Pediatrics 2007;119:e484; Endocrinol Metab Clin North Am 2008;37:235)
- Consider in any child dx'd w/ GH deficiency, anatomic abnormalities of pituitary or stalk on MRI, Hx of intracranial surgery, tumors, or trauma
- Can develop w/ cranial radiation, septo-optic dysplasia, autoimmune hypophysitis, PROP-1, Pit-1, or other transcription factor def

Clinical Manifestations (Lancet 2007;369:1461; Endocrinol Metab Clin North Am 2008;37:235)
- Pituitary lesions often present initially w/ visual impairment; can be classic bitemporal hemianopsia but more often unilateral
- Can present more acutely w/ dysfxn of vital hormones; adrenal insuff, hypoglycemia 2/2 GH deficiency (common presentation in newborns), diabetes insipidus, hypothyroidism, or as growth failure 2/2 growth hormone deficiency or pubertal delay 2/2 hypogonadism (gonadotropin def)
- Prolactin (Prl) is inhibited by dopaminergic signals from hypothalamus—failure of inhibition, inc prolactin and subsequent galactorrhea, hypogonadism

Diagnosis (Lancet 2007;369:1461; Endocrinol Metab Clin North Am 2008;37:235)
- Initial eval interrogate multi pituitary axes & peripheral responses: TSH, fT$_4$, IGF-1, IGFBP3, FSH, LH, AM cortisol, prolactin serum Na & urine Osm, sex steroids
- MRI focused on pituitary/hypothalamus needed to r/o mass lesion

Rx (Pediatrics 2007;119:e484; Endocrinol Metab Clin North Am 2008;37:235)
- Treat underlying etiology (i.e., surgery for amenable pituitary masses)
- Adequate replacement of deficient pituitary hormones

Complications (Pediatrics 2007;119:e484)
- Correction of hypothyroidism can precipitate adrenal crisis in patients w/ unrecognized adrenal insufficiency (inc need for cortisol and inc clearance)
- Growth hormone could precipitate adrenal insufficiency 2/2 decreased production of cortisol from precursors (or increased metabolism) (rare)

AMBIGUOUS GENITALIA

Pathophysiology
- SRY gene → testes development → testosterone
  - → wolffian ducts (vas deferens seminiferous tubules, epididymis)
  - conversion to DHT → scrotum, penis
  - Müllerian duct inhib substance (MIS or AMH—antimullerian hormone produced by Sertoli cells) → disappearance of müllerian ducts

Clinical Manifestations
- Overt genital ambiguity (cloacal exstrophy), ♀ genitalia w/ enlarged clitoris, post labial fusion, labial mass, or ♂ genitals w/ micropenis, b/l undesc testes, perineal hypospadias

Physical Exam
- Phallic length, presence/absence of palpable gonads

Diagnostic Studies
- FISH for Y chromosome material (quicker); karyotype:
  - Majority of 46 XX have CAH; only 50% of 46 XY receive definitive dx (GWAS may improve this)
- Abdominopelvic ultrasound
- 17-OH progesterone, testosterone, gonadotropins, MIS, inhibin B, lytes, and UA

Management (Pediatrics 2006;118:e488)
- General concepts of care
  - Avoid gender assignment until expert evaluation
  - Multidisciplinary team: Endo, surg, uro, psych, gyn, genetics, neonatology
- Gender assignment:
  - >90% pts w/ 46 XX CAH and all patients with 46 XY CAIS are assigned female
  - 60% of 5-α-reductase def pts assigned ♀ first & virilize at puberty & live as a male

PRECOCIOUS PUBERTY

Definition (Pediatrics 1999;104:936; Pediatr Ann 2006;35:916)
- Girls w/ thelarche (breast dev) or pubarche (pubic hair) before 7 yo in obese & before 8 yo in non-obese need eval. Obesity inc risk of early puberty In girls
- Girls w/ pubarche and no thelarche <8 yo usually dx'd w/ benign premature adrenarche
  - Further eval if evid ↑ androgen (linear growth accelerated, clitoral enlargement, acne)—bone age >1–2 yr advanced looks for late-onset CAH
  - Girls w/ thelarche after 7 yo need eval if:
  - Rapid progression of puberty w/ adv bone age (>2 yr above chrono age) and/or predicted adult ht >2 SD below genetic target ht (father's ht + mother's ht − 5)/2)
  - New CNS symptoms (headache, seizure, or focal neurologic deficits, underlying CNS disease including hydrocephalus, behavioral concerns)
- Boys <9 yo w/ signs of puberty other than pubic hair (e.g., penile and scrotal enlargement, acne, growth acceleration) w/ or w/o testicular enlargement need eval—if only hair, likely premature adrenarche and only bone age is needed

Pathophysiology
- In girls, breast tissue dev (thelarche) 1st signs of activation of pituitary–gonadal axis, testicular enlargement (gonadarche) in boys; pubic hair development (adrenarche) results from adrenal androgen production, different axis
- May be gonadotropin-releasing hormone (GnRH) dependent or independent

Etiology
- Majority of girls, central precocious puberty (CPP) is idiopathic
- Significant proportion of boys w/ CPP will have CNS disease
- Also consider obesity (girls), gonadal tumors, other sources of sex steroids

Diagnostic Evaluation
- Labs: Bone age, testosterone (males), estradiol (females), 8 AM 17-OH progesterone, LH/FSH, hCG, DHEAS, and DHEA. GnRH stim test
- Eval may also include TFTs, MRI brain (depends on H&P)
- Consider exogenous exposure to estrogen/androgens

Complications

- Precoc puberty may cause bone age accel, premat growth plate closure & ↓ adult ht
- In girls w/ idiopathic CPP, puberty may be longer, thus adult height not significantly adversely affected (slowly progressive precoc puberty)

Therapy

- Rx w/ GnRH-agonists (inhibit gonadotropin and sex steroid secretion) may improve adult height. Benefit to height greatest if Rx started before 8 yo

DELAYED PUBERTY

Definition (Pediatr Ann 2006;35:916)
- Lack of 2° sex characteristics by 13 yo (girls) or 14 yo (boys); no menarche by 16 yo

Etiology
- Includes: Hypogonadotropic (constitutional delay, chronic dz, malnut, Kallmann, pituitary, or other CNS dz) or hypergonadotropic (Turner, Klinefelter)

Diagnostic Studies
- If signs of puberty are present, AM testosterone (males) or estradiol (females)
- If not, FSH/LH, thyroxine, TSH, IGF-1, prolactin, bone age, test smell (Kallmann)
- Karyotype for hypergonadotropic hypogonadism, androgen insensitivity, Turner
- Pelvic U/S (girls)

Management
- Treat underlying cause if identified
- For male constitutional delay of puberty, low-dose testosterone can achieve 2° sexual characteristics and growth w/o premature epiphyseal closure
  - Cont hypogonadism off supplemental testosterone after age 18 suggests GnRH def
- For female constitutional delay of puberty, short courses of estrogen therapy (w/ trials of withdrawal) can achieve similar ends
  - After age 18, if cont hypogonadism, GnRH def is likely
  - Replacement doses of estrogen and progesterone should continue

SHORT STATURE

Definition
Below the 3rd percentile for height

Etiology
Familial short stature, constitutional delay, hypopituitarism, hypothyroidism, hypercortisolism, idiopathic short stature (ISS), deprivation dwarfism, syndromic (Turner, Prader–Willi, Noonan), skeletal dysplasia (hypo and achondroplasia), SHOX gene defect (Leri–Weill, etc.), chronic dz (cong heart dz, CF, celiac, IBD, SCD, RTA, JRA)

Diagnostic Studies
Guided by H&P; CBC, ESR, Chem20, celiac panel, UA w/ ph, karyotype (girls), TSH, free T$_4$, prolactin, IGF1, IGFBP3
Imaging: X-ray L hand for bone age; MRI if suspect midline defect or tumor

Idiopathic Short Stature (N Engl J Med 2006;354:2576)
Definition: Short stature in otherwise healthy child w/ exclusion of other causes, bone age w/i 2 SD of chronologic age, nml GH response on provocative testing
Evaluation:
- Hx, PE, labs to r/o: other pathology (as described previously)
- Left hand-wrist x-ray for bone age + patient's height + patient's age
  - Use Bayley–Pinneau table to predict future adult height
  - Compare with what is normal, and with parental height
Pharmacologic **treatment can be considered:** GH daily × several yr (4–7) → inc height 3–6 cm; can also use aromatase inhibitors/GnRH analogs to delay puberty (Horm Res Paediatr 2011;76(Suppl 3):27; Curr Opin Endocrinol Diabetes Obes 2011;1:3; Pediatr Endocrinol Rev 2011;9:579; J Clin Endocrinol Metab 2008;93:4210; J Clin Endocrinol Metab 2010;95:328; Pediatrics 2008;121:e975; Pediatr Clin North Am 2011;58:1167)

Growth Hormone Deficiency (GHD) (J Pediatr 2003;143:415)
- Suspect in child with persistently sub-nml growth rate and no identifiable cause
  - Classic GHD "cherub," high pitched voice, ↑ weight for height, truncal adiposity
- GH stim test : Approx 10% of people who do not respond to 2 tests, may still be nml
- If pt passes GH stim test, trial Rx recommended if it meets MOST of the following
  - Ht >2.25 SD below mean for age or >2 SD below mid-parental height percentile
  - Growth velocity <25th percentile for bone age
  - Bone age >2 SD below mean for age
  - Low IGF-1 and/or IGFBP3
  - Other clinic features suggestive of GHD
- MRI/CT— to rule out empty sella, pituitary hypoplasia, tumors, etc. However, true GHD is not assoc with a nml response to stimuli except if previous cranial irrad

FDA Approved Uses of Recombinant Human GH in Pediatrics (J Pediatr 2003;143:415)
- GHD/insufficiency, Turner syndrome, Noonan syndrome, Prader–Willi syndrome, SHOX gene defect
- Chronic renal insufficiency pre-transplantation
- Children with Hx of IUGR (SGA) who have not reached nml height by 2 yo
- ISS >2.25 SD below mean height & unlikely to catch up in height

Safety of GH
- Known adverse drug reactions (J Pediatr 2003;143:415)
- Raised ICP, edema, SCFE, hyperglycemia, worsening of scoliosis, gynecomastia
  Increased mortality (JCEM 2012;97:416; JCEM 2012;97:E213)
- Drug monitoring: Check IGF-1 and IGFBP3 qyr and with dose changes
  - Check TSH, free T_4 b/c hypothyroidism can develop during Rx; also check HgbA1c for glucose intolerance

AMENORRHEA

Definition
- Normal menses: Avg age menarche 12.8 yr (Pediatr Rev 1992;13:43)
- 2–2.5 yr after breast budding; 1 yr after growth spurt
- 1° amenorrhea: Any one of the following:
  - No menses by age 16 + nml pubertal growth and development
  - No menses by age 15 + abn pubertal growth and development
  - No menses 2 yr after completed sexual maturation
- 2° amenorrhea: Absence of menses for 6 mo or 3 cycles in pt w/ established menses

Evaluation of 1° Amenorrhea
- 4 groups based on pubertal maturation and internal genitalia
- **Breast (−)/uterus (+):** Lack of estrogen 2/2 lack of gonads, HPO axis problem, or defect in estrogen production. **Check FSH** to direct studies
- **Breast (−)/uterus (−):** Rare; suspect genetic male whose gonads produce MIS (suppresses internal F genital dev) but insuff testosterone to produce M genitals
- **Breast (+)/uterus (−):** Phenotypically female, but check karyotype for Ddx
  - **CAIS (testicular feminization):** Develop breasts 2/2 unopposed estrogen from gonad + adrenals. No/sparse axillary or pubic hair. Gonadal testes must be removed after pubertal dev is complete 2/2 ↑ rate malignancy
  - **Müllerian agenesis (Rokitansky–Küster–Hauser syndrome):** ↑ risk renal (30%), skeletal (12%), and cardiac problems
- **Breast (+)/uterus (+):** Eval HPO axis, U/S for obstruction (often cyclic pain)

Evaluation of 2° Amenorrhea
- **Multi causes:** Stress, anorexia nervosa, systemic dz (IBD, DM, thyroid dz, PCOS)
- **History:** Caloric intake, wt Δ, diet, meds, headaches, visual change, galactorrhea
- **PE:** BMI, anorexia stigmata, visual fields, CN, breast exam, androgen excess, pelvic
- **Labs:** β-hCG, LH, FSH, fT$_4$, TSH, prolactin (1/3 w/ galactorrhea), DHEA-S, and testosterone (if signs/symptoms) of virilization
  - **Prolactin:** Mild ↑ usually 2/2 meds, breast stim, stress, hypothyroid
- **Other labs:** Adol w/ nml uterus/vagina, FSH, LH if elevated
  - If ↑, check karyotype; r/o Turner mosaicism w/ ovarian failure vs. other causes of ovarian failure (autoimmune, galactosemia, etc.)
  - If ↓ or nml, think hypothalamus × image; if no tumor, consider stress, AN, etc.

- Progesterone challenge: Give PO medroxyprogesterone acetate 5–10 mg qd × 5–10 d
  - **+ withdrawal bleed:** Uterus nml & primed by estrogen, so ovaries intact; PCOS
  - **− withdrawal bleed:** Abn uterus or no estrogen, e.g., Asherman syndrome, AN, and other causes of hypothalamic amenorrhea
- Trial of combined estrogen/progesterone

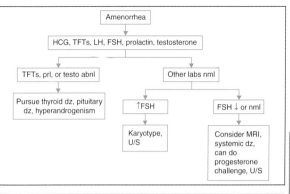

POLYCYSTIC OVARIAN SYNDROME (PCOS)

Pathophysiology (N Engl J Med 2005;352:1223)
- Associated w/ ↑'d intra-ovarian androgens & often associated with insulin resistance
- Visceral adiposity assoc w/ hyperandrogenemia, insulin resistance, glucose intolerance, dyslipidemia
- Hyperinsulinemia is also central. Insulin ↑ thecal androgen production, ↓ sex-hormone–binding globulin, which ↑ fraction of free testosterone

Epidemiology (N Engl J Med 2005;352:1223)
- Affects ~5–10% of women; 30–75% of women with PCOS are obese
- Currently considered a complex, multigenic disorder

Diagnosis (N Engl J Med 2005;352:1223)
- Rotterdam Criteria, 2003 (2 of 3): Oligo/amenorrhea; hyperandrogenism or hyper-androgenemia; radiographic evidence of polycystic ovaries OR
- Androgen Excess Society 2006 (all): Hyperandrogenism, ovarian dysfunction, exclude other androgen disorders/excess
- Polycystic ovaries are not necessary or sufficient to confirm dx (functional condition)
- Must r/o hyperprolactinemia, CAH, Cushing syndrome, acromegaly, androgen-secreting neoplasm
- Consider the following labs: HCG, prolactin, 17-OH P, DHEA, SHBG, LH/FSH, testosterone, fasting glucose, insulin, TFTs ("The Polycystic Ovary Syndrome: Current Concepts On Pathogenese And Clinical Care. Legro, RS 2007)
- Symptoms of hyperandrogenism include hirsutism, acne, and male-pattern alopecia
- Often disordered uterine bleeding & infertility 2/2 anovulation, acanthosis nigricans 2/2 hyperinsulin
- ↑ LH or LH:FSH ratio (>2) less reliable, as levels vary throughout menstrual cycle
- Risk assessment for endometrial carcinoma, glucose intolerance (OGTT, random glucose, A1c), dyslipidemia (fasting lipids), obstructive sleep apnea

Treatment (N Engl J Med 2005;352:1223)
- Hyperandrogenism (hirsutism and acne)
  - Combined estrogen–progestin contraceptives: Choose lowest androgen activity
  - Antiandrogens: Spironolactone; reserve steroids for marked androgen excess
- Oligomenorrhea and amenorrhea
  - Combined estrogen–progestin Rx or cyclic progestin administration may inhibit endometrial proliferation from chronic anovulation
  - Weight loss and lowering insulin levels are shown to improve ovulatory function
- Insulin resistance and glucose intolerance: Weight reduction, metformin

Composition of Basic Fluids and Replacement Solutions

	[Na] (mEq/L)	[Cl] (mEq/L)	[K] (mEq/L)	[HCO₃] (mEq/L)	pH
Gastric	70	120	5–15	0	Acidic
Pancreatic	140	50–100	5	100	Basic
Bile	130	100	5	40	Acidic
Diarrhea	50	40	35	50	Variable
Ileostomy	130	120	15–20	25–30	Basic
NS (0.9%)	154	154	0	0	5.5
½ NS (0.45%)	77	77	0	0	5.5
¼ NS (0.23%)	38	38	0	0	5.5
Ringer Lactate	130	109	4	28	6.5

Maintenance Fluids & Electrolyte Calculations (Pediatr Rev 2001;22:380)
- Basal state maintenance fluid needs determined by basal metabolic rate; amt of fluid needed to dissipate heat via respiratory tract and skin
- Multiple methods: BSA method, basal calorie method, and Holliday–Segar system. Only last (Holliday–Segar) does not require a table of values
- Holliday–Segar formula equates kcal with mL (1:1) of fluid needed for dissipation

Weight (kg)	kcal or cc (1:1 equivalence)	kcal/hr or cc/hr (1:1)
0–10	100/kg/d	4 cc/kg/hr
11–20	1,000 + 50/kg/d	40 cc + 2 cc/kg/hr
>20	1,500 + 20/kg/d	60 cc + 1 cc/kg/hr

Adapted from: Pediatrics 1957;19:823.

- Electrolyte maintenance needs (**not for neonates**): Na 2–4 mEq/kg/d, K 1–3 mEq/kg/d, Ca 2–3 mEq/kg/d, Phos 0.5–1.5 mEq/kg/d, Mg 0.1–1 mEq/kg/d
- D5 1/2 NS usually used for maintenance w/ 20 mEq/L KCl added once pt has urinated; for pts <1 yo consider D5 1/4 NS (now controversial; does not apply to neonate) (see NICU section) (Arch Dis Child 2008;93:335)
- Some authors recommend NS for maintenance due to risk of iatrogenic hyponatremia with hypotonic IVF (Curr Opinion Pediatrics 2011;23:186; Pediatrics 2011;128:857); postoperative patients appear to be at highest risk. However, evidence is weak for improved outcomes with NS compared with standard therapy (BMC Pediatrics 2011;11:82; Arch Dis Child 2008;93:335)

DEHYDRATION AND REHYDRATION

Definition (Pediatr Rev 2002;23:277; JAMA 2004;291:2746; Am Fam Phys 2009;80:692)
- Fluid deficit 2/2 imbalance btw fluid losses (nml or ↑) and fluid intake (nml or ↓)
- Dehydration is a leading cause of morbidity & mortality in kids, esp in the 3rd world
- Though often used interchangeably, strictly, dehydration ≠ hypovolemia
- Hypovolemia → ↑ ADH, susceptibility to hypoNa if repleted with hypotonic fluids/H₂O

History and Exam (JAMA 2004;291:2746)
- Hx fever (insensible losses), ↓ oral intake, types of intake, freq of urination (↑ UOP w/ dehydration → diabetes insipidus), diarrhea (frequency), other sites or sources of loss (ostomies, biliary tubes, etc.)
- Assessment of weight loss via H&P as above or from actual documented weights
  - Weight loss (kg) = fluid deficit (L); based on radio-labeled albumin experiments
  - Inaccurate in setting of "3rd spaced fluids" (nephrotic syndrome, CHF, cirrhosis) where patient is intravascularly deplete but weight is up
- Capillary refill; compress and release superficial cap bed (palmar finger-tip w/ arm heart level), varies as fxn of temperature, site, lighting, meds, & autonomic Δ
- Skin turgor (ST); skin pinch at lateral abd wall at umbilical level. Less accurate w/ HyperNa (false nml) and w/ malnutrition (falsely prolonged). Complicated in 1° skin dz
- Can assess dehydration clinically based on history, exam, & assessment of weight loss

Dehydration	Mild	Moderate	Severe	Sens/Spec[a]
Weight loss—infant	5%	10%	>15%	—
Weight loss—child	3–5%	6–9%	>10%	—
HR/BP	Nml	Nml-tachycardic and orthostatic	Tachycardiac and orthostatic-shock	0.52/0.58 (for inc HR)
RR	Nml	Nml-increased	Hyperpnea (deep rapid breathing)	0.43/**0.79**
Anterior fontanelle	Nml	Sunken	Very sunken	0.49/0.54
Mucous membranes	Nml	Dry	Cracked	**0.86**/0.44
Tears	Nml	Decreased	Dry, sunken eyes	0.63/0.68
Skin (less accurate if HyperNa or <2 yo)	Cap refill (CR) <2 sec	CR 2–4 sec, dec ST	CR <4 sec and skin tenting, cool and mottled	CR 0.60/**0.85** ST 0.58/**0.76**
Urine output and SG	>1.020	>1.020 +/– oliguria	Oliguria to anuria	
Behavior	Nml	Irritable	Lethargic/obtunded	**0.80**/0.45
Total fluid deficit	30–50 cc/kg	60–100 cc/kg	>100–150 cc/kg	

[a]Tested for assessment of 5% dehydration.

- **Most sens for dehydration are dry mucous memb & irritability/lethargy**
- **Most spec; poor CR, poor ST, hyperpnea** (rapid deep breaths w/o evidence resp distress)

Diagnostic Studies (Pediatrics 2004;114:1227)

- Chem 7, U/A w/ spec grav, serum pH, serum Osm, anion gap (AG), serum Osm, urine Osm, urine electrolytes, stool culture can help clarify complex situations but not recommended in most uncomplicated cases
  - One study showed $HCO_3 \leq 13$ mmol/L predicted admission in pts 6 mo–13 yo p/w acute gastroenteritis and dehydr receiving IVFs. (Ann Emerg Med 1996;28:318)
  - Another study looked at lytes in pts 2 mo–9 yo w/ acute gastro & dehydr; 1/10 had lab labs affecting care. Bicarb did not affect need for admit
    - Pts <1 yo had lower HCO_3 than older pts w/ equiv dehyd (Pediatrics 2004;114:1227)

Lab Parameters	Sensitivity	Specificity
BUN/Cr > 40	0.23	0.89
Bicarb < 17 mEq/L	0.83	0.76
Bicarb < 15 mEq/L	0.93	0.40
pH < 7.35	0.43	0.80
AG > 20 mmol/L	0.46	0.74

Adapted from: JAMA 2004;291:2746.

Management (Am Fam Physician 2009;80:692; Arch Dis Child 2007;92:546; MMWR 2003;52:RR-16; Pediatr Rev 2001;22:380)

- For severe dehydration, correct hemodynamics with 20 cc/kg boluses NS (or LR); repeat until stabilized (Crit Care Med 2009;37:666)
- If Hyper/HoNa, see mgmt sections on Hyper/HoNa below. In hypernatremic dehydration, intravascular volume is preserved, so degree of dehydration cannot reliably be estimated by physical signs. Therefore, correct fluid deficit as per HyperNa recs instead of per dehydration recs
- For mild/mod & for severe dehydration s/p NS or LR resuscitation, give aggressive ORT (50–100 cc/kg over 3–4 hr) followed by maintenance and replacement of ongoing losses
- PO ondansetron prior to ORT → ↑ cessation of vomiting, ↓ need for IVF, ↓ rate of immediate hospitalization (Cochrane Database 2011;9:CD005506)
- ORT promptly resolves [Na] abn; no need for IVF in 90% (Am J Clin Nutr 1980;33:637)
- ORT comparable to IVF, with lower rates of hospitalization (1/3 of ORT vs. 1/2 of IVF; Pediatr 2005;115:295) and acceptably low failure rates (4.9% PO vs. 1.3% IV; Cochrane Database 2006;3:CD004390)
- ORT used <30% of the time that it is indicated in U S

- Replacement of ongoing losses: For each emesis or diarrheal stool, give 60–120 mL ORS pt weight <10 kg; 120–240 mL ORS if >10 kg
- Continue breastfeeding or routine (undiluted) infant formula during ORT
- ORT composition (Cochrane Database 2002;1:CD002847; Oral Rehydration Salts: Production of the new ORS. WHO/UNICEF, 2006)

	Glucose (mmol/L)	Na (mEq/L)	Cl (mEq/L)	Citrate/HCO_3 (mEq/L)	K (mEq/L)
Pedialyte	140	45	35	30	20
WHO-ORS	75	75	65	10	20

- If ORT fails, remaining fluid deficit + maintenance given over 24 hr as D5 $^1/_2$ NS (with 20 mEq KCl added once UOP established) using 1 of 2 approaches, below

Classic approach:
- Remaining deficit = Total volume deficit (% weight loss) − initial boluses
- Provide $^1/_2$ of remaining deficit over first 8 hr + hourly maintenance rate
  - *If 5 kg pt w/ 10% wt loss, deficit = 500 cc, if given 20 cc/kg bolus, remaining deficit is 400 cc. Give 200 cc over 8 hr (25 cc/hr) + maintenance (4 cc/hr × 5 kg = 20 cc/hr); so 45 cc/hr for first 8 hr*
- Provide other $^1/_2$ of remaining deficit over next 16 hr + hourly maintenance
  - *For pt above, give remaining 200 cc over next 16 hr (12.5 cc/hr) + maintenance (20 cc/hr); so 32.5 cc/hr (round to 33 cc/hr) for next 16 hr*

Short hand approach:
- Remaining deficit calc as above, and all given over 1st 8 hr w/o maintenance
  - *For same pt above, give all 400 cc over 8 hr (50 cc/hr) and no added fluid for maintenance; so 50 cc/hr for first 8 hr*
- Then give total 24 hr maintenance over remaining 16 hr (accounts for that not included for 1st 8 hr); equivalent to 1.5× maintenance for 16 hr
  - *So for same pt above, give 1.5× maintenance for next 16 hr (maintenance 20 cc/hr); 1.5 maintenance is 30 cc/hr; so 30 cc/hr for 16 hr*
- Recent literature increasingly questions use of hypotonic IVF in gastroenteritis 2/2 ↑ risk of hypoNa (e.g., Pediatr Nephrol 2010;25:2303)
- Aggressive fluid resuscitation may increase risk of death in children with shock in the developing world (NEJM 2011;364:2483); use WHO recs or local guidelines

HYPONATREMIA

Definition (Pediatr Rev 2007;28:426)
- Serum sodium <135 mEq/L; most common electrolyte abnormality in pediatrics
- Pseudohyponatremia is lab abnormality 2/2 ↑ serum lipid or protein (nml P_{Osm}) if gas chromatography used to assess [Na]; diff than true dilutional hyponatremia 2/2 osmotic shifts (inc P_{Osm}) 2/2 hyperglycemia, IVIG, mannitol, etc.

Pathophysiology and etiologies (Rose & Post. Clinical Physiology of Acid-Base & Electrolyte Disorders 2001:696; Pediatr Clin N Am 58:1271)
- H_2O excess relative to total body Na. Mech is usually impaired by renal H_2O excretion; sometimes markedly excessive H_2O intake (or hypotonic IVF) w/ nml excretion
- Impaired H_2O excretion most often 2/2 volume loss, usually with replacement of lost volume by H_2O. Other causes of impaired H_2O excretion: Diuretics, channelopathies, SIADH, renal failure, ↑ collecting tubule (CT) permeability 2/2 hypothyroid or adrenal insufficiency (AI)
- Mechanism of HoNa in volume loss: ↓ volume → ↑ ADH → aquaporin channel insertion in CTs → ↑ H_2O resorption
- ↓ serum Osm → H_2O shift → tissue edema (esp brain); if rapid, ↑ risk herniation or apnea; if subacute or chronic, fluid shifts mitigated by loss of intracellular electrolytes (e.g., K+) and organic osmolytes

Clinical Manifestations (Pediatr Rev 2002;23:371)
- Symptoms: Neuro dysfunction 2/2 brain cell swelling (rare unless [Na] < 120 mEq/L). Even with [Na] < 120, often asymptomatic (or w/ subtle cognitive defects) if achieved slowly
  - **Can be nonspecific;** malaise/lethargy, N/V, HA, confusion/agitation, muscle cramps, sz (2/2 pressure against rigid skull), ↓ reflexes, muscle weakness, hypothermia, irregular resp (2/2 impending herniation), coma, and even death
- **Primary goal of clinical exam is assessment of volume status**

Etiologies and Diagnostic Studies (Pediatr Rev 2007;28:426; Pediatr Clin N Am 2011;58:1271)

- Attempt to define chronicity
- Hx of volume loss (source), fluid repletion (type of fluid used, how formula is made, esp w/ powdered formulas), meds (diuretics, IVIG, mannitol), underlying illness (DM, hypothyroid, AI, renal channelopathy)
- Check electrolytes, serum Osm, U_{Osm}, U_{Na}, can check lipids and protein (pseudohypoNa)
- If hyperglycemia, hyperlipidemia, or hyperproteinemia, can correct [Na]
  - Hyperglycemia: Correct up [Na] 2.4 mEq/L for each 100 mg/dL glucose above 200
  - Hyperproteinemia: Correct up [Na] 0.25 × (protein [g/dL] − 8); only if Tot Prot >8
  - Hyperlipidemia: Correct up [Na] 0.002 × (triglyceride [mg/dL])
- **1° polydipsia and water intoxication:** 2/2 excess water intake either in 2/2 psychiatric condition w/ excess H_2O consumption, or in populations unable to control intake (infants), admin of excess H_2O. Rx'd w/ free water restriction
- **SIADH** (Am J Med 1967;42:790): Release of ADH not stim by hypovolemia or hyperosmolality (pt cannot be hypovolemic & serum Osm >275 mOsm/kg for this dx), resulting in inapprop enhanced water reabsorpt (urine Osm >100 mOsm/kg) & natriuresis
  - Multiple etiologies
    - Neuro: Meningitis/encephalitis, SAH/subdural/epidural, brain abscess, stroke, neoplasm, pituitary surgery, psychosis, HIV, Guillain–Barré, TBI, SLE, MS
    - **Drugs:** Cyclophosphamide, vincristine, vinblastine, SSRIs, antipsychotics, carbamazepine, tricyclics, MAOIs, gen anesthesia, narcotics, nicotine, desmopressin, others
    - Pulmonary: PNA, TB, asthma, lung abscess, empyema, pneumothorax, PPV
    - AIDS, AI, hypothyroidism
    - Ectopic ADH 2/2 leukemia, lymphoma, sarcoma; small-cell lung CA (rare in peds)

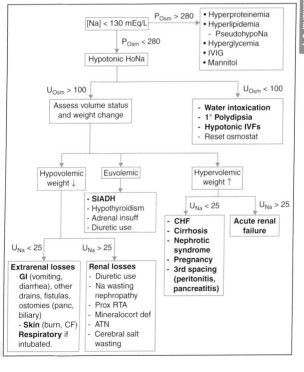

Management (Rose & Post. *Clinical Physiology of Acid-Base & Electrolyte Disorders* 2001:696)

- Correction of HoNa is driven by patient's symptomatology and chronicity of HoNa
- If hemodyn compromise 2/2 vol depletion, rx w/IV NS 20 cc/kg boluses until stable
- If HoNa occurred acutely, pt seizing, significant Δ MS, or impending resp arrest, then correct [Na] rapidly, otherwise slowly
- Overrapid HoNa correction (>~12 mEq/24 hr) can result in central demyelinating lesion (particular at pons; central pontine myelinolysis) presents days to weeks after correction w/ paraparesis/quadriparesis, dysarthria, dysphagia, coma, or sz. Confirmed by CT or MRI; can take 4 wk + before radiologically detectable
- **Hypovolemic HoNa:** Correct HoNa by providing sodium, do not need to normalize [Na] and do not correct >12 mEq/24 hr
  - Total Na deficit = (% body H$_2$O × lean body weight[kg]) × (goal Na – measured Na)
    - % body water as above; generally can use 60% (0.6) in pediatric patient
    - So for 25 kg pt w/ Na 110; total Na deficit = (0.6 × 25) × (120 – 110) = 150 mEqNa
  - Choose Na solution for repletion and do not replace at >12 mEq/24 hr
    - If asymptomatic, replace 0.5 mEq/hr over first 24 hr
    - If severe neuro sx, can replace at 1.5–2 mEq/hr for first 3–4 hr or till sx resolve, but still try not to correct >12 mEq over the first 24 hr total
    - 3% NaCl has 513 mEq/L; 0.9% NaCl (NS) has 154 mEq/L
      - So for above pt could give ~ 1 L NS over 24 hr (~40 cc/hr), or 292 cc of 3% NaCl over 24 hr (~ 12 cc/hr) for a rough correction of 0.4 mEq/L/hr, may round down to avoid over correction
      - Make sure to account for insensible losses and maintenance as well
      - **Rough correction of severe HoNa is w/ 0.5 cc/kg/hr 3% NaCl to achieve raise in Na of 12 mEq in 24 hr. 1 cc/kg/hr to achieve in 12 hr**
      - **Correction is never perfect, so serum [Na] should be followed q2–4h**
- **Hypervolemic HoNa:** Generally Rx'd w/ Na and free H$_2$O restriction, unless severe neurologic sx due to HoNa in which case replace Na as above
  - Can also use diuresis (CHF and cirrhosis), or if anuric in renal failure then dialysis
- **SIADH:** Eliminate underlying etiology (if any); free water restriction (if needed, can use $^1/_2$ maintenance or just restrict to replacement of insensible losses [40 cc/kg/d]). Isotonic IVF can make hypoNa worse if osmolarity of urine exceeds osmolarity of fluids given
- Chronic tx may include demeclocycline, lithium (contraindicated in young children), urea

HYPERNATREMIA

Definition (Pediatr Rev 2002;23:371)

- Sodium concentration >145 mEq/L; seen in hospitalized pts w/o access to free water or receiving hypernatremic IVFs, can also be seen in infants unable to obtain free water

Pathophysiology (Rose & Post. *Clinical Physiology of Acid-Base & Electrolyte Disorders* 2001:746)

- HyperNa is 2/2 either inappropriate water loss (>Na loss) or Na retention
- Free water loss can occur from skin and respiratory tract or w/ dilute urine (diuretics or osmotic diuretic agents [glucose, mannitol]), diarrhea is variable in composition but can see excess water loss w/ osmotic or malabsorptive diarrhea
- Body attempts to correct HyperNa w/ inc ADH release → concentrated urine (occurs at P$_{Osm}$ > 280 mOsm/L) & by driving thirst (rare for pt to be hypernatremic w/ access to H$_2$O)
- HyperNa (w/ resultant hyperosmolality) → cellular dehydration, particularly at brain resulting in the symptoms assoc w/ HyperNa
  - Acutely can be severe enough to cause subdural bleed or SAH (Pediatr Rev 1996;17:395)
  - Subacute or chronic HyperNa allows brain cells to adapt by production of intracellular osmoles to balance gradient (w/i 1 hr); overrapid correction → cerebral edema
  - Hypernatremia w/ [Na] >160 mEq/L has mortality of 10–15%

Epidemiology (Pediatr Rev 2002;23:371)

- High risk include debilitated pts w/ acute or chronic illness, infants, & particularly preterm (small mass: BSA ratio) and reliance on caretakers for fluids (ineffective breastfeeding)

- Assess patient's access to free H_2O, hx of polyuria (DI, DM, nephropathy), absence of thirst (in setting of HyperNa and inc P_{Osm}, this reflects hypothalamic lesion)
- Patients are generally irritable but can progress to lethargy, seizures, coma, or death
- Neurologic exam may reveal increased tone, brisk reflexes, or nuchal rigidity
- HyperNa can result in "doughy" skin texture; falsely normalizes ST

Etiologies and Diagnostic Studies
- Check basic electrolyte panel, U/A, serum Osm, **urine Osm,** urine sodium

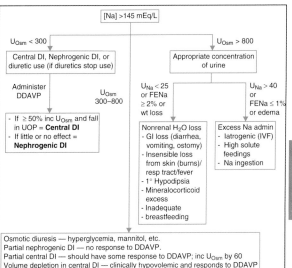

- **Diabetes insipidus** (Pediatr Clin N Am 2011;58:1271): Complete or partial failure in secretion of (central) or response to (nephrogenic) ADH
- Renal water absorption decreases, resulting in dilute urine
- P/w polyuria and polydipsia before developing HyperNa
- To establish diagnosis, do water deprivation test (fasting without fluids × 8–10 hr with regular monitoring of S_{Na}, S_{Osm}, U_{volume}, U_{Osm}). If $S_{Osm} > 300$ mOsm/kg and $U_{Osm} < 300$ mOsm/kg, pt has DI. Intermediate values may indicate partial DI. To distinguish central from nephrogenic DI, check AVP level then administer DDAVP (desmopressin) and monitor response in S_{Na}, S_{Osm}, U_{volume}, U_{Osm}
  - **Central DI** (responds to DDAVP) can be idiopathic, 2/2 neurosurgery (transsphe-noidal surg), neoplastic (craniopharyngioma), 2/2 hypoxic/ischemic encephalopathy (Sheehan syndrome, s/p arrest), congenital (2/2 hypothalamic/pituitary malformation or AVP-NPII gene mutation) or other (infectious, infiltrative or granulomatous diseases, anorexia nervosa, histiocytosis X)
  - **Nephrogenic DI** (no/minimal resp to DDAVP): Congenital (mutations in AVPR2 or AQP2), drugs (**Lithium,** ifosfamide, demeclocycline), obstructive uropathy, sickle cell, pregnancy, 2/2 hyperCa or hypoK
- Dehydration may be difficult to differentiate from salt poisoning based on urine [Na] alone; also consider history, clinical appearance (edema? signs of dehydration?), and FENa (= [UNa][PCr]/[UCr][PNa]; BMJ 2003;326:157)

Management (Pediatr Rev 1996;17:395)
- Rapid correction of HyperNa can result in cerebral edema, seizures, permanent CNS sequelae, or death; unless pt is significantly symptomatic, correct slowly
- If pt hemodyn unstable 2/2 hypovolemia, rx w/ IV NS 20 cc/kg boluses until stable
- Maximum safe rate for lowering [Na] is 0.5 mEq/L/hr over 24 hr or 12 mEq/L/d

- If significant sx from HyperNa (seizing), lower sodium more rapidly until sx resolve (1.5–2 mEq/L/hr for 3–4 hr), then try not to lower >12 mEq/L/d over all
- Calculation of water deficit as follows:

$$\text{Water deficit (L)} = 0.4 \times \text{lean body weight (kg)} \times \left[\frac{\text{Plasma [Na]}}{140} - 1 \right]$$

- Total body water calculated as 0.4 (40%) of lean body weight (instead of usual 60%) as assumes pt somewhat dehydrated (water deplete)
- So for 25 kg pt w/ [Na] 160; water deficit is $(0.4 \times 25) \times ((160/140) - 1) = 1.4$ L H_2O
- Assume correct 10 mEq/d; so needs to correct over 2 d; approx 30 cc/hr H_2O
- Seizure may occur during correction (may reflect cerebral edema); if occurs, rate of correction should be slowed or administer hypertonic saline. Usually self-limited and not reflective of long-term sequelae (Pediatr Rev 2002;23:371)
- Make sure to account for insensible losses and replacement as well
- A rough rule of thumb is that 4 cc/kg of free H_2O will dec [Na] by 1 mEq/L
- Water deficit is the amount of positive water balance needed to correct sodium to 140
- Provide such that correction is <0.5 mEq/L/hr; ideal w/ change [Na] <10–12 mEq/d
- If patient has central DI, cannot correct [Na] w/o administration of DDAVP
- If nephro DI, mgmt involves use of thiazide diuretic and low Na and low-protein diet
- Breastfeeding infants require lactation support & judicious provision of supplemental fluids

HYPOKALEMIA

Definition (Pediatr Rev 1996;17:395)
- Serum K <3 mEq/L; common finding in hospitalized children and not usually further evaluated, just repleted; if assoc with sx or if persists, warrants further eval

Pathophysiology (Pediatr Clin North Am 1990;37:419)
- Majority of body K intracellular; 1° ion responsible for cell's net negative charge
  - Acute changes in K do not reflect body stores; but chronic changes do
- As such, hypokalemia presents with nerve and muscle dysfunction.
- $[K^+]$ can be lost from the body through renal or GI secretion or can be shuttled in and out of cells mediated by certain hormones or in exchange for H^+

Etiologies (Pediatr Clin North Am 1990;37:419; Rose & Post. *Clinical Physiology of Acid-Base & Electrolyte Disorders* 2001:836; Pediatr Rev 2008;29:e50)
- ↑ **renal excretion** 2/2 primary tubulopathies (Bartter, Gitelman, Liddle, Fanconi, distal Type 1 RTA, proximal type 2 RTA), drugs (**diuretics**, cisplatin, amphotericin B), mineralocorticoid excess (**Hyperaldosteronism**, Cushing's, exogenous mineralocorticoid, high renin state (RAS), CAH due to 17α-hydroxylase or 11β-hydroxylase deficiency)
  - **Diuretic use** or w/ excretion of non-resorbable anions, which pull K w/ them in distal tube (i.e., bicarb, seen in alkalosis) & w/ **hypomagnesaemia**
  - **Bartter:** Rare p/w hypoK and met alkalosis early (<6 yo); assoc w/ multiple genes; often w/ stunted growth and MR
  - **Gitelman:** Rare p/w hypoK, generally normal Ca, hypoMg, met alkalosis; defect in Na–Cl channel in DT, more benign and incidentally dx'd in early adulthood, often p/w tetany (Q J Med 2010;103:741)
  - **Liddle:** (Rare AD) similar to presentation of 1° hyperaldosteronism; gain of fxn mutation in Na channel at CT, so eval w/ low renin and aldo levels, HTN
  - **Nonrenal losses:** GI losses: Vomiting, diarrhea (consider laxative abuse), NGT suction, fistulas, or ostomies. Rarely 2/2 clay ingestion or profuse sweating
  - **Shift of extracellular to intracellular fluid** can be mediated by hormones (insulin or $β_2$-catecholamines), by alkalosis (0.4 mEq/L per ↑ 0.1 pH), or w/ use of GM-CSF or treatment of megaloblastic anemias w/ B_{12} (settings of high-cell turn over). Transient hypoK also seen in trauma, concussions (J Trauma 2003;54:197)
  - **Pseudohypokalemia** w/ metabolically active cells (i.e., inc WBC in AML) can consume K following blood draw resulting in spuriously low value)

Clinical Manifestations (Pediatr Rev 1996;17:395)
- Significant symptoms are unlikely unless $[K^+]$ <2.5 mEq/L but significant variability
- Neuromuscular: P/w weakness, ↓ reflexes, paralysis, ↓ GI motility, even ileus
  - Can be severe enough to result in rhabdomyolysis
- Cardiac: Multi arrhythmias 2/2 ↑ automaticity and prolonged repolarization
  - Premature ventricular beats, sinus bradycardia, AV blocks, paroxysmal atrial and junctional tachycardias (prolonged depol sets up for SVT), even VT or VF

- Classic EKG: PR and QRS shortening, T wave flattening, development of U wave
- Renal: W/ loss of renal concentrating ability and decreased responsiveness to ADH p/w polyuria and polydipsia; requires 2–3 wk of K depletion

Diagnostic Studies (Rose & Post. *Clinical Physiology of Acid-Base & Electrolyte Disorders* 2001:746; Pediatr Rev 2011;32:65)
- Chem 10 (w/ Ca, Mg, Phos), U/A, urine lytes (K, Na, Cl, Osm, Cr), pH, and BP, S_{Osm}
  - Spot urine $[K^+]$ <15 mEq/L suggests extrarenal losses but less sensitive w/ hypovolemia or w/ polyuria; 24 hr urine $[K^+]$ <25 mEq more definitive
  - Transtubular potassium gradient (TTKG; can use if $UNa > 25$ & $U_{Osm} > P_{Osm}$) = $(UK)(P_{Osm})/(PK)(U_{Osm})$ is typically 8–9 given normal dietary K intake & normal renal fx. TTKG < 3 c/w GI losses or inadequate K intake. HypoK & TTKG > 3 c/w renal loss
- In more complicated cases or w/ significant symptoms can check CK, cortisol, plasma renin activity, aldosterone level, 17-OH ketosteroids, EKG
- Urine $[Cl^-]$ useful: U_{Cl} <25 mEq/L strongly suggests of vomiting or diuretic effect (even after drug effect passed), if >40 mEq/L should assay urine for diuretic and if neg & pt normotensive, consider Bartter's or Gitelman's syndrome

Management (Pediatr Rev 1996;17:395)
- W/ severe sx or EKG Δ's, IV repletion advised and accomplished with KCl (0.5–1 mEq/kg IV × 1, repeat as needed). Need CV monitoring and central access if repleted at >0.5 mEq/kg/hr or >10 mEq/hr or with concentration >10 mEq/100mL
- In the asymp pt, oral repletion preferred and choice of K salt depends on etiology
  - In metabolic acidosis (i.e., RTA) use K citrate
  - In metabolic alkalosis use KCl
  - If hypophosphatemic, use K phos
- If chronic K wasting, can require daily repletion for weeks w/ 3–5 mEq/kg qd
- Check and replete Mg, as K repletion is ineffective in the presence of hypoMg

HYPERKALEMIA

Definition (Pediatr Rev 1996;17:395)
- Hyperkalemia defined as $[K^+]$ >5.5 mEq/L and most commonly seen in pediatric pop as a spurious value ("**pseudohyperkalemia**") 2/2 diff blood draw w/ hemolysis. If pt stable, level should be repeated, ideally from a free-flowing venous sample
- If serum $[K^+]$ is truly elevated, this can be a real medical emergency

Pathophysiology (Rose & Post. *Clinical Physiology of Acid-Base & Electrolyte Disorders* 2001:888)
- As above, majority of K intracellular and responsible for cell membrane potentials; small changes can have serious effects on muscle and nerve tissue
- Acutely, body responds to ↑ serum $[K^+]$ by shifting excess K intracellularly via insulin and β_2-adrenergic. Over 6–8 hr, urinary excretion of K ↑ resolving imbalance
- Hyperkalemia develops secondary to inc intake, transcellular shift, or dec excretion

Etiology (Rose & Post. *Clinical Physiology of Acid-Base & Electrolyte Disorders* 2001:888)
- ↑ intake 2/2 PO's or hx of K rich foods, salt substitutes, low Na soups, and red clay (common in the SW United States) or w/ IVs (iatrogenic, w/ meds [i.e., K-PCN], stored blood xfn)
- Transcellular shift w/ metab acidosis, hypoinsulin and hyperglyc (DKA/HONKC), BB (usually minor and rare hyperK w/o other defect hypoaldo or ESRD)
- ↓ excretion. Most often 2/2 renal failure: HyperK w/ oliguria and subsequently anuria
  - HyperK in nonoliguric pt; eval other cause (↑ intake, hypoaldo, tissue breakdown)
  - Hypoaldosteronism: Results in decreased K excretion from principle cells of CT
  - ↓ activity renin–angiotensin axis 2/2 renal insuff, NSAIDs, ACEIs, cyclosporine, AIDS
  - ↓ adrenal synthesis w/ low cortisol levels (1° adrenal insuff or CAH), nml cortisol levels (heparin induced or isolated hypoald)
  - Aldosterone resistance 2/2 cyclosporine, tacrolimus, K-sparing diuretics, pseudohypoaldo
- Common clinical settings in pediatrics include:
  - Low-birth-weight preterm baby (50% w/ inc K) 2/2 extracellular shift and low effective GFR (J Pediatr 1997;131:81)
  - Infant w/ vomiting and virilized (CAH) or nml genitalia (pseudohypoaldo)
  - DKA or other metabolic acidosis

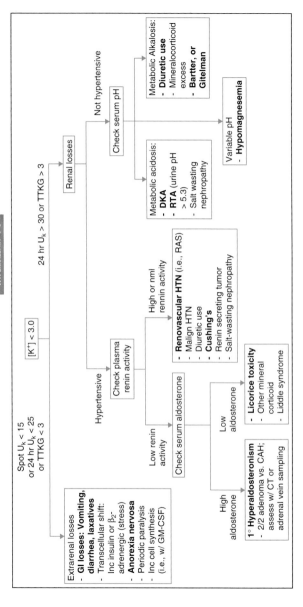

[K+] < 3.0

Spot U_k < 15 or 24 hr U_k < 25 or TTKG < 3

Extrarenal losses
- **GI losses: Vomiting, diarrhea, laxatives**
- Transcellular shift:
  Inc insulin or β₂-adrenergic (stress)
- **Anorexia nervosa**
- Periodic paralysis
- Inc cell synthesis
  (i.e., w/ GM-CSF)

24 hr U_k > 30 or TTKG > 3

Renal losses

Hypertensive

Check plasma renin activity

Low renin activity

Check serum aldosterone

High aldosterone

1° Hyperaldosteronism
- 2/2 adenoma vs. CAH; assess w/ CT or adrenal vein sampling

Low aldosterone

Licorice toxicity
- Other mineral corticoid
- Liddle syndrome

High or nml renin activity

- **Renovascular HTN** (i.e., RAS)
- Malign HTN
- Diuretic use
- **Cushing's**
- Renin secreting tumor
- Salt-wasting nephropathy

Not hypertensive

Check serum pH

Metabolic acidosis:
- **DKA**
- **RTA** (urine pH > 5.3)
- Salt wasting nephropathy

Metabolic Alkalosis:
- **Diuretic use**
- Mineralocorticoid excess
- **Bartter, or Gitelman**

Variable pH
- **Hypomagnesemia**

Clinical Manifestations (Pediatr Rev 1996;17:106)

- Clinical signs of hyperkalemia are not generally seen until $[K^+] > 7$ mEq/L (if weakness at lower levels, consider periodic paralysis hyperkalemic variant)
- Sx include muscle dysfunction (paralysis or ascending weakness, resp func spared)
- **Earliest EKG changes include peaked T waves, shortened PR, and shortening QT**; seen at lower $[K^+]$ levels than symptoms as above (at 5.5–6.5 mEq/L)
  - At levels of 6.5–7.5 mEq/L, may see widening of QRS and PR
  - At 7–8 mEq/L, see broad and low amp P's, prolonged QT and ST changes
  - At >8 mEq/L, P wave disappears, QRS widens; develops "sine" wave pattern; ↑ risk of VF or asystole significantly
  - Degree of hyperK & assoc EKG changes can be variable in some pts

Diagnostic Studies (Rose & Post. Clinical Physiology of Acid-Base & Electrolyte Disorders 2001:888)

- **If stable w/o EKG Δ, first step is to repeat value** (r/o pseudohyperK)
- Obtain hx focused on K intake, hx of kidney dz, DM, meds predisposing to hyperK (i.e., spironolactone), PE for muscle weakness, and obtain EKG
- Check Chem 10 (including Ca), serum pH, S_{Osm} and TTKG; can use if $U_{Na} > 25$, $U_{Osm} > P_{Osm}$, see below for formula
- In absence of other etiology, consider hypoaldosteronism
  - Aldosterone upregulates K^+ secretion in exchange for H^+ via principle cells in CT
  - Children w/ hypoaldo p/w dehydration, hyperK, hypoNa, met acidosis, inc U_{Na}
  - Check AM plasma renin, aldosterone, and cortisol (off interfering meds, NSAIDs, ACEIs, heparin, K-sparing diuretics)

HYPERKALEMIA 6-10

	Renin	Aldosterone	Cortisol	Resp to aldo
Hyporeninism	↓ to nml	↓	Nml	Nml
1° adrenal insuff	↑	↓	↓	Nml
CAH	↑	↓	↓	Nml
Isolated hypoaldo	↑	↓	Nml	Nml
Pseudohypoaldo	↑	↑	Nml	None to ↓

- **Can ↑ sensitivity by pretreating w/ Lasix; potentiates renin, ↑ aldo except in pts w/ hypoaldosteronism**
- Can also estimate aldosterone effect by checking TTKG

$$TTKG = \frac{(U_K \times (U_{Osm} / P_{Osm}))}{serum\ [k^+]}; \text{ value <7 suggests ↓ renal excretion (e.g., hypoaldo)}$$

Management

- Treat for EKG changes or K > 6
- **Calcium gluconate (10%);** stabilizes membrane, used if EKG changes or severe sx are present; fastest onset of action and shortest duration of action
  - 100 mg/kg/dose (1 mL/kg/dose) infused over 2–3 min under cardiac monitoring
  - Repeat q5min if EKG changes persist
  - Use carefully in pts on digitalis; can potentiate digitalis toxicity
- **Insulin and glucose:** Drives K into cells; acts over 30–60 min, effect for few hours
  - Regular insulin 0.1 U/kg w/ $D_{25}W$ glucose as 0.5 g/kg (2 mL/kg) IV over 30 min
  - Repeat dose q30–60min; can also begin regular insulin drip 0.1 U/kg/hr w/ $D_{25}W$ drip 1–2 mL/kg/hr w/ at q1h glucose monitoring
- **Bicarbonate:** Also drives K into cells and acts over 30–60 min, effect for few hours
  - 1–2 mEq/kg IV given over 5–10 min; minimal benefit in absence of acidosis, limited benefit in significant renal failure
- **β_2 adrenergic agonists:** Also drives K into cells, acts over 90 min w/ inhalation, 30 min if given IV, effect lasts for few hours
  - Albuterol neb 5 mg (adults 10–20 mg) ×1; less reliable than insulin/glucose
- **Diuretics:** Loop or thiazide diuretics; limited efficacy w/ significant renal failure, longer onset of action
- **Cation-exchange resins:** Cornerstone of longer term hyperK management; removes K from body. May be ineffective in preterm infants; risk of GI complications
  - Kayexalate 1–2 g/kg; has been mixed w/ sorbitol in the past but case-reports of intestinal necrosis in uremic pts
- **Dialysis:** Last line of defense if all of the above fail
- **Preterm infants:** Weak evidence suggests insulin/glucose may be preferred over rectal cation-exchange resins (Cochrane Database 2007;1:CD005257)

HYPOCALCEMIA

Definition (Clin Pediatr (Phila) 2001;40:305)
- Hypocalcemia is defined as a serum calcium level <7 mg/dL in preterm neonates, 8 mg/dL in term neonates, and 8.8 mg/dL in older children
- ~50% serum Ca^{++} albumin-bound, hyper/hypoalbumin Δ accuracy of serum $[Ca^{++}]$
- Corrected calcium = add 0.8 mg/dL to $[Ca^{++}]$ for every 1 mg/dL albumin <4 mg/dL
- Ca corrected for pH: Add 0.2 mg/dL to $[Ca^{++}]$ for every 0.1 pH <7.4

Epidemiology (CMAJ 2007;177:1494)
- Neonatal hypocalcemia is estimated at 50% in infants born to mothers w/ DM
- Moderately inc risk w/ spring and winter births, low maternal vit D intake during pregnancy, prolonged breastfeeding, and w/ lower socioeconomic status
- Children w/ darker pigmented skin have inc risk 2/2 dec vit D formation

Pathophysiology (Clin Pediatr (Phila) 2001;40:305)
- 98% Ca^{++} in bone; of remaining 2%, 50% bioactive (ionized), 50% protein bound
- Calcium plays an important role in muscle contraction and nerve activity
- Homeostasis by PTH and vit D acting on kidneys, intestines, bones, skin, and liver
- Hypocalcemia is sensed by the parathyroid gland via a membrane receptor calcium sensor → ↑ PTH
  - Kidney: ↑ PTH → ↑ Mg, Ca retention, ↑ phos excretion, ↑ vit D activation
  - Bone: ↑ PTH → release of Ca stores
- Vitamin D is formed by the skin through exposure to UV light (also the form of intake from dietary sources), hydroxylated to 25-OH vit D in the liver and activated to $1,25(OH)_2$ vit D in the kidney (stimulated by PTH)
  - Activated $1,25(OH)_2$ vit D acts on GI tract, (↑ Ca absorp is neg regulator of PTH)
- Dysfxn at any level (Ca sensor, end organs, hormone fxn) can result in hypocalcemia

Etiology (J Clin Endocrinol Metab 1995;80:1473)
- Multiple etiologies possible, approach based on physiology
- **Hypoparathyroidism:** 2/2 impaired production, function, or periph resistance
  - **DiGeorge anomaly:** 22q11 deletion w/ branchial dysembryogenesis; absent thymus, T-cell defect, facial abn, parathyroid hypoplasia, and cardiac anomalies (aortic arch defects, tetralogy of Fallot)
  - **Polyglandular autoimmune syndrome I:** Assoc w/ early candidiasis (chronic mucocutaneous), hypoPTH, later (adolescent) w/ adrenal insuff
  - Congenital absence or suppression (can suppression in neonate w/ maternal hypercalcemia suppressing PTH), isolated late onset, infiltrative dz (Wilson, hemochromatosis, thalassemia), postop, postradiation
  - **Pseudohypoparathyroidism:** Peripheral tissue resistance to PTH
    - **Type Ia: Albright hereditary osteodystrophy** w/ short stature, round face, obesity, short metacarpals/metatarsals, MR, SC calcifications
    - Type Ib: Normal phenotype w/ PTH resistance
- **Vitamin D abnormalities:** 2/2 deficiency or abn metabolism
  - **Vitamin D deficiency:** 2/2 nutritional def, malabsorption (CF, celiac dz, chronic pancreatitis, PBC, short bowel syndrome), anticonvulsants, ↓ UVB exposure
  - **Vitamin D deficient rickets:** Undermineralization of epiphyseal growth plate w/ flaring of ends of long bones, rachitic rosary (costochondral prominence), delayed fontanelle closure, leg bowing, frontal bossing
  - Vit D dependent rickets Type I: Def renal 1-α hydroxylase; Type II: Vit D resistance; **both very rare**
  - Congenital rickets: Maternal vit D def
  - **Chronic renal failure:** W/ resultant bone disease 2/2 phos retention, ↓ $1,25(OH)_2$ vit D, and 2° hyperPTH
- Acute pancreatitis: Ca deposition at site of fat necrosis
- **Tumor lysis syndrome:** ↑ phos → CaPhos precipitation

Clinical Manifestations (J Clin Endocrinol Metab 1995;80:1473)
- Symptoms: Abnormalities of sensation and neuromusc excitability; 2/2 not only absolute $[Ca^{++}]$ but rate of fall
- Early findings include distal digit and perioral tingling and numbness
- Tetany (spontaneous muscle contraction) 2/2 ↑ excitability, most commonly w/ carpopedal spasm, but can result in laryngeal stridor or bronchospasm as well
  - **Chvostek sign:** Tap on facial nerve → lip twitch (71% sens)

- **Trousseau sign:** Induction of carpal spasm by sustained compression of brachial artery by sphygmomanometer cuff at 20 mm Hg > SBP × 3 min (94% sens)
- CNS manifestations include seizure, change in mental status, and irritability
- Cardiac: Bradycardia, malign arrhythmias, prolonged QTc, HoTN (↓ smooth muscle tone and poor card contract; pressor and volume resistant till hypoCa corrected)
- Chronic hypoCa: Cataracts, coarse hair, brittle nails, hypoplastic teeth; if 2/2 vit D def → rickets (rachitic rosary, wide wrists, bow legs)/osteomalacia

Diagnostic Studies (Clin Pediatr (Phila) 2001;40:305; J Clin Endocnnol Metab 1995;80:1473)
- Chem 7, Ca^{++}, Albumin, ionized Ca^{++}, Phos, Alk Phos, 25-OH vit D, $1,25(OH)_2$ vit D, Mg, Urine calcium/creatinine/phosphorus, and possibly long bone films

	Phos	Alk Phos	PTH	25-OH D_3	1,25-OH D_3	Mg	UCa
HypoPTH	↑	Nl	↓	Nl	↓	Nl	↓
PseudohypoPTH	↑	Nl	↑	Nl	↓	Nl	↓
Ca-sensing receptor def	↑ – nl	Nl	Var	Nl	↓ – Nl	Nl	↑
Vit D def rickets	↓ – nl	↑	↑	↓	Var	Nl	↓
Vit D dependent rickets type I	↓ – Nl	↑	↑	Nl	↓	Nl	↓
Vit D dependent rickets type II	↓ – Nl	↑	↑	Nl	↑	Nl	↓
Rickets of prematurity	↓ – Nl	↑	↑	Nl	↑ – Nl	Nl	?
Chronic renal failure	↑	↑	↑	Nl	↓	↑ – Nl	↓
Mg deficiency	Nl	Nl	Var	Nl	↓	↓	↑

Management (Clin Pediatr (Phila) 2001;40:305; Pediatr Rev. 2009;30:190)
- Acute mgmt hypoCa++ szr w/ slow 10% Ca++gluc IV (usual pedi dose 200–500 mg, do not exceed 200 mg in infant) w/ CV monitor. Can use CaCl if pt has central line
- Symptomatic hypoCa: 20 mg/kg elemental Ca IV (=2 mL/kg 10% CaGlua via secure PIV or 0.7 mL/kg 10% CaCl via central access) over 20 min; monitor for arrhythmias
- After sx resolution, for neonates infuse 500 mg/kg 10% CaGluc over 24 hr; for older infants/children infuse 200 mg/kg 10% CaGluc over 24 hr & titrate to nml Ca
- [Ca] × [Phos] product >70 can result in soft-tissue calcification
- If hypoMg associated; give 6 mg/kg elemental Mg IV
- For asymptomatic hypoCa, replete orally; consider repleting vit D
- Long-term management
  - HypoPTH: Maintain Ca levels at lower level of normal; supplement Ca and calcitriol (0.25 mcg/d); monitor for evidence of hypercalcemia
- Vit D def rickets. Stoss rx w/ vit D 600,000 IU PO × 1 in 6 divided doses q2h (vit D stored in fat and converted to active form for weeks), w/ Ca supps 500–1,000 mg elemental PO until levels nml. Start vit D 400 IU qd 12 wk later

HYPERCALCEMIA

Definition (Am Fam Physician 2003;67:1959; Curr Opin Pediatr 2010;22:508)
- In newborns, serum Ca (corrected for albumin) normal up to 11.3 mg/dL. In children up to 5 yr, normal up to 10.8 mg/dL. In older children and adults, mild hyperCa 10.5–12 mg/dL; mod 12–14 mg/dL, and severe (life-threatening >14 mg/dL

Pathophysiology (Lancet 1998;352:306)
- As above, 1° control of body Ca++ mediated by PTH, $1,25(OH)_2$ vit D, and calcitonin
- ↑ serum Ca++ 2/2 ↑ bone resorption, ↑ GI absorption, and ↓ renal excretion and can be mediated by inapprop ↑ PTH levels, and ↑ vit D levels (vit D toxicity)
- Renal excretion is 1° means for dealing w/ large fluxes of Ca++ but limited (only 10% of Ca reabsorp controlled by vit D and PTH, rest coupled to Na reabsorp). Regulation of intestinal absorp provides long-term homeostasis

Etiology (Am Fam Physician 2003;67:1959; Curr Opin Pediatr 2010;22:508)
- Ddx at all ages includes hyperPTH, ↑ vit D activity, ↑ bone turnover, ↓ renal clearance, increased Ca intake, malignancies; see chart for details

- Malignancy can cause hyperCa by 2/2 osteolytic lesions (e.g., sarcoma, neuroblastoma, rhabdomyosarcoma, other metastatic disease) or humoral production (e.g., PTHrP from squamous cell Ca, RCC, dysgerminoma, leukemia; or calcitriol from Hodgkin's)
- ↑ vit D activity: Toxicity 2/2 vit D O/D, excess vit D 2/2 granulomatous dz (sarcoidosis, TB, berylliosis, *P. jiroveci* PNA, Wegner dz)
- ↑ bone turnover; i.e., thyrotoxicosis, vit A toxicity, pheochromocytoma, immobility
- ↓ renal clearance; AI, thiazide diuretics

Clinical Manifestations (Lancet 1998;352:306)
- Symptoms include "stones, bones, moans (abdominal), and psychiatric overtones"
  - **"Stones":** Nephrolithiasis 2/2 increased urinary calcium excretion, can result in nephrocalcinosis and nephrogenic diabetes insipidus
  - **"Bones":** Osteoporosis, osteitis fibrosa cystica (2/2 hyperPTH w/ subperiosteal resorption, bone cysts), arthritis
  - **"Abdominal moans":** N/V, abdominal pain, anorexia, and weight loss; extreme manifestations include pancreatitis and peptic ulcer disease
  - **"Psychiatric overtones":** ↓ concentration/memory, confusion, Δ MS, lethargy, coma. Muscle weakness. Impaired vision 2/2 to corneal calcifications
- Cardiac sequelae include HTN, ↓ QTc, and rarely cardiac arrhythmias

Diagnostic Studies (Lancet 1998;352:306; Am Fam Physician 2003;67:1959)
- Check serum Ca++, albumin, ionized Ca++ (where available), phosphate, Alk Phos, basic serum electrolytes w/ BUN/Cr, TSH, PTH (and if suspected PTHrP), 1,25(OH)$_2$ vit D, 25-OH vit D, 24 hr urine calcium/creatinine, and EKG
- Consider U/A, KUB, and renal US if concern for nephrolithiasis

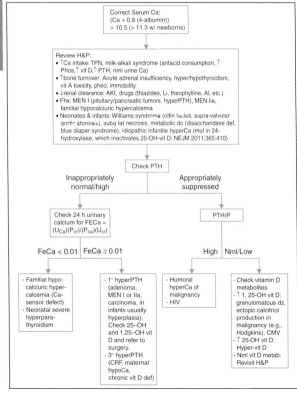

Management (Am Fam Physician 2003;67:1959; Curr Opin Pediatr 2010;22:508)
- Mild asymptomatic hyperCa: IVF (with KCl), mobilization
- Symptomatic or severe hyperCa: IVF followed by furosemide (monitor K^+), calcitonin (short-acting; tachyphylaxis after 24 hr), cardiac monitoring
- HyperCa resistant to IVF and loop diuretics: Consider bisphosphonates (but long-term effects on bone metabolism poorly studied in children) or glucocorticoids (dec vit D and Ca absorption)
- Williams syndrome, IHH, or FHH: Low-Ca, low-vitamin-D diet (consider Calcilo XD low-Ca, low-vitamin-D infant formula)
- 1° hyperPTH: Consult endocrine surgery for parathyroidectomy
- **In resistant situations, can use dialysis w/ low Ca^{++} bath or EDTA chelation**

HYPERMAGNESEMIA/HYPOMAGNESEMIA

(Lancet 1998;352:391)

Definition: Normal serum [Mg] ranges from 1.7–2.2 mg/dL
- 50–60% of total body Mg is in bone; only 1% is extracellular (measured in serum)

Pathophysiology
- Daily Mg homeostasis depends on GI absorption and renal excretion of Mg
  - 50–60% renal reabsorption at loop of Henle; 10% at DT but site of regulation
  - Regulated by multiple hormones but major controller is serum [Mg]
- Magnesium is essential for the function of multiple enzymes, particularly all reactions requiring ATP and every step in transcription of DNA and translation of mRNA
- It is also involved in membrane stabilization, nerve conduction, and ion transport

Hypomagnesemia
- **Definition:** No one level is accepted as a cut off for hypoMg, some argue serum [Mg] does not accurately reflect total body Mg stores
- **Etiology**
  - GI losses: **Diarrhea,** NGT suction, malabsorption syndromes (celiac, CF), steatorrhea, acute pancreatitis, **malnutrition/refeeding,** intestinal fistulae or resection
  - Renal losses: ↑ urine output for any cause (**osmotic diureses** in DM, w/ mannitol, etc.), **diuretics,** hyperCa w/ hypercalciuria, RTAs, hyperPTH, drugs (**aminoglycosides, cisplatin, amphotericin B,** cyclosporine), phosphate depletion, ATN, Gitelman syndrome (see hypoK)
- **Clinical manifestations:** Often asymp or sx 2/2 assoc electrolyte disturbances. Often presents w/ assoc hypoCa and hypoK, both resistant to rx w/o Mg repletion
  - **Cardiac:** Widened QRS (inc risk for Torsades), PR prolongation, inc risk for severe ventricular arrhythmias, inc sensitivity to digoxin
  - **Neuromuscular:** Tetany (w/ Trousseau and Chvostek signs), seizure, vertigo, ataxia, muscle weakness (diaphragm weakness), psychosis, and depression
  - **Metabolic:** Can result in hyperinsulinemia and carbohydrate intolerance
  - **Skeletal:** Osteoporosis/osteomalacia
- **Evaluation:** 24 hr urine Mg or Frac excretion of Mg can distinguish renal from GI losses
  - Check serum electrolytes (spec Ca^{++} and K^+), and renal function (BUN/Cr)
- **Treatment**
  - Oral therapy preferred over IV (IV bolus can dec renal reabsorption w/ wasting of Mg); still, in severe or symptomatic hypoMg use IV rx
  - Acutely provide 25–50 mg/kg/dose IV q4–6h (max 2 g/dose) w/ rate of infusion not to exceed 150 mg/min; need cardiac monitoring
  - Chronic depletion, rx w/ MgOxide 5–10 mg/kg PO divided bid–tid, can also use MgGluconate or MgSulfate PO **(remember, oral Mg is a cathartic)**
  - Treat concurrent electrolyte deficiencies

Hypermagnesemia
- **Etiology:** Iatrogenic (IV repletion, asthma treatment, peripartum use for preeclampsia or tocolysis, cathartics [e.g., Epsom salts], antacids), renal failure
- **Clinical manifestations**
  - **Neuromuscular:** Nausea/vomiting, weakness, delta MS, hyporeflexia, lethargy, paralysis
  - **Cardiac/respiratory:** HoTN, long QTc, wide QRS, wide PR, bradycardia, respiratory depression or failure, complete heart block
- **Evaluation:** Serum electrolytes and renal function, review medication list
- **Management:** D/c supplements, IV hydration (NS blouses), consider diuresis w/Lasix

- W/ signs & sx, slow infusion of 10% CaGluconate IV (usual pediatric dose is 200–500 mg, not to exceed 200 mg in infant) w/ concurrent cardiac monitoring
- In resistant disease, consider dialysis

HYPOPHOSPHATEMIA/HYPERPHOSPHATEMIA

(Lancet 1998;352:391)

Definition: Nml serum [Phos] 2.8–4.5 mg/dL w/ slightly $\uparrow$ concentration in children vs. adults.

Pathophysiology
- Homeostasis by balance btw GI absorption (60–80% dietary Phos absorbed) and renal excretion (80% Phos reabsorbed in proximal tubule, coupled to Na)
- Controlled by PTH (inc renal secretion) and vit D (inc GI absorp, dec urine excretion)

Hypophosphatemia
- **Etiology**
  - $\uparrow$ urinary excretion: **HyperPTH, vit D deficiency,** renal tubule defects (Fanconi, hereditary hypophosphatemic rickets [formerly known as vit D dependent rickets] caused by mutations in PHEX [X-linked], FGF23 [autosomal dominant], DMP1 [autosomal recessive], SLC34A3 [autosomal recessive hypophosphatemic rickets with hypercalciuria] etc.), metab or resp acidosis, acetazolamide (Nat Rev Nephrol 2010;6:657; Curr Opin Pediatr 2007;19:488)
  - $\downarrow$ intestinal absorption: Dietary restriction, **chronic antacid use,** vit D def, chronic diarrhea, steatorrhea
  - Internal redistribution: **Hungry bone syndrome,** respiratory alkalosis, recovery from DKA or malnutrition, **refeeding syndrome (Pediatr Clin N Am 2009;56:1201),** sepsis
- **Clinical manifestations**
  - Rarely symptomatic unless severe (**<1 mg/dL**); generally due to ATP deficiency
  - Muscle dysfunction w/ prox myopathy, dysphagia, and ileus; rarely rhabdo
  - Respiratory failure 2/2 weakness of respiratory muscles
  - Cardiac involvement w/ impaired contractility and CHF
  - Heme abnormalities w/ hemolysis, thrombocytopenia, and impaired phagocytosis
  - Renal dysfunction w/ calcium and magnesium wasting
  - Neurologic dysfxn w/ metab encephalopathy, seizures, lethargy, confusion, coma
- **Evaluation:** Chem 7, Ca (iCa), Phos, Mg, vit D, PTH, U_{Ca}, U_{Phos}, U_{Cr}, and urine pH
- **Management**
  - Acute onset w/ severe depletion (<1 mg/dL) and/or symptoms treat w/ IV
    - KPhos contains 4.4 mEq K^+ and 3 mMol phosphate/mL. NaPhos contains 4 mEq Na^+ and 3 mMol phosphate/mL
    - Administer 0.1–0.2 mMol/kg phosphate over 6 hr, then maintenance infusion 15–45 mg/kg/d; observe for HypoCa and follow [Ca] × [Phos] product
  - Chronic onset: NeutraPhos contains 250 mg (= 8 mMol) phosphate per packet, half as the Na salt and half as the K salt
    - Cow's milk has 1 mg Phos/mL

Hyperphosphatemia
- **Etiology**
  - Inc exogenous load: Cow's milk intake in infants, vit D intoxication, phosphate containing enemas, supplements
  - Inc endogenous load: Tumor lysis syndrome, rhabdomyolysis, malignant hyperthermia (w/ anesthesia), hemolysis, acidosis
  - Dec renal excretion: Renal failure, hypoPTH, Mg def, acromegaly, thyrotoxicosis
- **Clinical manifestations**
  - Rapid increase in [Phos] can result in hypoCa and assoc symptoms
  - [Ca] × [Phos] >70 results in soft-tissue deposition of calcium
- **Evaluation:** Serum electrolytes, BUN/Cr, Ca (iCa), Phos, Mg, vit D, PTH, ABG, U_{Ca}, U_{Phos}, U_{Cr}, and urine pH
- **Management**
  - **Most effective therapy is reduction of intestinal absorption** 2/2 dec dietary intake and use of phosphate binders (calcium carbonate, calcium acetate [PhosLo], Renagel [binding resin])
  - If 2/2 cell lysis, management as per management of tumor lysis syndrome or rhabdomyolysis (IV fluid, consider mannitol)
  - If severe symptoms and 2/2 renal failure, consider dialysis

Definition (Pediatr Rev 1996;17:395)
- Acids are substances that donate protons (H^+) and bases accept protons
- The pH of blood is tightly regulated to remain between 7.35 and 7.45
  - Average value: **Arterial pH** 7.37–7.43 and **Venous pH** 7.32–7.38
- **Acidemia** is defined as serum pH <7.36; **acidosis** indicates a process whereby acid is added to or base is removed from the body
- **Alkalemia** is defined as serum pH >7.44; **alkalosis** indicates a process whereby base is added to or acid is removed from the body
- If the pH is brought out of range by a 1° process (metabolic or respiratory), the body tries to restore pH to nml via activities of lungs and kidneys on body's main buffer HCO_3
  - **Respiratory compensation;** lungs control the ratio of partial pressure of CO_2 to HCO_3; used to counteract 1° metabolic processes and **occurs in minutes**
  - **Renal compensation;** kidneys control the rate of excretion of HCO_3; used to counteract 1° respiratory processes and **requires hours to days**
  - There are other extracellular and intracellular buffers but HCO_3 is the major one

Pathophysiology (Rose & Post. Clinical Physiology of Acid–Base & Electrolyte Disorders 2001:535)
- Myriad of etiologies for each 1° process; all distinguished by following table
- The body will attempt to correct the pH deviation as described above
- More than one process (acidosis and alkalosis; though not both resp acidosis and alkalosis) can be present at once, assessed by calculating approp expected compensation and checking if it matches with what is objectively measured

1° Disorder	Formula to Calculate Compensation (assumes nml HCO_2 24, PCO_2 40)
Metabolic acidosis	1 mm Hg decrease in $PaCO_2$ expected for every 1 mEq/L decrease in $[HCO_3]$
Metabolic alkalosis	10 mm Hg increase in $PaCO_2$ expected for every 7 mEq/L increase in $[HCO_3]$
Respiratory acidosis	
Acute	1 mEq/L $[HCO_3]$ increase expected for every 10 mm Hg increase in $PaCO_2$
Chronic	3.5 mEq/L $[HCO_3]$ increase expected for every 10 mm Hg increase in $PaCO_2$
Respiratory alkalosis	
Acute	2 mEq/L $[HCO_3]$ decrease expected for every 10 mm Hg decrease in $PaCO_2$
Chronic	4 mEq/L $[HCO_3]$ decrease expected for every 10 mm Hg decrease in $PaCO_2$

- Of note: Corrections assume nml HCO_3 24 and PCO_2 40; but in pts w/ underlying resp dz (CLD, BPD, etc.) use HCO_3 and PCO_2, they live at as nml
  - Also of note, infants maintain a lower average HCO_3 (21.5–23.5 mEq/L) than older children (23–25 mEq/L) (Pediatr Rev 1996;17:395)
- If change in $PaCO_2$ or HCO_3 is > or < expected, there may be a 2nd 1° process
  - $PaCO_2$ too low implies a concomitant respiratory acidosis
  - $PaCO_2$ too high implies a concomitant respiratory alkalosis
  - HCO_3 too low implies a concomitant metabolic acidosis
  - HCO_3 too high implies a concomitant metabolic alkalosis
- **Suspect presence of two, 1° acid–base processes if serum pH nml but:**
  - Increased $PaCO_2$ and increased HCO_2; respiratory acidosis and metabolic alkalosis
  - Decreased $PaCO_2$ and decreased HCO_2; respiratory alkalosis and metabolic acidosis
  - Nml $PaCO_2$ and nml HCO_2 w/ + AG; AG met acidosis and met alkalosis
  - Nml $PaCO_2$ & nml HCO_2 w/ no AG; Nml or nonanion gap (NAG) met acid & met alk

METABOLIC ACIDOSIS

Definition (Pediatr Rev 2004;25:350; Pediatr Rev 2011;32:240)
- Net gain of H^+ or loss of HCO_3 and can be divided into AG or NAG
- AG acidosis: Implies presence of unmeasured anions; ↑ organic acids from ingestion, production, inborn errors of metab, or ↓ excretion 2/2 renal failure
  - AG = $[Na^+] - ([Cl^-] + [HCO_3^-])$; normal defined as 8–12 w/ normal values believed to be higher in pts <2 yo (some use 16 +/– 4 mEq/L as normal for this group)

- Figge formula corrects AG for albumin: Adjusted AG = observed AG + 2.5 (nl albumin − observed albumin)
- NAG acidosis: 2/2 inability to excrete H^+ or loss of HCO_3 from GI or urinary tracts
- Severe met acidosis: $HCO_3 \leq 8$ mEq/L (if nl resp compensation)

Clinical Manifestations (Pediatr Rev 1996;17:395; Pediatr Rev 2011;32:240)

- Nl response to met acidosis is **hyperpnea** (deep, pauseless respirations) w/ resultant 4–8×'s increase in minute ventilation. As acidosis worsens, resp muscle strength decreases and WOB increases → resp failure
- At pH <7–7.1, cardiac contractility can be impaired and the risk of malignant arrhythmias is increased. Can p/w arteriolar dilation, HoTN, pulmonary edema
- CNS: Cerebral edema, lethargy, coma
- Other: Oxyhemoglobin dissociation curve shifts right, hyperK, insulin resistance, protein denaturing

Etiologies (Rose & Post. Clinical Physiology of Acid-Base & Electrolyte Disorders 2001:535; Pediatr Rev 2011;32:240)

- AG acidosis: Due to exogenous and endogenous H^+ excess: **MUD PILES**
  - **M**ethanol: Found in wood alcohol, varnishes, shellac, and sterno, metabolized to formaldehyde, Osm gap >10; p/w sx 12–36 hr after ingestion w/ weakness, N/V, can result in blindness, coma, and death
  - **U**remia (2/2 renal failure w/ decreased clearance of sulfate, urate, phosphate)
  - **D**iabetic ketoacidosis, starvation ketosis
  - **P**araldehyde (solvent, anticonvulsant and hypnotic, not available in the United States but still used elsewhere)
  - **I**ron, **i**soniazid, and **i**ngestions (other): Toluene (glue sniffing), sulfur, etc.
  - **L**actic acidosis: Most common, 2/2 anaerobic metab, can be 2/2 ↑ production (severe hypoxia, ischemia, shock, CO or cyanide poisoning, szr, inborn errors of metab) or ↓ clearance (hypoperfusion, liver disease)
  - **E**thylene glycol (in antifreeze, w/ glycolate, oxalate, and Osm gap >10; Ethylene glycol ingestion p/w drunkenness or even coma, then pulmonary edema and then renal failure, consider fomepizole and/or dialysis for rx), **E**thanol (alcoholic ketoacidosis)
  - **S**alicylate: Results in combination resp alkalosis and met acidosis, tinnitus
  - If concern for ingestions, check Osmolar gap = Measured Osm − Calculated Osm
    - Calculated Osm = $2[Na^+]$ + [glucose]/18 + [BUN]/2.8 + [EtOH]/4.6
    - If Osm gap >10, presence of unmeasured Osm; methanol, ethylene glycol, etc.
  - W/ +AG; to check if >1 cause for low HCO_3 can check $\Delta/\Delta = \Delta$ **AG**/Δ **HCO_3**
    - Δ/Δ <1: loss of HCO_3 greater than expected (AG acidosis + NAG acidosis)
    - Δ/Δ = 1–2: typical AG acidosis as almost 1:1 buffering of H^+ w/ HCO_3
    - Δ/Δ >2: loss of HCO_3 less than expected (AG acidosis + metabolic alkalosis)
- NAG acidosis: 2/2 ↑ GU or GI loss of HCO_3 or inability to excrete H^+: **HARD UP**
  - **H**yperalimentation, **H**ypoaldosteronism, **H**yperPTH
  - **A**cetazolamide, **A**mmonium chloride
  - **R**TA (see later), **R**enal loss 2/2 **r**apid correction of chronic resp alkalosis
    - **RTA II** (proximal RTA): Dec HCO_3 reabsorption, p/w normal or low serum $[K^+]$, variable urine pH, fractional excretion of HCO_3 (Fe_{HCO3}) >15–20%
      - Can result in rickets or osteomalacia
      - Carbonic anhydrase inhibitors (e.g., acetazolamide) impair HCO_3 reabsorption
      - Treat w/ 10–15 mEq/kg HCO_3 divided multiple times a day
      - Renal dysfunction: Some cases of renal failure and RTA
    - **RTA IV** (hypoaldosteronism): W/ normal or inc serum $[K^+]$, urine pH < 5.3, Fe_{HCO3} < 3%, check serum aldo; treat w/ HCO_3 1–3 mEq/kg qd
    - **RTA I** (distal RTA): Dec H^+ secretion w/ urine pH >5.3, low serum $[K^+]$, and fractional excretion of HCO_3 <3% in adults but can be 5–10% in children
      - Can be 2/2 autoimmune process, hyperPTH, amphotericin
      - Can result in nephrocalcinosis or nephrolithiasis
      - Treat w/ daily HCO_3 4–14 mEq/kg qd in children, 1–2 mEq/kg qd in adults
  - **D**iarrhea (most common cause) and other GI losses (ostomy, etc.)
  - **U**reteral diversion (ureteroenterostomy/ureterosigmoidostomy → intestinal HCO_3^- loss)
  - **P**arenteral NaCl (common cause, due to rapid dilution of HCO_3^- by Cl^-; similar effect from KCl or $MgCl_2$), **P**ancreatic fistula
- Urine AG can distinguish between situations w/ intact NH_4^+ secretion (GI losses RTA II, rapid correction of chronic resp alkalosis) vs. those where secretion of NH_4^+ is impaired (renal failure, RTA I, and IV)
  - UAG is inaccurate w/ high AG acidosis or w/ significant volume depletion

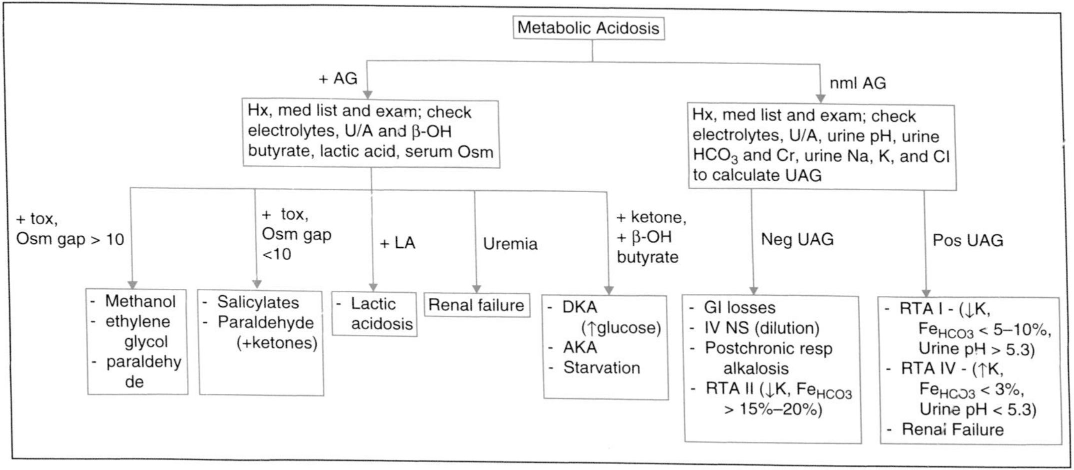

Metabolic Acidosis

+ AG

Hx, med list and exam; check electrolytes, U/A and β-OH butyrate, lactic acid, serum Osm

- **+ tox, Osm gap > 10**
  - Methanol
  - ethylene glycol
  - paraldehyde

- **+ tox, Osm gap <10**
  - Salicylates
  - Paraldehyde (+ketones)

- **+ LA**
  - Lactic acidosis

- **Uremia**
  - Renal failure

- **+ ketone, + β-OH butyrate**
  - DKA (↑glucose)
  - AKA
  - Starvation

nml AG

Hx, med list and exam; check electrolytes, U/A, urine pH, urine HCO₃, and Cr, urine Na, K, and Cl to calculate UAG

- **Neg UAG**
  - GI losses
  - IV NS (dilution)
  - Postchronic resp alkalosis
  - RTA II (↓↓K, Fe$_{HCO3}$ > 15%–20%)

- **Pos UAG**
  - RTA I - (↓K, Fe$_{HCO3}$ < 5–10%, Urine pH > 5.3)
  - RTA IV - (↑K, Fe$_{HCO3}$ < 3%, Urine pH < 5.3)
  - Renal Failure

Management (Pediatr Rev 2004;25:350)
- Correct underlying abnormalities as described above
- Sodium-bicarb is the agent of choice for severe metabolic acidosis (especially NAG) but controversial as evidence of improved outcomes is weak
  - Amt bicarb to infuse = (weight in kg) × (15 − [measured HCO₃]) × (0.5)
  - Mix amount calculated in hypotonic solution and infuse over 1 HR
  - Provides enough bicarb to correct pH >7.2 or bicarb concentration >15 mEq/L
- Rapid correction can result in acidification of CSF (w/ worsening symptoms); volume overload; development of alkalemia, hypocalcemia, and respiratory depression

METABOLIC ALKALOSIS

Definition (Pediatr Rev 2004;25:350; Pediatr Rev 2011;32:240)
- Processes resulting in net loss of H^+ or gain of HCO_3^-; alkalemia is a serum pH >7.44

Pathophysiology (Pediatr Rev 2004;25:350; Pediatr Rev 2011;32:240)
- Gain of HCO_3^- can be 2/2 ↑ intake, ↓ renal excretion, or volume contraction around stable amount of bicarbonate
- Healthy kidneys can excrete a large load of bicarbonate rapidly, so to maintain a metabolic alkalosis renal bicarbonate excretion must be impaired
- Renal bicarbonate excretion is impaired when prox tubule bicarb reabsorp is inc 2/2, dec effective circ volume and chloride depletion (results in 2° hyperaldo, dec tubular Cl^- inhibiting Cl^-/HCO_3^- exchanger), $[K^+]$ depletion (creates intracellular acidosis, stimulates H^+/Na^+ exchanger), or posthypercapnia adaptation

Clinical Manifestations (Pediatr Rev 1996;17:395; Pediatr Rev 2011;32:240)
- Can present w/ lethargy, confusion, and eventually seizures
- Can see tissue hypoxia, CNS effects, and muscular irritability
- Body compensates w/ respiratory acidosis and some w/ dec respiratory excursion

Etiologies (Pediatr Rev 2004;25:350; Pediatr Rev 2011;32:240)
- Can be divided into chloride responsive and chloride-unresponsive etiologies
- Chloride responsive (urinary Cl^- <10 mEq/L)
  - GI (emesis [pyloric stenosis], diarrhea, laxative abuse, villous adenoma, NGT suction)
  - Diuretics (loop and thiazide), PCN, CF, posthypercapnic
- Chloride unresponsive (urinary Cl^- >10 mEq/L)
  - Adrenal dysfunction (hyperaldosteronism or Cushing syndrome)
  - Exogenous steroids (glucocorticoids, mineralocorticoids, and licorice)
  - Inherited channelopathies (Bartter syndrome and Gitelman syndrome)
  - Alkali ingestion, large volume blood transfusions (due to citrate in blood)
  - Edematous states Rx'd w/ diuretics (e.g., CHF, cirrhosis, nephrotic syndrome)
  - Refeeding alkalosis
  - Hypokalemia

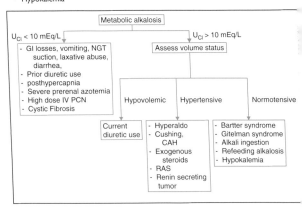

Management (Rose & Post. *Clinical Physiology of Acid-Base & Electrolyte Disorders* 2001:551; Pediatr Rev 2011:32:240)
- Rx underlying condition and correct met alkalosis by renal secretion of HCO_3^-
- For saline responsive etiologies, provide IV saline (monitor efficacy via urine pH [which is <5 before therapy and rises to >7 w/ repletion] and U_{Cl} [which rises above 10mEq/L with tx]) and replete K as needed
- For saline unresponsive etiologies
  - If edematous state (CHF, cirrhosis, nephrotic syndrome): Withhold diuretic if possible, acetazolamide, HCl, Arginine Chloride or dialysis
  - Hypokalemia: Replete K
  - Hyperaldosteronism: K-sparing diuretics/aldo antagonists or removal of parathyroid adenoma

Complications (Pediatr Rev 2004:25:350; Pediatr Rev 2011:32:240)
- Cardiac: Arteriolar constriction, refractory SVT, and ventricular arrhythmias
- Cerebral: Reduction of cerebral blood flow, tetany, seizures, lethargy, stupor
- Respiratory: Hypoventilation w/ hypercapnia and hypoxia
- Metabolic: HypoK, hypoMg and hypoPhos, stimulation of glycolysis, oxyhemoglobin dissociation curve shifts left

RESPIRATORY ACIDOSIS AND ALKALOSIS

Definition (Pediatr Rev 2004:25:350; Pediatr Rev 2011:32:240)
- Respiratory acidosis and alkalosis result from a $1°$ increase or decrease in PCO_2
  - Resp acidosis = PCO_2 >40 mm Hg, Resp alkalosis = PCO_2 <40 mm Hg)
  - Renal compensation takes about 3–5 d

Etiology (Pediatr Rev 2004:25:350; Pediatr Rev 2011:32:240)

Causes of Acute Respiratory Acidosis	Causes of Respiratory Alkalosis
Acute CNS Depression Drug O/D (benzos, narcotics, barbiturates) Head trauma, CVA, CNS infections	Hypoxia
	Mechanical ventilation
	Hyperventilation syndromes
Acute Neuromuscular Disease Guillain–Barré syndrome, myasthenic crisis Botulism, organophosphate poisoning Spinal cord injury	**Pregnancy** (2/2 progesterone)
	Parenchymal Lung Disease PNA, asthma, diffuse interstitial fibrosis Pulmonary embolism, pulmonary edema
Acute Airway Disease Status asthmaticus, upper airway obstruction	**Medications** Salicylate, xanthines (caffeine, theophylline), nicotine, catecholamines
Acute Parenchymal and Vascular Disease Pulmonary edema, acute lung injury Multilobar PNA	**Metabolic disorders** Sepsis, pyrexia, hepatic disease
Massive Pulmonary Embolism	**CNS Disorders** Meningitis, encephalitis, CVA
Acute Pleural or Chest Wall Disease Pneumothorax, hemothorax, flail chest, severe scoliosis, obesity hypoventilation syndrome	Head trauma Space-occupying lesion Anxiety

ACUTE ABDOMINAL PAIN

Definition (Silen W. Cope's Early Diagnosis of the Acute Abdomen. 20th ed. New York, NY: Oxford Univ. Press, 2000; Pediatr Rev. 2010;31:135)
- Abd pain 2/2 activation of visceral nerves (innervate hollow viscera & mesentery; poorly localizing), or somatic nerves (innervate parietal peritoneum; focal)
  - Parietal inflammation can be 2/2 worsening underlying visceral inflammation; presenting w/ generalized abd pain, which progressively localizes (i.e., appendicitis)
- Pain can be referred to abd from other structures (i.e., pleuritis in lower lobe PNA, *Strep.* pharyngitis) (Pediatr Clin North Am 2006;53:107)

Clinical Manifestations (BMJ 1969;1:284; Pediatr Rev. 2010;31:135)
- History w/ assoc sx, signs, & physical exam are important to narrow differential
- Concerning sx: Anorexia (appendicitis), bilious emesis (obstruction), rebound or guarding (peritonitis), assoc findings of palpable purpura (HSP) or ecchymosis on abdomen or back (pancreatitis). Fever can be concerning but nonspecific
- Localized pain can be helpful for localization, but is often nonspecific
  - RUQ: Gall bladder (GB) or hepatic/perihepatic disease, RLL PNA
  - LUQ: Stomach, LLL PNA, splenic dz (often w/ L shoulder pain)
  - Epigastrium: Stomach, small bowel, pancreatitis, mesenteric ischemia
  - RLQ: Appendicitis (starts periumbilical), ovarian disease in female, ileitis, colitis
  - LLQ: Colitis, ovarian disease in female
  - Suprapubic: UTI, PID
  - Radiating pain: To testicles or labia (nephrolithiasis), to back (pancreatitis, GB)
- Administration of analgesia does not impair clinical exam (Arch Dis Child 2008;93:995)

Etiology (Pediatr Clin North Am 2006;53:107)
- Etiologies and working differential varies based on age. See specific topics for Rx
  - **Gastroenteritis** (viral) & **constipation** most common benign causes for all ages
  - **Appendicitis** (see ED chapter); dx in 82% of children admitted w/ abd pain
    - Higher rates of perforation in children. Often mistaken for gastroenteritis
  - **Intussusception** (see ED chapter); most frequent btw 3 mo and 5 yr, 60% w/i 1st yr
    - Peak btw 6 and 11 mo. 60% p/w 2 of 3: Abd pain, vomiting, bloody mucous stool
  - **Small bowel obstruction:** Multi etiologies, most common 2/2 adhesions from prior surgery or incarcerated hernia; p/w abd pain, vomiting (bile), distention
  - **Incarcerated hernia:** 60% inguinal (R side) in 1st yr; p/w groin bulge
  - **Malrotation w/ midgut volvulus:** Highest incidence in 1st mo; often abd pain and bilious vomiting, but can be insidious. Surgical emergency
  - **Necrotizing enterocolitis:** Preterm but in full term as well; present in extremis
  - Consider systemic illnesses such as **sickle cell disease** and **DKA**

Diagnostic Studies
- Evaluation is dependent on history (associated symptoms & signs) & physical exam
- PMH of abd surgery raises risk of incarcerated hernia or obstruction 2/2 adhesion
- Always consider the possibility of child abuse

PEPTIC ULCER DISEASE (PUD)

Definition
- Damage to mucosal lining of upper GI tract 2/2 imbalance btw protective fxn of mucus and bicarb secretion and damage from gastric acid and pepsin, +/− external factors (NSAIDs, EtOH, other mucotoxic agents) or *H. pylori* infection

Pathology (Pediatr Rev 2001;22:349)
- Acid secretion is mediated by stimulation of parietal cells by acetylcholine (vagal), histamine, and gastrin (Zollinger–Ellison syndrome)
- *H. pylori* (gram-neg spiral rod) adapted to mucous layer; infxn possibly resulting in damage of intestinal mucosa 2/2 urease secretion (hydrolyzes urea to ammonia and bicarbonate) disrupts epithelial cell fxn; +/− vacuolating cytotoxin
- Non-*H. pylori*–related PUD on the rise, though ulcer disease in childhood still rare

Epidemiology (J Pediatr 2005;146:S21)
- *H. pylori* w/ ~50% prevalence worldwide (from 10% [US avg] to 80% w/ higher rates in lower socioeconomic groups); only 10–15% infected develop PUD
- Evidence suggests acquisition of *H. pylori* infection occurs in childhood (by 5–10 yo)
- Often FHx of PUD w/ evidence of vertical transmission; (Helicobacter. 2011;Supp 1:59)
- Other etiologies less common overall (can be more prevalent in inpts); stress related (severe illness, burn), 2/2 ↑ ICP (Cushing ulcer) or 2/2 NSAID and other drugs

Clinical Manifestations (Pediatr Rev 2001;22:349)
- Generally p/w recurrent epigastric pain and can be assoc w/ postprandial or nocturnal abd pain, vomiting or food regurgitation
- In severe cases can present with failure to thrive, upper GI bleed, or chronic anemia
- Controversial whether *H. pylori* infxn can cause acute abd pain; NSAID- and drug-induced gastritis and ulcer formation can (Pediatrics 1999;103:192)

Diagnostics (J Pediatr 2005;146:S21; Helicobacter 2011:Supp 1:59)
- Initial eval w/ CBC diff (assess for anemia), ESR (IBD), LFTs, electrolytes (if recurrent vomiting), and stool evaluation for O and P (if exposure/diarrhea)
- If PUD suspected, send *H. pylori* **IgG;** cannot distinguish btw current & prior infxn.
  - Sens 54–94%, spec 59–97% (assay dependent); neither sens nor spec in children 2/2 lower titer cutoffs, shorter durations of infection
- **Stool antigen** testing is highly sensitive (98–100%) and specific (99–100%) when using locally validated cutoff points for a given population
- **Urea breath testing (UBT):** Radio-labeled urea ingested, then CO_2 exhalation measured; good functional test and can be used to assess for cure. Sens 83.4%, Spec 99%
  - Less widely used in children 2/2 concerns about radiation
  - Can see false +, especially <3 yo, 2/2 discoordinated swallow (oral bacteria w/ urease too) Can see false neg if patient is already on Rx (acid suppression)
- Gold standard: Upper GI endoscopy and bx, radiographic UGI studies less sensitive

Treatment (J Pediatr Gastroenterol Nutr 2000;31:490)
- If *H. pylori* +; rx w/ PPI (1–2 mg/kg/d) w/ any 2 of the following: Amoxicillin 50 mg/kg/d, clarithromycin 15 mg/kg/d, and/or metronidazole 20 mg/kg/d
- Studies show 75–80% cure rate w/ 7 d of triple therapy, suggesting rx for 14 d
- Rx failure likely 2/2 abx resistance: Clarithro (18–35%), metro (15–20%)

Complications (J Pediatr 2005;146:S21)
- Atrophic gastritis +/– metaplasia; high risk if PPI use w/o eradication; gastric CA risk
- Gastric CA: 1% of *H. pylori* infected in adults; not reported in childhood
- Gastric mucosa-associated lymphoid tissue lymphoma (MALT): Rarer, only 0.1%

VOMITING

Definition (Pediatr Rev 2008;6:183)
- Reverse peristalsis 2/2 activation of vomiting center (VC) in medulla or chemoreceptor trigger zone (CTZ) in area postrema (floor IVth ventricle)

Etiology (Pediatr Rev 2008;6:183)
- See chart on next page.

Clinical Manifestations
- Assess for dehydration; Mod (5–10% BW) w/ irritability, cool ext, dry mucous membranes, sunken eyes, dec skin turgor (1–2 sec skin pinch), Severe (>10% BW) w/ lethargy, >2 sec skin pinch, cold ext, deep acidotic breathing, HoTN, tachycardia

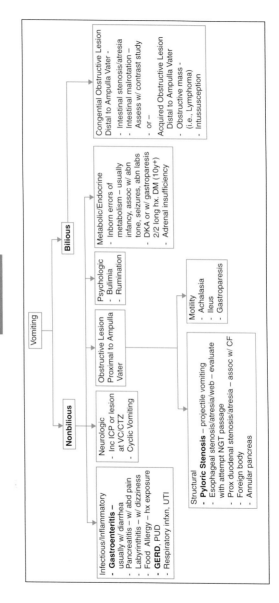

Vomiting

Nonbilious

Bilious

Infectious/Inflammatory
- **Gastroenteritis** –
  usually w/ diarrhea
- Pancreatitis – w/ abd pain
- Labyrinthitis – w/ dizziness
- Food Allergy – hx exposure
- **GERD**, PUD
- Respiratory infxn, UTI

Neurologic
- Inc ICP or lesion
  at VC/CTZ
- Cyclic Vomiting

Obstructive Lesion
Proximal to Ampulla
Vater

Psychologic
- Bulimia
- Rumination

Metabolic/Endocrine
- Inborn errors of
  metabolism – usually
  infancy, assoc w/ abn
  tone, seizures, abn labs
- DKA or w/ gastroparesis
  2/2 long hx. DM (10y+)
- Adrenal insufficiency

Congential Obstructive Lesion
Distal to Ampulla Vater -
- Intestinal stenosis/atresia
- Intestinal malrotation –
  Assess w/ contrast study
- or –
Acquired Obstructive Lesion
Distal to Ampulla Vater
- Obstructive mass -
  (i.e., Lymphoma)
- Intussusception

Structural
- **Pyloric Stenosis** – projectile vomiting
- Esophageal stenosis/atresia/web – evaluate
  with attempt NGT passage
- Prox duodenal stenosis/atresia – assoc w/ CF
- Foreign body
- Annular pancreas

Motility
- Achalasia
- Ileus
- Gastroparesis

Diagnosis & Treatment (Am Fam Physician 2000;61:2791; J Pediatr Gastroenterol Nutr 2001;32:S12; Pediatr Rev 2008:6:183)

- Definitive management as well as diagnostic testing depends on underlying etiology
- **Nonbilious emesis:** Generally less concerning; some emergencies, pyloric stenosis
- **Bilious emesis** is almost always concerning sx warranting further evaluation
  - NGT placement for decompression if obstruction suspected
  - Diagnostic evaluation varies but generally includes KUB and/or UGI
  - W/ neonate, bilious emesis can indicate surgical disease
  - **Duodenal atresia:** Congenital obstruction of 2nd part of duodenum, 2/2 failure to recanalize in utero, vomiting w/i hrs; pregnancy often w/ polyhydramnios
    - 1 in 5,000–10,000 and M > F, seen in 1/4 Down's syndrome pts, 20% w/ CDH
    - Membranous or interrupted lesion at papilla of Vater (PV), 80% w/ PV open to proximal duodenum resulting in bilious emesis.
    - KUB w/ "double bubble": Gastric air bubble and distended prox duodenum
    - Surgery necessary but not urgent (<48 hr) if decompressed w/ NGT and IVFs
  - **Midgut malrotation and volvulus:** Midgut rotated clockwise around SMA/V, can cause obstruction/ischemia/infarction
    - Usually p/w volvulus in 1st 3–7 d w/ bilious emesis +/– abd distention; majority w/i 1st yr of life but can present at older age (recurrent abd pain)
    - Imaging: U/S w/ jejunal "spiral" or UGI w/ malpositioned SMA/V or ligament of Treitz (normally to L of spine)
    - Needs urgent surgery (separation of Ladd band); if early, excellent prognosis
    - Complications: 2/2 gut ischemia → resection and short gut syndrome
  - **Jejunoileal atresia:** Mesenteric vascular accident in utero → segmental infarct
    - 4 types of abnormalities: Membranous, interrupted, apple peel, and multiple
    - All w/ same sx; abd distention and bilious emesis w/i first 24 hr
    - Abdominal films w/ air-fluid levels proximal to obstruction
    - Can be complicated by meconium peritonitis; intense inflammation resulting in calcifications, vascular fibrous proliferation, and cyst formation
  - **Meconium ileus:** 90–95% have CF, but only 15% CF pts have hx of mec ileus
    - KUB w/ distended loops, thickened wall, filled w/ "ground glass"
    - Can rx w/ Gastrografin (successful in 16–50%)
- **Treatment of nausea:** Based on etiology (N Engl J Med 2005;352:817)
  - GI tract irritation or distention: Via vagal and/or glossopharyngeal afferents (i.e., 2/2 constipation, NSAIDs, mucositis 2/2 chemo, stimulated via $5HT_3R$; rx with ondansetron, ($5HT_3R$ blocker) steroids to dec inflammation (mucositis)
  - Vestibular tract irritation (i.e., labyrinthitis): Stimulated via H_1R and muscarinic receptors; rx w/ antihistamine or anticholinergics
  - CTZ; sampling blood for emetogens (BBB absent here): Stimulated via D_2R
    - Emetogens can be endogenous (tumor, azotemia, HoNa) or exogenous (opioids, chemo); rx w/ haloperidol > phenothiazines (compazine)
  - Higher CNS center involvement: Can activate or suppress; rx anxiolytics
  - All stimulate VC (final common pathway): Stimulated by parasymp and H_1R, acts via parasymp and motor efferents

GASTROESOPHAGEAL REFLUX DISEASE (GERD)

Definition (J Pediatr Gastroenterol Nutr 2009;49:498)
- Passage of gastric contents to esophagus, nml & w/o sx (GER), or pathologic (GERD)

Pathophysiology (Pediatr Rev 2007;3:101)
- Intermittent relaxation of LES, acid refluxing to esophagus w/ esophagitis, chronically causes change from columnar to squamous (Barrett)

Epidemiology
- Prevalence physiologic reflux ~50% at 0–3 mo, 67% by 4 mo, 5% at 12 mo, and in children 3–17 yo, rates vary from 1.4–8.2%

Clinical Manifestation: Varies By Age
- **Infants:** Vomiting, FTT, irritability, congestion, ALTE, recurrent PNAs
- **Children/adolescent:** Abd pain, retrosternal CP, dysphagia, regurg, asthma/cough

Diagnostic Studies
- H&P only, unless complications present or dx in question; in infants H&P not diagnostic
- UGI: Not sensitive or specific for GERD but identifies malrotation, esophageal/antral webs, pyloric stenosis, Schatzki rings, hiatal hernia

- Esophageal pH probe: Checks freq and duration of acid exposure. Reflux index (RI) = % time pH <4 (most valid tool), upper nml 0–11 mo 11.7%, 1–9 yo 5.4%, adults 6%
- Endoscopy: Visualize and bx esophagus and duodenum for inflamm and complications
- Empiric Rx: For older children/adolescents widely used (up to 4 wk) but not validated

Treatment (J Pediatr Gastroenterol Nutr 2005;41:S41)
- Evidence for 2 wk trial of hypoallergenic hydrolyzed protein formula for formula-fed infants
- Thickening does not improve RI, does dec # of vomiting events (Pediatrics 2008; 122:e1268)
- Positioning (if >1 yr): Left-side positioning and elevation of head of bed in sleep
- Lifestyle Δ (adoles): No caffeine, chocolate, spicy food, tobacco, EtOH; not data-driven
- Acid suppression: **PPIs > H$_2$RAs;** if long-term PPI, check for H. pylori (risk of atrophic gastritis w/ chronic >6 mo PPI use and untreated H. pylori) (Pediatr Rev 2003;24:12)
  - **Space dosing of PPIs and H$_2$RAs** as PPI require acidic environment for activation
  - Majority of children develop tachyphylaxis to H$_2$RAs w/i 2 wk
  - There is evidence we are over prescribing (Pediatrics 2007;120:946)
- Prokinetic: Aside from cisapride (limited access 2/2 side effects) no prokinetics w/ benefit
- Surgical Rx: Case series show generally favorable outcomes

Prognosis: Most outgrow sx by 12 mo; poorer prognosis w/ neuro impairment, esophageal atresia, prematurity.

Complications
- Respiratory (asthma, apnea, ALTE, cough), ENT (sinusitis, dental erosions, laryngitis), esophageal strictures, Barrett, adenoCA, UGI bleeding, FTT, Sandifer syndrome
- ~$^2/_3$ of children w/ asthma improve to some degree w/ rx for GERD
- Neurologically impaired at high risk of recurrent aspiration (PNA, pulm fibrosis)

PYLORIC STENOSIS

Definition (Pediatr Rev 2000;21:249; Adv Pediatr 2011;58:195)
- Gastric outlet obstruction 2/2 hypertrophy and edema of pyloric canal, and antropyloric distension and muscle spasm → vomiting, dehydration, and hypochloremic, hypokalemic, metabolic alkalosis; thought to be an acquired condition

Epidemiology
- Incidence of 1 in 250–1,000, M 4–8× > F, Caucasian predilection

Clinical Manifestations
- Mean age 3 wk, but anytime birth to 5 mo; begins w/ regurgitation → nonbilious vomiting +/- projectile vomiting
- Classically w/ "olive-like" mass palpated in epigastric region, pathognomonic; not always appreciable; exam enhanced by NGT decomp and prone positioning

Diagnostic Studies
- U/S is study of choice, pyloric thickness >4 mm, length >16 mm w/ sens 89%, spec 100% may need repeat U/S given operator variability
- Most common cause of metabolic alkalosis in infancy; hypochloremic metabolic alkalosis 2/2 acid loss from vomiting and decreased HCO$_3$ secretion
- Excess bicarb can be excreted in urine w/ obligate Na loss, followed by H$_2$O, also 2° hyperaldo 2/2 inc renin release causes distal H$^+$ secretion and paradoxic aciduria
- Can have low or nml K but usually total body K depletion

Treatment
- Reverse metabolic derangements and volume status
- Pyloromyotomy is curative, incision through serosa and mucosal layer. Essentially 100% success rate

GASTROINTESTINAL BLEEDING

Definition (Pediatr Rev 2008;29:39)
- Intraluminal bleeding at any site from oropharynx to the anus; definition of upper GI bleed as proximal to the ligament of Treitz and lower GI bleed as distal

- Can p/w bloody vomit (hematemesis), "coffee ground" emesis, hematochezia (BRBPR; LGIB, or rapid UGIB [>20% blood volume]) or melena (tarry black 2/2 digestion, darkness correlates w/ time to pass); r/o other site (nasopharynx)
- Check for false coloring; red food coloring, fruit juice, beets can make vomit or stool red. Pepto-Bismol, iron, grape juice, spinach, and blueberry can make it black

Etiology of Upper GI Bleed (Clin Pediatr (Phila) 2007;46:16)

Differential of UGIB

	Common	Uncommon
Neonate	• Swallowed maternal blood (use Apt–Downey test w/ KOH, color Δ w/ maternal blood) • Milk protein allergy • Traumatic NGT placement	• Hemorrhagic dz of newborn • Esophagitis • Vascular malformation • Sepsis w/ coagulopathy • Congenital coagulopathy
Infant	• Esophagitis 2/2 GERD	• Stress ulcer/gastritis • Acid peptic disease • GI duplication • Gastric/esophageal varices
Child	• Esophageal varices • Acid peptic dz • Gastritis (H. pylori, NSAID) • Caustic ingestion, Mallory–Weiss	• Bowel obstruction • Crohn's disease • Hemobilia • Vasculitis

Etiology of Lower GI Bleed (Pediatr Emerg Care 2002;18:319)

- **Anal fissure:** Most common cause LGIB <2 yo. Blood coated stool. Painful. Constipation
- **Nodular lymphoid hyperplasia:** Painless rectal bleeding, usually after viral illness, can be associated with immunodef (IgA def, hypogamma)
- **Food allergy:** 3 different mechanisms; cow's milk and soy most likely offenders
  - Enterocolitis: Vomiting, bloody diarrhea; +/– malabsorption, FTT
  - Colitis: 1st few mos of life, healthy, normal weight w/ blood in stool
  - Eosinophilic gastroenteritis: Infiltration w/ eos, peripheral eos, no vasculitis, p/w postprandial N/V, abd pain, watery diarrhea +/– blood, anemia, FTT
- **Necrotizing enterocolitis:** Risk factors, prematurity, sepsis, LBW, HoTN, asphyxia
- **Infectious enterocolitis:** Bacterial, viral, or parasitic pathogens. C. diff w/ abx hx
- **Hirschsprung disease:** 10–30% develop enterocolitis w/ fever, bloody diarrhea
- **Meckel diverticulum:** 2/2 incomplete obliteration of omphalomesenteric duct
  - Painless passage of large amt of blood; otherwise healthy (2/2 heterotopic gastric mucosa in diverticulum causing adjacent ileal mucosa ulceration)
  - "Rule of 2s"; 2% pop, 2 in. long, 2 cm diameter, w/i 2 ft of ileocecal junction, w/ types of ectopic tissue (gastric and pancreatic), 2:1 M:F, and 50% w/ sx before 2 yo
  - Duplication of bowel same as Meckel but on mesenteric side, not antimesenteric
- **Intussusception:** Usually <2 yo, colicky abd pain, "sausage-shaped" abd mass w/ late finding of "currant jelly stool." See ED chapter
- **Polyps:** Outside of infants these are **most common source for painless LGIB**
  - **Painless rectal bleeding**
  - Juvenile polyps (95% of polyps in children) are 90% hamartomatous (benign) usually singular but multiple (>5 polyps) seen in juvenile polyposis, Peutz–Jeghers (mucocutaneous pigmentation; higher rate GI CA but not 2/2 polyps) and Cowden syndrome
  - Adenomatous polyps can be premalignant; found in familial polyposis (AD but 1 in 3 new mutation; sx after 10 yo), Gardner syndrome (AD; soft tissue/bone tumors) and Turcot syndrome
- **IBD:** Almost all UC and ¼ of Crohn have LGIB, 1 in 4 present before 20 yo
- **Angiodysplasia:** Vascular ectasia; assoc syndromes (Osler–Weber–Rendu, Turner)
- **Hemorrhoids:** Rare in childhood, assess for portal HTN; common after adolescence
- **Henoch–Schönlein purpura:** Typically 4–7 yo (but any age) systemic small vessel vasculitis w/ abd pain and bloody stools, "palpable purpura." +/– renal and joint
  - GI involvement in 45–75% cases and can precede skin findings in 15% of cases
  - IgA immune complex mediated
- **HUS:** Microangiopathic hemolytic anemia, thrombocytopenia, ARF usually preceded (3–16 d) by bloody diarrhea. (90% D + HUS w/ shiga-like toxin vs. atypical HUS/D – HUS w/o)
- **Ischemia:** 2/2 midgut volvulus, intussusception, etc.; generally ill appearing

Clinical Manifestations

Tachycardia most sensitive sign of acute, severe blood loss; orthostasis w/ >20 bpm ↑
HoTN and decreased capillary refill are ominous late findings (>30% blood vol loss)

- With infants who are breast-feeding, ask mother about presence of breast lesions
- Hemorrhagic disease of newborn; hx – child born athome, no vit K presents DOL 1–5
- Variceal bleed 2/2 extrahepatic portal HTN; no cirrhotic stigmata, + splenomegaly
  - Extrahepatic portal HTN 2/2 omphalitis 2/2 neonatal umbilical vein catheter or spontaneous inflammation of umbilical vessels
- Check skin for petechiae or purpura (coagulopathy or HSP), spider angiomata (liver dz), hemangiomas or telangiectasias (Osler–Weber–Rendu)

Diagnostic Studies (Pediatr Rev 2008;29:39)
- Confirm w/ hemoccult for stool guaiac or gastroccult w/ vomitus
- False pos w/ vit C, red meat, veg w/ peroxidase (broccoli, radish, turnips)
- NGT lavage useful if returns blood/coffee grounds = UGIB; can miss duodenal ulcer; if clears w/ lavage, then likely active bleeding has ceased
- Isolated increase in BUN can be a sign of gastric bleeding and absorption
- Plain films: KUB/upright for free air (perforation), pneumatosis intestinalis (NEC), air–fluid levels (obstruction)
- For LGIB w/ sx of colitis check stool cx for Yersinia, Salmonella, Shigella, Campylobacter, Aeromonas, E. coli (including O157:H7), Klebsiella oxytoca, C. diff, perirectal swab for N. gonorrhoeae (if sexually active), & O&P for E. histolytica & T. trichiura (if appt travel hx)
- Upper GI and small bowel follow through best for structural lesions
- Endoscopy: Indicated w/ acute UGIB necessitating transfusion or recurrent bleeding or as first step in diagnosis and evaluation of any GIB; contraindicated in clinically unstable patient
  - Retrospective studies show w/ EGD 5 most common dx = duodenal ulcer (20%), gastric ulcer (18%), esophagitis (15%), gastritis (13%), and varices (10%) in children and adolescents (Pediatrics 1979;63:408)
- Rectosigmoidoscopy/colonoscopy: Useful if not active major bleeding
  - Most helpful to assess IBD, angiodysplasia, polyps, pseudomembranous colitis
- Barium enema: For Hirschsprung dz, dx and rx of intussusception
- Nuclear medicine (Technetium-99 pertechnetate): Labels ectopic gastric mucosa, best for Meckel diverticulum or intestinal duplication
  - Can also do Technetium-99 RBC scan for bleeding (0.05–0.1 mL/min)
- Angiography: Must be >0.5 mL/min for detection
  - Can be used for guiding therapeutic approach, i.e., coiling
  - Indicated over EGD for hemobilia (bleeding from biliary tract)
- Abdominal U/S +/– Doppler: For specific evaluation (i.e., liver dz or portal HTN)
- In immune compromised consider assessment for CMV, HSV, or Candida esophagitis

Treatment
- **Acute management:** Volume resuscitation w/ 2 large bore IVs, IV bolus w/ NS or LR transfusion, if present, correct coagulopathies (FFP, platelets)
- **UGIB:** Basically 2 sources (1) Mucosal (-itis, ulcers, Mallory–Weiss) (2) Variceal
  - Mucosal: Neutralize/decrease acid production (PPIs > H_2RA); w/ Mallory–Weiss can coagulate w/ thermal probe or inject dilute epinephrine
  - Variceal: Acute bleeding stops spontaneously in 50% w/ rebleed in 40%
    - Stop bleeding (band ligation > sclerotherapy by risk profile)
    - Decrease portal pressure and splanchnic blood flow: Octreotide > vasopressin
- **LGIB:** Etiology specific (stool softener for fissure, abx for infectious colitis, rsxn for polyps)

ACUTE DIARRHEA

Definition (Pediatr Rev 1989;11:6)
- > nml stool output (>10 cc/kg/d) or Δ in character, usually ↑ # BMs/d; WHO crit >3 stools/c
- Young infants have intestinal mucosa permeable to water; have greater net fluid loss
- 80% fluid absorption at small bowel; processes affecting SB have rapid dehydration
- Generally duration <14 d; longer than 14 d considered persistent/chronic diarrhea

Pathophysiology (Arch Dis Child 1997;77:201)
- 4 basic processes: Secretory, cytotoxic, osmotic, and inflammatory
- **Secretory:** 2/2 infectious enterotoxin (cholera, ETEC), metabolic/endocrine (hyperthyroid VIPoma, ZES), or exogenous toxic agent (colchicines)
  - Enterotoxin → ↑ secretion fluids/lytes via mucosal crypt cells or blocks villi absorp
- **Cytotoxic:** 2/2 destruction of mucosal cells of small intestine, generally 2/2 viral infection (rota, Norwalk), similar changes in celiac disease, can result in 2° osmotic diarrhea

- **Osmotic:** Seen in malabsorptive conditions, unabsorbed substance in lumen reaches osmotically active concentration causing water influx (i.e., lactose intolerance)
  - Determined by fecal osmotic gap (FOG) = serum osm − 2(stool Na + stool K)
  - FOG >100–120 is osmotic diarrhea; use serum osm to avoid error 2/2 transit time. If serum osm unavailable, can use stool osm but less accurate
- **Inflammatory:** 2/2 damage to intestinal lining w/ bloody stools, fecal leukocytes, and tenesmus, generally involves large intestine and terminal ileum
  - Invasive organisms: *Yersinia, Campylobacter, Salmonella, Shigella,* EHEC

Etiology

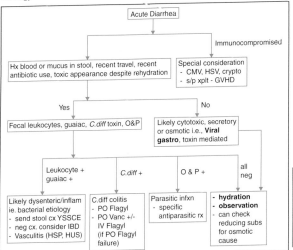

History
- Hx recent consumption raw milk, salad, undercooked meat/poultry, unpurified H_2O, recent Abx, immunocompromised, sick contacts, FHx GI dz (IBD), blood in stool

Clinical Manifestation
- In absence of bloody stools, hydration is $1°$ determinant of severity
  - Check glucose (r/o DKA), and U/A (r/o UTI)
- With bloody diarrhea, need to rule out life-threatening conditions, surgical disease
  - Intussusception: 6–12 mo (up to 2 yr), intermittent severe abd pain; "currant jelly stool" (late finding, vascular congestion/ischemia), palpable "sausage" on exam
  - *C. diff* colitis: Hx of recent antibiotic use, labs w/ inc WBC, fever, abd distention

Diagnostic Evaluation
- **Fecal leukocytes:** W/ methylene blue >1 WBC/HPF; 52% sens, 88% spec for +stool cx (outpts only), for *C. diff* 14% sens, 90% spec (J Clin Microbiol 2001;39:266)
- **C. diff toxin:** ELIZA; 73.3% sens, 97.6% spec, PCR 93.3% sens, 97.4% spec (Clin Infect Dis 2007;45:1152). Pts <1 yr generally w/ asymp carriage
- **O&P:** Single test sens 72%, but 93% NPV if prevalence of infxn <20% in pop; gold std 3 samples (Clin Infect Dis 2006;42:972)
- **Stool culture:** Gold standard but important to assess which agents involved
- **Fecal Osm Gap** = Stool Osm − 2([stool Na] − [stool K]), >100–120 osmotic diarrhea; <100 secretory diarrhea
- **Stool-reducing substances:** Benedict test w/ hydrolysis assesses for reducing sugars (malabsorption) in stool; 72% sens, 73% spec (Arch Dis Child 1997;77:201)
- **Fecal elastase-1:** Test to differentiate pancreatic from nonpancreatic steatorrhea; only 68% sens and 59% spec for pancreatic insufficiency (Neth J Med 2004;62:286)
- **Rotavirus ELISA:** 70–98% sens, 71–100% spec (Pediatr Rev 2007;28:183)

- Etiology dependent; generally supportive mgmt always a component
- ORT is as effective as IVF in >95% of cases for mild to moderate dehydration
- Early refeeding w/ milk or food after rehydration does not prolong diarrhea (CD007296); may reduce duration of diarrhea by $1/2$ d though not proven
- Routine use of antidiarrheals is not supported and may have serious consequences
- Bacterial/presumed bacterial colitis; abx if severe dz or if pt immunocompromised, hx of chronic GI disease (Infect Dis Clin North Am 2005;19:585)
  - Abx shorten course Shigella, no effect on Campylobacter, may prolong Salmonella
  - Reported inc risk of HUS following abx for EHEC, not seen in meta-analysis
  - C. diff: Rx w/ metronidazole +/- PO Vanco × 10 d beyond other abx; 40% need re-Rx

Complications
- Hemolytic uremic syndrome: Microangiopathic hemolytic anemia, ↓ plts, fever, ARF, after bloody diarrhea 2/2 E. coli O157:H7; 5–10% ~5–10 d after diarrhea
- Shigella assoc w/ CNS sx (incl szr, obtundation, death, Ekiri syndrome), reactive arthritis (HLA-B27+) and myocarditis
- Campylobacter associated w/ Guillain–Barré syndrome
- Postenteritis enteropathy: Loss of intestinal digestive and absorptive functions
  - Can be of variable severity from lactose intolerance to total dysfunction
  - Hx of recurrent diarrhea and FTT in infant
  - ↑ risk if no breast-feeding, use of hypotonic rehydration or restriction of intake
  - Rx w/ lactose-free, sucrose-free, full strength formula, support volume status w/ IVF, may need TPN/PPN as well; usually w/ complete recovery

CHRONIC DIARRHEA

Definition (Pediatr Rev 2005;26:5)
- No consistent duration separates chronic from acute; generally >2 wk to 1 mo

Etiology (Curr Opin Gastroenterol 2011;27:19; Pediatr Rev 2005;26:5)
- Studies demonstrate persistent/chronic diarrhea account for 5–18% of diarrheal cases
- **Congenital:** Rare, generally presents w/i 1st yr of life if not sooner
  - Structural abnormality: Chronic SBO or malrotation. Dx w/ radiology
  - Microvillus inclusion disease: Presents on DOL 1 w/ large volume watery diarrhea (continues w/ NPO); no cure, need TPN/PPN, death in infancy
- **Acquired:** More common, higher risk w/ immune compromise
  - **Viral diarrhea:** Mean duration is 6 d in absence of immune dysfunction
  - **Bacterial diarrhea:** Mean duration is 14 d but some agents much longer
    - Nontyphoid Salmonella in neonates can cause several mos of diarrhea
    - Exposure to untreated water, shellfish: Aeromonas spp, Plesiomonas
  - **Parasitic:** Immunocompetent or -compromised, often occult fecal exposure
    - Giardia is most common in US, 2/2 exposure to feces
      - Associated sx: Malaise, flatulence, abd distention, only $1/3$ w/ vomiting
      - ~$1/4$ w/ intermittent symptoms; avg duration in immunocompetent $1^1/2$ mo
      - Small % immunocompetent get prolonged sx, FTT, stunting up to 2+ yr
    - Cryptosporidium: 2+ wks. Rarely found on O&P, need fecal antigen test, generally assoc w/ immunosupressed
    - Cyclospora: Generally w/ immunocompromised; classically unpasteurized apple cider or imported raspberries
- Immune mediated: Food allergy or celiac disease; + exposure and IgE or Ab testing
- Immunodeficiency states often present w/ chronic diarrhea 2/2 chronic infection w/ one of the above agents, CVID, SCID, HIV, X-linked Bruton agammaglobulinemia, CGD (looks like Crohn's), Wiskott–Aldrich (IBD-like)
- Complication of acute gastroenteritis seen mostly in developing world; generally due to resulting malnutrition and micronutrient deficiencies

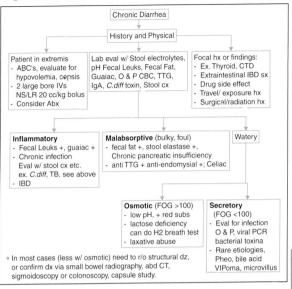

Treatment
• Highly dependent on etiology; see specific etiology subheadings where included

CELIAC DISEASE

Definition (N Engl J Med 2007;357:1731)
• Autoimmune enteropathy caused by a reaction to gluten in the diet resulting in effacement of the small bowel absorptive surface with resultant malabsorption

Pathophysiology
• Gliadin is the alcohol-soluble portion of gluten, is poorly digested in humans, and can pass through epithelial barrier of intestines (2/2 genetic susceptibility or infection)
• Adaptive immune (CD4 + T cells) and innate immune (NK cells) systems recognize gliadin bound HLA class II; trigger inflam w/ villous injury and crypt hypertrophy
• Tissue transglutaminase (TTG) enzyme deaminates gliadin, increasing inflammation

Epidemiology (J Pediatr Gastroenterol Nutr 2004;39:S601)
• Prevalence reaches 1 in 100–250 in some countries; classically thought most prevalent in Caucasian population (European ancestry), but dz worldwide

Clinical Manifestations (Gastroenterology 2005;128:S68)
• Classic picture malabsorption w/ bulky stools, abd distention and flatus, FTT, muscle wasting and hypotonia presenting in first 6 mo to 2 yr of life
  • Celiac crisis; now rare, acute explosive watery diarrhea and severe dehydration
• Silent disease; likely the large majority given prevalence rates
• Nonclassic sx; presents later (5–7 yo) w/ range sx, recurrent abd pain, N/V, constipation, aphthous ulcers, arthritis, skin dz (dermatitis herpetiformis), enamel defects, delayed puberty, short stature, or abnormal LFTs
• Syndrome of epilepsy w/ occipital calcifications and celiac disease
• Noted associations with other autoimmune diseases: DM type I, thyroiditis, Sjögren
• Down, Turner, (Williams pts w/ 3–10% prevalence of celiac)

Diagnostic Studies (N Engl J Med 2007;357:1731)
- European Society of Pediatric Gastroenterology and Nutrition requires a single small bowel bx w/ crypt hyperplasia, villous atrophy and intraepithelial lymphocytes as well as + response to a gluten-free diet (Gastro 2005;128:S98)
  - Limitations: Patchiness of disease (limitation of bx), lack of compliance w/ diet
  - Villous atrophy also seen w/ Crohn's, food allergy, HIV enteropathy, TB, giardia, intestinal lymphoma, CVID, and radiation enteritis
  - May not need bx; anti-TTG >100 U/mL w/ symptom improvement w/ gluten-free diet predicted 127 of 128 bx proven cases (J Pediatr Gastroenterol Nutr 2011;52:554)
- Most specific serologic marker is **antiendomysial antibody**; approaching 100%
- Combined sensitivity of anti-TTG and antiendomysial antibodies is >90%; **TTG** is less operator-dependent and cheaper; **best single study to send**
- Antigliadin antibodies not sensitive enough, except in <18 mo
- Assoc of HLA-DQ2/DQ8 & serologic markers w/ sens 98.8%, spec 96.2%, (J Pediatr Gastroenterol Nutr 2011;52:729)
- Check IgA levels as IgA deficiency is 10× more common in celiac patients
  - IgA deficiency has false negative anti-TTG and antiendomysial Abs; can check IgG

Treatment
- Eliminate all gluten (wheat, rye, and barley); very difficult, oats can be contaminated

Complications (N Engl J Med 2007;357:1731)
- Osteoporosis: Initially thought to be 2/2 vit D and Ca++ deficiency; now felt may be 2/2 associated inflammation as lifelong gluten-free diet is preventative
- Cancer: Overall rates are 2× rest of populations but decrease rate of breast CA
  - Specifically ↑ risk of adenoCa of small intestine and enteropathy assoc T-cell lymphoma as adults; risk ↓ w/ diet adherence
- Refractory sprue: 5% w/ continued symptoms and histology regardless of diet
  - Inc risk of enteropathy associated T-cell lymphoma if w/ clonal expansion

INFLAMMATORY BOWEL DISEASE (IBD)

Definition (Pediatr Rev 2005;26:314; Pediatr Rev 2011;32:14)
- **Crohn's dz (CD):** Transmural inflam anywhere w/i alimentary tract mouth to anus
- **Ulcerative colitis (UC):** Consists of contiguous mucosal inflammation of the colon
- **Indeterminate colitis (IC):** Unique subset of patients who tend to present with aggressive disease limited to the colon, w/ rapid progression to pancolitis
- Not uncommon for these distinct dzs to present diagnostic dilemma

Pathophysiology
- Onset and progression likely involve inherited susceptibility to aberrant immune response (excess Th1 in CD, excess Th2 in UC) to various intralumenal antigens
- Multiple susceptibility loci (NOD2/CARD15, IBD5, IBD3, DLG5, IL23R, ATG16L1)
- **CD** w/ "skip lesions," transmural extension of inflam & architectural distortion, cryptitis, edema, and noncaseating granulomas (pathognomonic, seen <25% biopsies)
- **UC** w/ rectal inflam that spreads proximally and may involve entire colon (10% ulcerative proctitis; 50% pancolitis), accumulation of PMNs in colonic crypts (cryptitis), concomitant ulceration, edema, and hemorrhage

Epidemiology (Gastroenterology 2004;126:1550; J Pediatr 2005;146:35)
- ~20–25% of pts w/ IBD present <18 yo, M = F. (Slight male preponderance in CD)
- In CD, ♀s tend to more severe dz; ♂ ↑ chance of growth failure (Pediatrics 2007;120:e1418; Pediatr Rev 2011;32:14)
- #1 risk factor is having a 1st-degree relative with IBD (~25% of pts; w/ 10–13× ↑ risk)
- Incidence 5 to 11 per 100,000 children w/ mean age of dx in US of 12.5 yo
- Highest incidence in Ashkenazi Jews, ↑ingly dx'd in blacks, ↓ in Asians; recent pediatric studies show no differences in rates of IBD due to ethnicity (J Pediatr 2003;143:525)
- Smoking positively correlated with CD and can worsen dz activity
- Smoking, hx of appendectomy (N Engl J Med 2001;344:808) negatively correlated w/ UC

Disease	0–2 yr	3–5 yr	6–12 yr	13–17 yr	Total
CD	36%	35%	60%	66%	58%
UC	31%	47%	28%	25%	29%
IC	33%	18%	12%	9%	13%
p value	0.814	<0.0001	<0.0001	<0.0001	

Adapted from the Pediatric IBD Consortium Registry (1/1/00 – 11/1/02) [n = 1370].

Clinical Manifestation

- **UC:** Bloody diarrhea, peri-defecatory abdominal pain, tenesmus, N/V
- **CD:** Abd pain, diarrhea, weight loss, N/V, oral & perianal dz (fistulae, abscesses)
- Growth failure may be presenting symptom (5%); impaired linear growth in >35%
- **Extraintestinal manifestations may precede GI symptoms by yrs in 1/3 of patients**
  - **Const:** Fever (CD >> UC), weight loss, growth retardation, delayed puberty
  - **HEENT:** Uveitis, scleritis, episcleritis, keratitis, retinal vascular dz, aphthous ulcers, glossitis (B_{12} deficiency)
  - **CV:** Pericarditis, myocarditis, heart block, thrombophlebitis, vasculitis (including arteritis and arterial occlusion)
  - **Pulmonary:** Bronchitis, pulmonary fibrosis, abnormal PFTs
  - **GI:** Fatty liver dz, primary sclerosing cholangitis → cholangiocarcinoma (UC >> CD), chronic autoimmune hepatitis, portal fibrosis, cirrhosis, cholelithiasis, Budd-Chiari syndrome, pancreatitis, anal fissures, and fistulae
  - **Renal:** Nephrolithiasis (oxalate stones in ileal dz), enterovesical or enteroureteral fistulae (**CD**), immune complex GN, renal tubular dz
  - **Musculoskeletal:** Arthralgias, arthritis, ankylosing spondylitis, sacroiliitis, hypertrophic osteoarthropathy, osteopenia, osteoporosis, AVN, polymyositis
  - **Hematologic:** Anemia (iron, B_{12}, folate def, or AIH), leukocytosis, TTP, thrombocytosis/thrombocytopenia, hypercoag, and portal vein thrombosis
  - **Neurologic:** Peripheral neuropathy, myelopathy, myasthenia gravis, cerebrovascular disorders (venous sinus thrombosis)
  - **Skin:** Erythema nodosum (CD > UC), pyoderma gangrenosum (<5% UC), acrodermatitis enteropathica, purpura, hair loss, brittle nails

Diagnostic Studies

- Dx rests on clinical, radiologic, endoscopic, serologic, and histologic data
- Lab eval w/ CBC, LFTs, amylase, lipase, ESR, CRP (10–15% w/ nml ESR, CRP), nutrition studies (albumin, total protein, Fe panel, Ca/Mg/Phos, Zn, AP, folate, B_{12}), stool studies (fecal α1-AT, leukocytes, culture, O&P, *C. diff*)
- Nml ESR or CRP do not r/o IBD; however, abn ESR, albumin, platelets, Hgb, or blood in stool 94% sensitive (Pediatrics 2007;119:1113)
- In **CD**, abnormal studies do not correlate with extent of dz
- In **UC**, direct correlation btw severity, extent bowel inflam, # abn labs (Pediatrics 2007;119:1113); severity score like PUCAI may predict response to Rx (Gastroenterology 2010;138:2282)
- Serological studies w/ poor sens, but good spec. May help distinguish CD vs. UC. ASCA highly spec for CD, pANCA more suggestive UC (vs. colon-limited CD)
- Imaging; abd plain films, UGI w/ SBFT, contrast abd CT, CT colo, WBC scan, DEXA
  - MRI w/ ↑ing role (no radiation) w/ sens & spec >90% for small intestine CD
- Endoscopic studies include EGD, colonoscopy, capsule endoscopy, double-balloon enteroscopy. EGD should be considered even in absence of UGI symptoms
- Mucosal biopsies provide invaluable information, often needed to clinch dx

Treatment (Pediatr Rev 2000;21:291)

- Involves nutrition, pharmacotherapy, psychological therapy, surgery, and surveillance
- Dietary manipulation is a cornerstone to sx management (highly variable; some may need to avoid lactose, caffeine, fatty foods, fresh fruits and vegetables, nuts, seeds)
- Screen and treat growth failure and malnutrition, including micronutrient deficiencies— esp Fe, folate (methotrexate, mesalamine), B_{12} (gastric, ileal dz), zinc, vit D
- Complementary/unconventional therapies with positive or mixed data include fish oil/omega-3 fatty acids, probiotics, fecal bacteriotherapy, helminthic therapy

Therapy for Active Disease (See Table on next page)

- Medical approach includes induction (see chart below) and maintenance therapy, take into consideration disease severity, location, and previous therapies
- Some favor early aggressive rx (early use of biologics) w/ subseq "step-down," (theory that critical window exists before irreversible damage and perpetuating inflammatory cascade). Risks of aggressive rx weighed against dz severity
- Rx w/ evidence of effective maintenance in CD; 6-MP/AZA, MTX, and anti-TNF
- Rx w/ evidence of effective maintenance in UC; oral or topical 5-ASA, 6-MP, AZA
- Surgery may be curative in **UC**, weigh risks of early surgery against those of increasingly potent immunosuppressive agents
- Surgery not curative for CD; reserve for refractory cases or dz complications (stricture, abscess). Continue maintenance therapy postop
- Colitis requires initiation of surveillance colonoscopy 8–10 yr after dx

Prognosis

- **CD** is a chronic, incurable disease, characterized by recurrent exacerbations and remissions. Postsurgical recurrence is the rule
- **UC** w/ recurrent exacerb. Surgery curative, but postop pouchitis in up to 50%
- Small, but increased mortality risk for patients with IBD (related to primary dz complications, carcinoma, thromboembolic dz)
- Risk for colon CA assoc w/ duration of dz (esp >10 yr) and extent involved

Therapy for Active Disease (Pediatr Rev 2011;32:14)

Agent	Basics	Advantages	Disadvantages
• **Enteral nutrition** (elemental diet, oligomeric or polymeric formulas) • **TPN**	• "Bowel rest" • Enteral elemental or polymeric formula • TPN if cannot use gut	• Effective for induction (similar to steroids) • Provides nutri support • Steroid-sparing	• Adherence may be challenging, can try diff recipes for taste • Higher cost relative to steroids
• **Corticosteroids** (prednisone, methyl-prednisolone, budesonide – enteric coated)	• Staple of anti inflam rx in the United States • In CD, 20% steroid-resistant, 36% steroid-dependent at 1 yr. (J Pediatr Gastroenterol Nutr 2001;33:S27)	• Highly effective • Budesonide with fewer AEs but only for ilial dz (Cochrane Database: CD000296)	• AEs: Osteopenia, impaired growth, HTN, cushingoid facies, acne, infection, cataracts • Budesonide somewhat less effective than conventional steroids
• **Purine analogs** (6-MP azathioprine)	• Steroid-sparing, evidence for both induction and maintenance	• Well-tolerated • Effective in fistulizing dz • ↓ surgery in CD (Gut 2010;59:1200)	• Hepatotoxicity, marrow suppression, pancreatitis, infect
• **Immuno-suppressants** (MTX, tacrolimus, cyclosporine)	• Multiple mechanisms of action, often used for steroid-sparing	• MTX effective for maintenance in CD • Oral tacrolimus effective in steroid-resistant UC (J Pediatr Gastroenterol Nutr 2007;45:306)	• Nausea, myelosuppr, pulm abn, hepatitis, mucositis, • Tacrolimus and cyclosporine use limited by infliximab
• **Biologic agents** (infliximab, adalimumab, natalizumab)	• Ab that target inflammatory mediators (TNF, integrin) • Earlier use w/ "top-down" approach	• Highly effective for fistulizing dz • Effective for CD induction & maintenance • Ada/nata may be less allergenic	• Infusion reactions, sensitization, infections (√PPD), lymphoma (rare) • Natalizumab assoc w/ JC virus leukoencephalopathy
• **5-ASAs** (Mesalamine; sulfasalazine; balsalazide, olsalazine)	• Historical first-line drugs for mild-mod active UC and CD • Site of action dependent on delivery system (i.e., coating or carrier molecule)	• Effective for mild active UC & CD • Topical rx benefit for proctitis, L-sided UC • Sulfasalazine w/ added benefit of combating arthropathy	• HA, n/v, rash, inc diarrhea, pancreatitis, severe nephrotoxicity (rare) • Not as useful for maintenance therapy in CD; meta-analysis showed no diff from placebo
• **Abx** (metronidazole, cipro, rifaximin)	• Used in mild-mod active CD (adjunct rx), complications (abscesses), fistulizing CD, pouchitis	• Many theoretical benefits (alter microflora, dec translocation, bacterial overgrowth)	• Concern for antibiotic-assoc colitis in UC • Nausea, neuropathy, fungal overgrowth, dysgeusia

IBD 7-13

JAUNDICE

Definition (Pediatr Rev 2011;32:341; Pediatr Rev 2007;28:83)
- Neonatal Hyperbili (>35 wk): TSB >95th %ile for hrs of age on Bhutani nomogram
  - Visible on exam at TSB 4–5 mg/dL, progressing from head down
- Older children/adults: Generally TSB >2–3 mg/dL with yellow sclera +/− skin
- Direct hyperbilirubinemia: >2 mg/dL or >20% of TSB; marker of cholestasis

Pathogenesis
- Heme catabolism in liver and spleen results in unconj bili bound to albumin in blood
- Circulating bili travels to hepatocytes → conjugated (UGT) and excreted in bile via biliary sys to small intestine → majority excreted, some (more in neonates) deconjugated by gut bacteria and reabsorbed/recycled (enterohepatic circulation)

Differential and Evaluation
- **Neonatal unconjugated** (indirect) bilirubin excess can be a result of:
  - Increased production: Isoimmune-mediated hemolysis, hereditary RBC abn (hereditary spherocytosis [HS]/elliptocytosis [HE]), G6PDD, PKD, polycythemia, resorbing cephalohematoma, sepsis/UTI
  - Decreased clearance: Normally dec in neonate, Crigler–Najjar I and II, Gilbert
  - Increased enterohepatic circulation: Breast-feeding, breast milk, SBO
  - Evaluation: Based on response to light therapy and adequate fluid intake
    - H&P, CBC w/ diff, retic count, periph blood smear, type, Coombs, f/u NBS
    - Consider UA/Ucx, blood cx given presentation, risk factors
- **Neonatal conjugated** (direct) hyperbilirubinemia (Pediatr Rev 2004;25:388)
  - Obstruction: Biliary atresia (30%), Alagille syndrome, choledochal cyst
  - Infection: Sepsis, TORCH (5%; Toxo, syphilis, HBV, CMV, HSV, rubella) parvo
  - Metabolic/genetic (30%): Alpha-1-antitrypsin def (10%), galactosemia, tyrosinemia, Rotor, Dubin–Johnson, CF
  - Misc: Idiopathic neonatal hepatitis, hypopituitarism, hypothyroidism
  - Turner, Trisomy 18, Trisomy 21
  - Toxin mediated, TPN cholestasis
  - Evaluation: Focused w/u based on maternal screening/risks, H&P, need to r/o emergencies, sepsis, biliary atresia, galactosemia
    - LFTs w/ GGT, albumin, PT, ammonia, CMP, CBC, TSH/T4 (newborn screen), alpha-1-AT, urine reducing substances (galactosemia)
    - RPR, HSV serology, blood and urine cx, UA, serum bile acids, iron studies, transferrin, serum AA, urine OA (tyrosinemia), sweat chloride
    - Stool color cards effective screen for biliary atresia (Pediatrics 2011;128:e1209)
    - Abdominal U/S, HIDA scan (pretreat with phenobarbital)
    - Liver biopsy
- **Children/adolescent with unconjugated bilirubin excess** (Pediatr Rev 2001;22:219)
  - Overproduction: Hemolysis (PKD, G6PDD, HS, HE, autoimmune hemolysis), sickle cell or thalassemia, resorption of hematoma
  - Impaired conjugation: Gilbert (AR), Crigler–Najjar (AR)
  - Eval: H&P, CBC diff, bilis, periph smear, Coombs, haptoglobin and retic count, G6PD level, Hgb electrophoresis
- **Children/adolesc w/ conjugated (direct) bilirubin excess** (Pediatr Rev 2001;22:219)
  - Extrahepatic cholestasis: Biliary tract disorders (cholelithiasis, cholecystitis, TPN)
  - Intrahepatic cholestasis: Rotor, Dubin–Johnson
  - Hepatocellular injury: See Hepatitis, viral, metabolic, autoimmune, drugs, toxin
  - Eval: Focused by H&P, risk factors; LFTs, synthetic labs (PT, albumin), abd U/S +/− Doppler (? Budd–Chiari), hep serologies, alpha-1-antitrypsin level, ceruloplasmin, 24-hr urine copper, ANA, ASMA, antiLKM Ab, liver bx
- **Red flags:** Encephalopathy, ↑ing Cr, vit K resistant ↑ PT, bili >18 mg/dL, hypoglycemia

ABNORMAL LIVER FUNCTION TESTS

Individual Lab Tests (Pediatr Rev 2011;32:333; Gastroenterology 2002;123:1367; N Engl J Med 2000;342:1266)
- **Aspartate aminotransferase (AST) and alanine aminotransferase (ALT)**
  - Together they are sensitive markers of acute/ongoing hepatocyte injury
  - AST alone is less specific; released from heart, skeletal muscle, kidney, brain, RBCs as well as liver; ALT more specific
  - ↑ in nonhepatic dz as well; hypo/hyperthyroidism, muscle dz, celiac dz

- **Lactate dehydrogenase (LDH):** Multi sources (heart, muscle, neoplasm, liver), not spec/sens, ↑ in hepatocellular damage
- **Alkaline phosphatase (AP)**
  - Released from liver, bone, and intestines; use GGT, 5NT, or isozymes to distinguish
  - If seen with increased direct bili, indicative of biliary obstruction or cholestasis
  - Isolated elevation seen with infiltrative processes of the liver or bone (infection, tumor)
  - Levels are decreased in hypothyroidism and Wilson disease
  - Can see 2× nml adult levels in rapidly growing adolescents 2/2 bone turnover
- **Gamma-glutamyltransferase (GGT) and 5'-nucleotidase (5NT)**
  - GGT is from liver and biliary tract, 5NT is from liver, muscle, heart, kidney
  - Neither are from bone so can be used to distinguish if AP from bone/not bone
- **Albumin:** Marker of the liver's synthetic function assuming adequate nutrition
  - Abn in hepatic dysfxn, malnut, protein loss (nephrotic, enteropathy), and w/ inflam
  - Decrease is seen only with chronic states as ½ life is 20 d; markers such as prealbumin (½ life 2 d) or transferrin (½ life 10 d) reflect more acute change
- **Prothrombin time (PT):** Marker of liver synthetic function, assess extrinsic pathway (Factors I, II, V, VII, X)
  - Can be prolonged with liver dysfunction, congenital or acquired bleeding states, consumptive coagulopathies, Coumadin, and vitamin K deficiency
  - Liver produces all clotting factors aside from VIII, so with severe hepatocellular dysfxn can see prolonged PT as well as a PTT
- **Bilirubin:** From heme catabolism in liver and spleen, marker of liver excretory fxn
  - Elevations seen in cholestasis, biliary obstruction, and impaired conjugation
  - Not specific or sensitive for liver disease

Patterns of Liver Injury

	AST	ALT	Bili	AP
Hepatocellular	++	++	+/-	+/-
Cholestatic	+/-	+/-	++	+
Infiltrative	Nml	Nml	Nml	++

- **Hepatocellular:** Elevated AST and ALT with or without increased bili and AP
  - <5× nml levels w/ ALT > AST: Chronic viral hepatitis w/ HCV, HBV, hereditary hemochromatosis, NASH (nonalcoholic steatohepatitis), Wilson, chronic autoimmune hepatitis, celiac disease, some drugs
  - <5× nml w/ AST > ALT: EtOH, cirrhosis, nonhepatic (hemolysis, myopathy, drugs)
  - >15× nml; acute viral hepatitis, drug or toxin mediated, ischemic hepatitis, acute bile duct obstruction, acute Budd–Chiari
- **Cholestasis:** Inc direct (>20% TSB) and indirect bili and AP w/ or w/o inc AST/ALT
  - Biliary tract obstruction (cholelithiasis, choledocholithiasis, etc.), PSC, meds (ceftriaxone, erythromycin, TMP–SMX, carbamazepine, anabolic steroids, estrogen), TPN, metabolic diseases (CF and A1AT)
  - Isolated elevation of indirect bilirubin; consider hemolysis and see Jaundice section
- **Infiltrative:** Increased AP with near normal bili/AST/ALT
  - Lymphoma, other neoplasm, sarcoidosis, TB, histoplasmosis

HEPATITIS

Definition (Pediatr Rev 2011;32:333)
- Multiple etiologies w/ liver inflammation and hepatocyte death w/ ↑ serum AST/ALT
- Etiology, evaluation, and treatment varies per age groups and risk factors/exposures

Etiology (Pediatr Rev 2011;32:333; Pediatr Rev 2001;22:219)
- Neonatal: Usually p/w cholestasis; DB >20% TSB (Clin Liver Dis 2006;10:27)
  - 25% 2/2 biliary atresia, 25% bile acid synthetic defect, Alagille, etc.
  - 30% metabolic diseases of which 10% are alpha-1-antitrypsin deficiency
    - Hereditary hemochromatosis, galactosemia, tyrosinemia, hereditary fructose intolerance, mitochondrial diseases
  - 5% congenital infections (TORCH infections)
  - 15% idiopathic neonatal hepatitis
- Older infants, children, and young adults (Pediatr Rev 2001;22:219)
  - Viral hepatitis is most common; accounts of 70–80% liver failure in children
    - Hepatitis A (HAV), HBV, HCV, HDV, HEV, EBV, CMV, HSV, VZV

- Biliary tract obstruction/disease (see later discussion)
  - Cholelithiasis (sickle cell), cholecystitis, sclerosing cholangitis (IBD)
- Metabolic liver disease: Alpha-1-antitrypsin deficiency, Wilson dz, CF
- Autoimmune liver disease: Generally progresses to cirrhosis; types 1 and 2
- Hepatotoxins: Acetaminophen and EtOH most common but many others
  - Antiepileptics (carbamazepine, phenytoin, valproic acid)
  - Antibiotics (sulfonamides, INH, azoles)
  - Other drugs of abuse (ecstasy, PCP, cocaine)
  - Over-the-counters and herbals (NSAIDs, amanita mushroom)
- Vascular disease: Budd–Chiari syndrome, ischemia, veno-occlusive disease
- Infiltrative disease: Steatohepatitis (NASH), sarcoidosis, TB

Selected Clinical Manifestations, Evaluation, and Treatment
- Presentation can vary from asymptomatic to fulminant hepatic failure
  - Sx may include, abdominal pain (particularly RUQ), hepatomegaly, nausea and vomiting, fever, acholic stools, jaundice, encephalopathy, tremor (asterixis)
- **Hepatitis A:** RNA virus, acute and self-limited infection w/ fever, jaundice, fatigue, N/V and diarrhea; at risk for fulminant hepatic failure if underlying liver disease
  - Most common cause of acute viral hepatitis
  - Symptomatic in ~30% <6 yo (rarely w/ jaundice), 70% symptomatic in older pts
  - Transmission is fecal–oral, blood-borne, and vertical transmission rare; travel hx
  - Check serology for IgM (lasts 4–6 mo after acute infection) and IgG
  - Treatment is supportive; 2 dose vaccination for prevention
  - Pt <1 yo and likely future exposure; give immunoglobulin (Pediatrics 1996;98:1207)
- **Hepatitis B:** DNA virus, acute or chronic, or just abn labs (Clin Liver Dis 2006;10:133)
  - Asymptomatic, anicteric seroconversion is the norm if young, more sx if older
    - Vertical transmission patients usually w/ nml ALT for yrs, mild histopath Δ's
  - Risk of chronic HBV inverse to the age of infection. 90% w/ vertical transmission, 25–50% btw ages 1–5, and only 5–10% in older (Clin Liver Dis 2006;10:133)
    - 25% of infants/older children w/ HBV develop cirrhosis or HBV-related HCC
  - HBeAg+, HBeAB negative usually w/ high HBV viral load, inc infectivity
    - Endemic regions (Asia, Africa, S. America); vertical transmission most common
    - Mother HBsAg and HBeAg+, vertical inf rate 70–90%; HBeAg neg 5–20%
  - Transmission through infected body fluids, percutaneous, or permucosal
    - If mom HBsAg+/unknown, give HBV vac and HBIG w/i 12 hr at diff sites
    - No risk associated w/ breast-feeding
  - Check HBsAg, HBeAg, anti-HBsAb, anti-HBcAb, anti-HBeAB, HBV viral load

	HBsAg	anti-HBsAb	HBeAg	anti-HBeAb	anti-HBcAb
Vaccinated	–	+	–	–	–
Acute infection (high infective)	+	–	+	–	+ (IgM then IgG)
Acute infection (low infective)	+	–	–	+	+ (IgM then IgG)
Chronic infection	+	–	+/–	+/–	+ (IgG only, if IgM – flare)

- Management of chronic HBV in children (Pediatrics 2009;124:e1007)
  - Prove chronicity (HBsAg+ >6 mo)
  - In addition to above obtain baseline ALT, CBC, AFP, liver U/S, and FHx of liver dz
    - HBeAg+, Anti-HBe–, ALT nml, HBV DNA >20,000 IU/mL = immune tolerant
      - Follow ALT and HBeAg q6–12 mo and HBeAg/Anti-HBe q12mo; if ALT elevated (above nml or >40 IU/L) or AFP >10 ng/mL – refer to hepatologist
    - HBeAg–, Anti-HBe +/–, ALT nml, HBV DNA <2,000 IU/mL = inactive carrier
      - Follow ALT and AFP q6–12mo and HBeAg/Anti-HBe and ALT q12mo; if ALT-elevated or AFP >10 ng/mL, or if HBV >2,000 IU/mL – Refer
    - ALT elevated, AFP >10 ng/mL, HBeAg– with HBV >2,000 IU/mL &.or +FHx liver dz or HCC then immediate referral to hepatologist
  - Immunize all household contacts, immunize/check immune status of pt for HAV
  - Immunize for hepatitis A, check yearly AFP and liver U/S
  - Hepatology will follow q1–2yr liver U/S, obtain liver bx and consider treatment if patient >2 yo and ALT 1.5–2× nml for >3 mo, active HBV replication (+HBeAg or HBV DNA >4 log) w/o seroconversion and bx w/ evidence chronic hepatitis
- No treatment of proven efficacy in the pediatric population
  - INF-alpha w/ seroconversion in 20–58% (used in children for last 10 yr)

- Lamivudine w/ seroconversion in 23–35% (N Engl J Med 2002;346:1706)
  - Requires 1 yr of therapy and can develop resistance, well-tolerated
  - Rx options in lamivudine-refractory pts include entecavir, adefovir
- Chronic HBV infection as infant confers a 15–25% chance early death 2/2 liver dz
- **Hepatitis C:** RNA virus; acute disease mild, insidious, often asymptomatic
  - <20% w/ jaundice but 50–60% w/ persistent infection (less than in adults)
  - Transmission is primarily from exposure to infected blood
    - Now vertical xfr >> transfusion as risk; since 1992 (universal blood screening)
    - Vertical risk ~5–6%; inc w/ HIV coinfection (~20%) (Clin Liver Dis 2006;10:133)
    - No inc risk of xfr w/ breast-feeding unless w/ bleeding or cracked nipples, in which case advisable to hold breast-feeds (Adv Exp Med Biol 2004;554:211)
  - Usually asymptomatic in 1st 20 yr, w/ mild inflam, necrosis, and fibrosis on bx
    - Risk of cirrhosis and HCC in adulthood exists; but low (~5%)
  - Check HCV RNA viral load and genotype if RNA is positive; best prognosis for genotypes 2 and 3 as best response to therapy, though type 1 is most common
  - Treatment: Few contraindications to INF, higher frequency of response, less relapse, shorter duration of disease, but natural history of disease unclear
    - FDA approved rx include INF-alfa-2b w/ ribavirin (age 3–17) w/ 49% SVR (Hepatology 2002;36:1280) & PEG-INF-alfa-2b w/ ribavirin w/ 48% SVR (Hepatology 2005;41:1013). New agents under study (telaprevir & boceprevir).
      - Consider for genotypes 2 and 3, also if bx w/ significant injury or fibrosis
    - Genotype 1 w/ minimal inflammation or fibrosis can be followed
    - Vaccinate all patients against hepatitis A and hepatitis B
    - Need for surveillance AFP and screening U/S unknown at present
- **Hepatitis D:** Only can infect pts w/ HBV, at initial infection or afterwards; usually w/ acute illness and 5% risk of fulminant hepatitis; rx is supportive care
- **Hepatitis E:** Acute illness, developing world, severe in pregnant pts (10% mortality)
- **Epstein–Barr virus (EBV):** Acute hepatitis and jaundice in adolescents w/ mononucleosis; acute jaundice, pharyngitis, LAD, splenomegaly
- **CMV, VZV, HSV, toxo:** Usually w/ systemic presentation in immunocompromised
- **Alpha-1-antitrypsin disease:** (AD genetics), AAT opposes proteolytic enzymes
  - Only 20% of PiZZ homozygous patients present with liver disease
  - In 1st 20 yr, liver dz > respiratory (COPD/emphysema); can present w/ neonatal jaundice, or later w/ acute jaundice, chronic hepatitis, or cirrhosis
  - Smoke exposure is major determinant of lung fxn; can be mistaken for asthma
  - Check alpha-1-antitrypsin level (dz if <11 μmol/L) and genotype study
  - Rx for significant liver disease is transplant; curative so makes A1AT
- **Wilson disease:** (AR genetics), dysregulation of copper metabolism w/ excess accumulation in liver, CNS, kidney, corneas (Pediatr Rev 2001;22:219)
  - Acute hepatitis or fulminant liver dz (mod ↑ AST/ALT, low/nml AP, w/ Coombs neg hemolytic anemia, coagulopathy), to chronic hepatitis and cirrhosis
  - Often w/ marked neuropsychiatric sx, motor disturbance, depression, psychosis, if present will also have Kayser–Fleischer ring (gold discoloration from copper deposit in Descemet membrane of cornea seen on slit lamp)
  - Renal involvement w/ proximal tubule dysfunction, proteinuria, glucosuria, RTA
  - Diagnosis by 24-hr urinary copper excretion >100 mcg (Hepatology 1992;15:609)
    - Urine copper ↑ in other liver dz, check w/ penicillamine challenge test; 500 mg at start and at 12 hr of collection, level >1,600 mcg (per 24 collection) urinary copper diagnostic of Wilson (large validation study in children)
    - Ceruloplasm low in disease, and can be variable, poor positive predictive value
- **Autoimmune hepatitis:** Chronic inflammatory disease, unknown etiology, generally resulting in cirrhosis; 2 types (Clin Liver Dis 2006;10:89)
  - 40% type I (mean age 10 yr) and 80% of type II (6.5 yo) dx'd before age 18 yr
  - Usually presents as acute hepatitis w/ F > M; usually evidence of chronic dz already present at dx; spider nevi, ascites, palmar erythema, splenomegaly
  - AST/ALT inc, usually w/ hypergammaglobulinemia
  - Type I: + anti-smooth muscle Ab and ANA+; other sx IBD, vasculitis, arthritis, ↓ plts, GN, hemolytic anemia, fibrosing alveolitis
  - Type II: More rapidly progressive, +anti–liver-kidney microsome Ab and or +anti–liver-cytosol Ab; DM, thyroiditis, vitiligo, alopecia, AI enteropathy
  - Rx w/ immunosuppression; generally prednisone and then Imuran complete/sustained response in 95% patients
- **Hepatotoxins:** Acetaminophen OD is 1° cause of acute hepatic failure in childhood
  - Treatment (except for acetaminophen OD; see ED chapter) is supportive usually w/ improvement after withdrawal of hepatotoxin. (Pediatrics 2004;113:1097)
  - AST/ALT 8–20+ × nml: Acetaminophen, ASA, halothane, INH, VPA

- AST/ALT >3× nml: Augmentin, 6MP, carbamazepine, ketoconazole, minocycline, phenobarbital, PTU, sulfonamides
  - AST/ALT <3× nml: Cyclosporine, erythromycin, estrogens
- **Budd–Chiari:** Any blockage of blood outflow from liver resulting in congestion
  - Acute, subacute, chronic, or fulminant; dx w/ U/S + Doppler, CT, MRA, venogram
- Rx may involve meds (anticoag, thrombolysis), IR (stent, angioplasty, TIPS), or surgery (shunts, transplant).

BILIARY TRACT DISEASE

Definition
- Impaired bile sec by the liver w/ subseq ↑ serum total and direct bili; often w/ jaundice
- Biliary hepatic congestion → chronic hepatic inflammation → fibrosis and cirrhosis

Etiology (Pediatr Rev 2004;25:388; Pediatr Rev 2007;28:83)
- Neonatal obstructive cholestasis: Biliary atresia, choledochal cysts, bile duct paucity (Alagille syndrome as well as nonsyndromic), neonatal sclerosing cholangitis, inspissated bile syndrome, cholecystitis, bile sludging, CF
- Child and young adult: Choledochal cyst, cholecystitis, tumor, primary biliary cirrhosis, primary sclerosing cholangitis, missed neonatal diagnosis (Alagille, nonsyndromic bile duct paucity, Caroli disease)

Selected Clinical Manifestations, Evaluation, and Treatment
- Presentation varies based on age, etiology, severity, and duration of illness
- **Biliary atresia:** Most common cause of extra-hepatic cholestasis in 1st mo of life (33%)
  - Complete blockage of bile outflow 2/2 complete or partial destruction or absence of extrahepatic bile ducts. (Clin Liver Dis 2006;10:73; Pediatr Rev 2006;27:243)
  - Results in ~50% of all pediatric liver transplants; most freq hepatic cause of death
  - P/w jaundice at 3–6 wk of life, otherwise healthy; rare embryonic form at birth
    - Subclinically, BA pts w/ T/D bili ↑ on DOL 1-2 (Pediatrics 2011;128:e1428)
    - Rapidly progressive process w/ continuing inflammation and fibrosis/destruction
    - Prenatal form (less common) assoc w/ polysplenia, malro, CDH in 10–15%
  - Etiology unknown, proposed viral association; reovirus, CMV, HPV, rotavirus C
  - Evaluation: Can screen generally w/ stool color cards (Pediatrics 2011;128:e1209)
    - Most p/w elevated direct bilirubin and evaluated for other causes (above)
    - Abd U/S: R/o other structural disease, looking for the absence of gall bladder though nonspecific finding, pathognomonic finding is triangular cord sign
    - HIDA scan: If tracer to intestines, argues against dx, but may need ×repeat as biliary atresia is a progressive disease; most people use phenobarb ×5 d prior
    - MRI cholangiography and liver bx also good but sensitivities too low to exclude biliary atresia if strongly suspected
    - Intraoperative cholangiogram (or ERCP where available) necessary to rule out if above equivocal; if present, surgical correction at time of study
  - Rx w/ Kasai hepatic portojejunostomy (anastomosis of porta hepatis to Roux en Y), which allows for small patent bile ducts to drain restoring bile flow
    - Success related to pt age at correction w/ 80% <2 mo but only 20% >3 mo
    - Kasai is essentially palliative and these patients eventually go on to transplant
- **Cholelithiasis:** Rare in pediatrics (0.15–0.22%) except sickle cell, other hemolytic dzs, CF, obesity, OCP use, chronic TPN, ileal resection. Has 4:1 ♀:♂ predominance, inc to 11–22:1 in adolescence (Curr Opin Pediatr 1997;9:276; Pediatr Rev 2009;30:368)
  - Pigment stones (hemolytic dz, TPN, ileal resection), cholesterol stones in others
  - Acalculous cholecystitis almost always post-op or assoc w/ other severe illness
  - Asymptomatic generally but can develop **cholecystitis, choledocholithiasis, or pancreatitis,** w/ jaundice, RUQ pain, vomiting +/- fever
  - Do not always see elevated bilirubin with uncomplicated cholecystitis; if present, consider cholangitis (pus under pressure), choledocholithiasis (stone in CBD)
  - Radiographs demonstrate radiopaque stones in 36–47% (vs. 15% adults)
  - Abd U/S check for + Murphy sign (tender RUQ), and thickened wall (4–5 mm)
    - Sens 84% and spec 95% in adults; likely higher in children given habitus
    - HIDA scan: If dx suspected clinically but U/S equivocal; sens 97%, spec 90%
    - Rx: IVFs, Abx (ceftriaxone or quinolone + flagyl), surgery or ERCP once patient is stable and infection/inflammation has quieted on antibiotics
- **Primary sclerosing cholangitis:** Progressive chronic inflam of intra & extra hepatic biliary ducts (small or large ducts). (Curr Gastroenterol Rep 2010;12:195)

- Mean age of dx is 13 yr (2:1 M:F), 80% assoc w/ IBD (UC in 85% cases)
- $^2/_3$ pts w/ sx at dx; intermittent abd pain (40%) & fatigue (25%) w/ subseq anorexia & weight loss. 20% w/ fever; other signs – HSM, jaundice, and pruritus. Other AI dz 5%
- Labs w/ elevated GGT/AP +/– AST/ALT, but 90% w/ nml bilirubin, also w/ + ANCA staining peripheral nucleus (>70%), + ANA (50%), and SMA (25%)
  - See high serum and urine copper (2/2 bile flow obs), ceruloplasm high/nml
  - Diagnosis: Cholangiography or ERCP can visualize large duct narrowing/dilation but not w/ small ducts, need liver bx to dx small duct predominant PSC
  - MRCP excellent option for noninvasive imaging of intra/extrahepatic ducts
  - No specific rx; ursodiol for sx relief, no mortality benefit w/ anti-inflammatories, if cirrhosis and liver failure then liver transplant; w/o xplt mean lifespan 12 yr
  - Increased incidence of colorectal CA and cholangiocarcinoma in later adult life

ACUTE PANCREATITIS

Etiologies (J Pediatr Gastroenterol Nutr 2011;52:262)
- Idiopathic (13–34%)
- Trauma (10–40%): Blunt abdominal, postsurgical, post-ERCP
- Biliary tract disease/structural dz (10–30%): Divisum, annular pancreas, choledochal cysts, duct stricture, choledocholithiasis, duplication cyst, sphincter of Oddi dysfunction
- Multisystem disease (14–33%): Sepsis, SLE, HSP, HUS, Crohn's, Kawasaki
- Drugs/toxins (12–25%): Corticosteroids, VPA, carbamazepine, sulfonamides, metronidazole, pentamidine, tetracycline, furosemide, chlorothiazides, azathioprine, 6-MP, L-asparaginase, scorpion stings, ethanol
  - Recent study w/ 25.6% acute pancreatitis 2/2 drugs; most commonly VPA and steroids, L-asp and 6-MP (J Pediatr Gastroenterol Nutr 2011;53:423)
- Infection (10%): Mumps, Coxsackie B, CMV, HAV, VZV, EBV, HBV, Flu A/B, mycoplasma, leptospirosis, ascariasis, malaria
- Hereditary (2%) – see Chronic Pancreatitis for etiologies
- Metabolic (2%) → DKA, hyperlipidemia, hypercalcemia, organic acidemia, malnut/refeed

Clinical Presentation (J Pediatr Gastroenterol Nutr 2011;52:262)
- Abd pain (87%), classically epigastric/LUQ radiating to back but <10% in children; worse after eating, N/V (40–80%), anorexia, and altered sensorium
- Exam: abd pain, +/– distention, +/– guarding (29–37%)/rebound, ↓ BS, fever, ↑ I IR
- Retroperitoneal hemorrhage (Cullen – periumbilical, Grey Turner – flank)
- Wide spectrum of presentation from normal exam to hypotension and shock

Diagnostic Studies
- Laboratory testing (Am J Gastroenterol 2002;97:1309)
  - Amylase: Spec highest when >3× nml limit, rises w/i hrs, no correlation btw rise and severity of dz, 20% false neg, can fractionate pancreatic vs. salivary
  - Lipase; spec highest if >3× nml, more spec than Amy, ↑ up to 14 d, 85–95% sens
- Imaging studies
  - Abd U/S: W/ pancr enlargement, ↓ echogenicity, dilated ducts, pseudocyst, gallstones. Can be used for guided aspiration of pseudocyst
  - CT: W/ diffuse enlarge, +/– hemorrhage, necrosis, pseudocyst. 20% w/ nml CT, rapid bolus better identify necrosis. Used when U/S not adeq to identify anatomy
  - MRCP: Can define anatomy for therapeutic intervention but not therapeutic
  - ERCP: Indications include recurrent or prolonged pancreatitis, abn MRCP, trauma, sphincterotomy, gallstone extraction. Growing pediatric experience. Most sensitive and specific test for divisum and choledochal cyst, sphincter of Oddi dysfunction

Indicators of Severity (Am J Gastroenterol 2002;97:1726)
- Multiple scoring systems are used in adults (Ranson criteria, Glasgow, APACHE, CT-severity index) but none have been validated in children
- Some widely agreed upon indicators for severe disease include:
  - Clinical: Altered sensorium, hypotension, renal failure, pulmonary edema, shock
  - Labs: ↓ Ca, ↑ gluc, hypoxemia, ↑ BUN and Cr, ↑WBC, alb, CRP 48 hr into course
  - Imaging: Amount of necrosis correlates w/ risk of infection and severity of disease

Treatment (N Engl J Med 2006;354:2142)
- Classic approach was initial fluid resuscitation, pain management, and bowel rest
  - Enteral (NGT) vs. parenteral nut: Recent adult data w/ ↓ in infxn and dz severity w/ enteral feeding. (BMJ 2004;328:1407). PO should begin once pain improved

- Pain mgmt: Meperidine often used over MSO$_4$; no studies show advantage
- NGT decomp: Often used but lack of published evidence (not in mild disease)
- Antibiotic: Use is controversial (some studies show benefit, others do not)
  - May be reserved for cases with severe necrotizing disease
- ERCP papillotomy: Diagnostic and therapeutic, indications discussed above
- Surgery: Indicated if infected necrosis (may be confirmed by FNA), trauma w/ duct rupture. Relative indications – sterile necrosis with more than 50% involved

Complications (N Engl J Med 2006;354:2142)
- Systemic: Shock, metabolic derangement (hypoCa, hyperglycemia, hyperK, hyperlipidemia, GI hemorrhage, ileus, stress ulcer, obstruction, colonic wall erosion, splenic hematoma, pericarditis, pleural effusion, ARDS, Δ MS, psychosis, coma, $\downarrow$ plts, hemolysis, DIC
- Local:
  - Pseudocyst; expanding, organized fluid collection; diagnosed by abd U/S
    - Asymptomatic cysts do not require intervention
    - Some require drainage (endoscopic, IR, surgical) need 4–6 wk for maturity
    - Complications include rupture, hemorrhage, infection
  - Necrosis: Diffuse or focal, can develop early in course. Suspected w/ fever, leukocytosis, and failure to improve. Dx by CT (rapid bolus technique)
    - Complications: Infected necrosis/abscess (can dx by FNA). Rx w/ abx or surgery

CHRONIC PANCREATITIS

Etiologies (Gastroenterology 2001;120:682)
- TIGARO classification
- **T**oxic/metabolic: EtOH, hypercalcemia, hyperlipidemia, organic acidemias, CRF
- **I**diopathic
- **G**enetic (PMID: 22094894)
  - PRSS 1 (24%) (serine protease 1); cationic trypsinogen; $\uparrow$ trypsin act/block inactivation
  - SPINK 1 (27%) (serine protease inhib Kazal type 1); AR, blocks trypsin inhibition, early onset
  - CFTR (48%); highest risk in compound heterozygotes
  - Hereditary pancreatitis; (AD genetics), onset age 10–12, strong risk for pancreatic Ca, most w/ some genetic mutation (PRSS 1 most common)
- **A**utoimmune: Isolated autoimmune pancreatitis, Sjogren, IBD, PBC
- **R**ecurrent acute
- **O**bstructive: W/ pancreatic divisum, choledochal cysts, stricture, trauma, idiopathic

Clinical Presentation
- Repeated episodes of acute pancreatitis
- Chronic abdominal pain: Generally w/ epigastric pain, radiating to back, +/– emesis
  - Worse after meals (particularly fatty foods)
  - Fluctuates and may improve as exocrine glands "burn out"
- Insidious onset often with less pain
  - Malabsorption (protein and fat); w/ greasy, loose, foul-smelling stools, FTT
  - Diabetes mellitus/glucose intolerance (high risk for hypoglycemia, rarely DKA)

Diagnosis
- Often clinical diagnosis with repeated episodes of acute pancreatitis
- Laboratory: $\uparrow$ amylase and lipase (can be nml early or late), hyperglycemia (late and w/ endocrine pancr damage), ADEK and Vit B$_{12}$ def (late), $\uparrow$ fecal fat (72-hr collection vs. Sudan III stain spot test), $\downarrow$ fecal elastase, gene test PRSS I, SPINK I, CFTR
- Imaging: KUB (pancreatic calcifications), abd US ($\uparrow$ pancr duct diameter, pseudocyst), abd CT (calcification, dilated ducts, atrophy), MRCP (sens $\uparrow$ w/ secretin), ERCP (therapeutic as well; stricture dilation, stone extraction, stents)

Treatment
- Treat flares as you would episodes of acute pancreatitis (see previous section)
- Special considerations
  - Pain control w/ narcotic/non-narcotic analgesia, avoid triggers
  - Nutrition; low-fat diet, pancreatic enzyme replacement, adequate protein, fat soluble vitamins, NJ/J-tube feeds if severe growth failure
  - Islet cell autotransplantation: Total pancreatectomy followed by reimplantation of islet cells into liver; may improve glycemic control and pain

Definition (Am Fam Physician 2010;81:12)
- RBC volume as a fraction of whole blood (hematocrit) or hemoglobin concentration <5th percentile for age (e.g., <11 g/dL for age 2–35 mo)
- Hematologic parameters vary w/ age (interpret using age-specific indices)
- "Physiologic anemia of infancy": Incr tissue oxygen level at birth depresses production of erythropoietin (reaches nadir at 1 mo); RBC production is lowest during 2nd wk and reaches max at 3 mo. Hgb nadir occurs at 6–9 wk of age
- Microcytic anemia is the most common category of anemia in children

Clinical Manifestations
- Can be asymptomatic or p/w fatigue, irritability, dyspnea, heart failure, growth delay
- Pica, pagophagia (craving and eating ice; common with iron deficiency)
- Signs or symptoms of blood loss: Hematochezia, melena, heavy menses
- Signs or symptoms of hemolysis: Jaundice, scleral icterus, change in urine color
- History: Diet Hx (nutritional iron def is the primary cause of microcytic anemia in children), medications (including herbal), birth, growth/development, menstrual hx
- FHx: Eval hemoglobinopathy in African-Americans, Mediterranean region/Southeast Asia
- Exam: Pallor when examining conjunctivae, tongue, palm, nail beds (correlates well with severe dz; 94% sens for Hgb <5/dL); tachycardia or flow murmur; splenomegaly

Diagnostic Studies
- CBC, MCV, MCHC, RDW, retic, hemolysis labs (Coombs, bili, haptoglobin, LDH), smear
- Absolute reticulocyte count = retic% × RBC count/L; Reticulocyte index (to correct for low Hct) = retic% × (patient Hct/Normal Hct) × (1/retic maturation factor) nml 1–2% (<1: Decr pdtn >2: Incr loss)
- Hemoglobin and mean corpuscular volume by age (J Pediatr 1979;94:26)
- Exam: 6 mo MCV nml range 71–94 fL, 18 yo MCV nml range 78–98 fL
- Hgb does not detect early/mild anemia as RBC life span reflects marrow iron content up to 120 d prior; retic Hgb count more accurate due to 1–2 d life span

	Normocytic		Macrocytic
Microcytic	**Retic < 3%**	**Retic > 3%**	
Iron deficiency (bleed or dietary)	*Normal WBC/platelets* Hypoplastic anemias, infxn (congenital parvo B19, HIV, sepsis), Diamond–Blackfan, renal dz, drugs, bleed transient Erythroblastopenia of childhood	• Hemorrhage	*Megaloblastic marrow* (Hyperseg PMNs)
Lead tox		• Membranopathies (spherocytosis, elliptocytosis)	• B₁₂, folate def
Anemia chronic dz		• Enzymopathies (G6PD, PK def)	• Medication (anticonvulsants, AZT, immunosuppressants)
Thalassemias		• Hgb'pathies	• Hereditary orotic aciduria
Hgb'pathies		• Autoimmune	*Non-megaloblastic*
Sideroblastic	*Nml/decr WBC/platelet* Drug, infxn, renal dz, splenomegaly	• Isoimmune (ABO, Rh)	• Reticulocytosis, hypothyroid, liver dz, post-splenectomy, Downs syndrome
	Decr WBC/Platelets Leukemia, aplastic, infxn, Fanconi	• Microangiopathic (HUS, TTP, DIC, Kasabach–Merritt, mec valves)	• MDS, aplastic/ dyserythropoietic anemia

Microcytic Anemia (Pediatr Rev 2007;28:5; N Engl J Med 1999;341:1986)
- Mentzer index (MCV/RBC): >13 consistent w/ iron def; <13 with β-thal trait
- **Iron studies**
  - Iron deficiency: Decr Iron, incr TIBC, decr ferritin
  - Chronic disease: Decr Iron, decr TIBC, incr ferritin
  - Thalassemia/lead: Incr nml Iron, decr TIBC, incr ferritin
- **Iron deficiency anemia:** Most common form of microcytic anemia (Pediatrics 2010; 126:e874). Risk factors: Low SES, premature, low birth wt, lead exposure, exclusive breast-feed over 4 mo without supp, weaning to iron-poor foods, feeding problems
  - Requirements: Birth—6 mo 0.27 mg/d; 6–12 mo 11 mg/d; age 1–3yo 7mg/d
  - Preterm infants may miss 3rd tri accretion of iron stores; may need 2–4 mg/kg PO daily
  - Term infants taking breast milk >50% daily feeds: 1 mg/kg/d oral Fe starting at 4 mo
    - Universal screening at 12 mo: Check risk factors and serum Hgb. If + anemia, measure ferritin and CRP levels or retic Hgb conc; OR empirical trial of iron supps (retest Hgb after 1 mo; should incr by 1 g/dL)

- Rx: 6 mg/kg elemental Fe × 6 wk in 2–3 doses, IV Fe in severe def; RBC xfusion
- Vit C increases iron absorption. Tea, phytates (e.g., corn) decr iron absorption (see AAP statement Pediatrics 2010 for advised foods)
- Typically improvement in retic count in 2–3 d, MCV and Hgb in 1–4 wk
- **Anemia of chronic disease:** Can be microcytic or normocytic. (N Engl J Med 2005;352:1011); hepcidin (incr w/ inflam) blocks Fe release
  - Treat underlying disorder (i.e., epo for renal disease)

Normocytic Anemia (Pediatr Rev 1988;10:77)
- Low retic: Diamond–Blackfan, trans-erythroblastopenia of childhood, aplastic crisis (see later section on pure RBC Aplasia)
- High retic: **Hemolytic anemias**
  - Intrinsic: Inh abnl Hgh (for sickle cell & thalassemia see below, unstable Hgb mutations e.g., congenital Heinz body anemia, Hgb Hasharon); abnl RBC membrane (e.g., spherocytosis, elliptocytosis); abnl RBC enzymes (e.g., pyruvate kinase or G6PD deficiency)
  - Extrinsic: Autoimmune hemolytic anemia (warm-reactive or cold agglutinin), liver disease, hypersplenism, oxidant agents, microangiopathies, paroxysmal cold hemoglobinuria, paroxysmal nocturnl hemoglobinuria
- **Hereditary spherocytosis:** ~75% autosomal dominant, deficient, or abnl membrane structural protein (usually spectrin); splenomegaly, jaundice, chronic anemia; dx: smear, FHx, osmotic fragility
- **G6PD deficiency:** X-linked, lack of G6PD allows oxidant metabolites of drugs to denature Hgb, acute hemolysis occurs with exposure to sulfa, antimalarials, naphthoquinones, or fava; hemoglobinemia and hemoglobinuria within 24–48 hr of ingestion, self-resolution in 3–4 d
- **AIHA:** Ab against intrinsic membrane Ag, positive DAT (Coombs); pallor, jaundice, hemoglobinuria, splenomegaly; may be a/w resp infxn or chronic dz, e.g., SLE or lymphoma

Macrocytic Anemia (Ped Rev 1988;10:77; N Engl J Med 1999;341:1986)
- **Vit B_{12} deficiency:** Rare in kids, 2/2 pernicious anemia and ileal disease (Crohns)
  - Assoc w/ pancytopenia w/ macrocytosis, hyperseg PMNs
  - Exam: Glossitis and decreased vibration and position senses
  - Neuro manifestations → can be irreversible if untreated
  - Rx: Oral or parenteral Vitamin B_{12} supplementation
- **Folate deficiency:** Rare 2/2 incr in folate supplementation for pregnancy
  - Found in malabsorption syndromes, EtOH use, chronic hemolysis, drugs (MTX)
  - R/o Vit B_{12} def (folate supps fix RBC parameters; B_{12} def can be missed)

HEMOGLOBINOPATHIES

Sickle Cell Disease (SCD) (Pediatr Rev 2007;28:259; Am J Hematol 2010;85(S):346)
- **Definition:** Chronic hemolytic anemia; includes Hgb variants SS, SC, S-β thal, SO Arab, SD, and other rare S-Hb genotypes
- **SS disease:** Both β-globin genes w/ mutation (valine for glutamate at AA 6 on β-chain)
- **SC disease:** 1 β-globin chain w/ mutation (lysine for glutamate at AA 6); longer survival of Hgb SC; milder anemia, 50% less pain crises, lower risk of silent infarcts/stroke, lower rate of fatal bacterial infxn, later osteonecrosis; splenic infarct/sequestrum at any age
- **CC disease:** Relatively mild-microcytic anemia
- **Sickle-β-thal:** 1 β-globin gene w/ S mut, other nonfxnl. Similar course as SS dz
  - **AS (sickle cell trait):** Normal lifespan and protective carrier trait, but a/w rare fatal medullary cancer in adults, exercise-related deaths, splenic infarction, hematuria, hyposthenuria, venous thromboembolism (VTE), complicated hyphema, and fetal loss (Am J Med 2009;122(6):507)
- **Pathophysiology**
  - Nucleotide sub (GTG for GAG; codon 6) of β-globin gene (chromo 11); valine for glut acid; HbS polymerizes on deoxygenation, distorts RBC into crescent
  - Sickled cells less deformable and incr adherence to vasc endothelium; lead to vascular occlusion, organ ischemia, and chronic end-organ damage
- **Epidemiology**
  - African-American: 1 in 375, 9% carrier prev in US; Hispanics: 1 in 1,200
  - Sickle cell–related death decr 42% 1999–2002, coinciding with pneumococcal vaccine. In Dallas Newborn Cohort, 93.9% HbSS and Hb SB0 pts survived to adulthood. Most recent deaths in pts >18 yo after transition to adult care (Blood 2010;115(17):344)
  - No consistent early predictive factors identified for morbidity or mortality

- **Clinical manifestations:** Appear in first yr as fetal Hb concentrations decline (see table)
  - Fetal Hb protective because it inhibits deoxy-HbS polymerization in the RBCs
  - Those w/ persistence of fetal Hb (HbF >30%) have mild or no symptoms
- **Diagnostic studies:** Newborn screening (NS) performed in 44 states and DC
  - If NS not offered, high risk infants tested by electrophoresis before 3 mo
  - Sickledex (rapid test based on solubility) inappropriate in newborns, does not identify Hgb C or β-thal
  - Lab monitoring: CBC/retic annually, Hgb electrophoresis at 1–2 yo, RBC Ag at 1–2 yo or before first transfuse, LFT/bili/BUN/Cr/UA annually
  - Screening: PFTs baseline when adolescent (earlier if severe/recurrent ACS); EKG/echo as needed, Ophtho exam annually after age 10, Transcranial Doppler (TCD) (see below)
- **Prophylaxis:** (Pediatrics 2002;109(3):526)
  - PCN birth—36 mo: 125 mg PO bid 3–5 yo: 250 mg PO bid >5 yo: Discontinue unless splenectomy (alt: Erythromycin 20 mg/kg divided bid)
  - Vaccination: Hib, pneumococcal, meningococcal (after age 2), influenza
- TCD: If flow velocity >200 cm/sec, incr risk for stroke
  - Screening all kids w/ Hb-SS and Hb-S-β every 6–12 mo at 3–16 yo. D/c of Rx after 36 mo of Rx resulted in reversion to abn TCD velocity or stroke in 45% of pts
- **Treatments:**
  - Transfuse with sickle negative, CMV-irradiated, leukoreduced, extended phenotype cross-matched (if available)
  - Folate 400 mcg–1 mg PO daily
  - Hydroxyurea: Induces Hgb F; decr VOC, ACS, dactylitis, admission, transfusion; incr Hgb and Hgb F; used in children as young as 9 mo, 20 mg/kg per d; a/w mild–mod neutropenia, mild decr plts, rash (Pediatrics 2008;122:1332, BABYHUG trial. Lancet 2011;377(9778):1663)

Complications and Management

Complication	Features	Evaluation and Management
Vaso-occlusive pain crises	70% of all pts; 5% (Hb-SS) account for 30% of admissions (#1 cause of hospitalizations) Triggered by cold, stress, infxn, menses, EtOH, dehydration but majority w/o identifiable cause 50% w/ fever, swelling, tenderness, tachypnea, N/V	Sickle cell care plan at home • Trial of oral analgesia prior to parenteral narcotics at home or in acute care setting w/ opioids/ toradol • PO regimen: Long-acting opioid (for basal rate) and short-acting opioid (for bolus); NS bolus if dehydrated, then 1.25 maintenance (IV + PO), if concern for acute chest limit to 2/3–3/4 maintenance, consider ↓ after 24 hr Labs: CBCD, Retic Monitor: CV, SaO₂ (keep >95%) Manage side effects: Bowel regimen, itch, GI discomfort/nausea, incent spiro
Infection *Strep pneumo* sepsis/meningitis Osteomyelitis	Fever >101.5°F (38.5°C) Assume functional asplenia Pts with acute chest may not present with resp sx Reduced by vaccination and expedient abx *Salmonella, Staph aureus* (<25%), *Strep pneumo* (joint)	CBC diff, retic, UA, blood/urine culture, CXR. If focal sx, then throat cx, LP, stool, viral panel. Rx w/ Ceftriaxone, Azithromycin (if new infiltrate on CXR), Vancomycin (for sepsis, meningitis, toxic, CVL, h/o resistant organisms) Consider admit: Age <6, toxic, sepsis, poor perfusion, h/o resistant organism, unable to PO, hypoxia or positive CXR, RAD exacerbation, Hct <18, reliable f/u

SICKLE CELL 8-3

Aplastic crisis	Arrested erythropoiesis, retic < 1 Often with Parvo B_{19} infxn	Transfusion, reticulocytopenia 2–14 d, recurrence rare
Splenic sequestration	HbSS <3 yr, HbSC/Sβ-thal any age. Vaso-occlusion in spleen and pooling of RBC → acute splenomegaly and Hgb decr >2 g/dL from baseline Presenting sx in 20% SCD pts, 1/3 under age 2. 10–15% mortality, 50% recurrence	CBC diff, retic, serial exam Transfuse Splenectomy if recurrent
Hyperhemolysis syndrome	Severe sudden anemia, a/w drugs, ACS, infxn, enzyme deficiencies, transfusions (rare)	CBC diff, retic, DAT, LDH, Bili; IVIG & Solu-medrol cover for transfusions (Expert Rev Hematol 2009;2(2):111)
Stroke	Likelihood of first CVA by age 20, 30, & 45 yr is 11, 15, & 24%. 25% kids have silent ischemic lesions. Often large arterial risk HbSS >Sβ-thal0 >Sβ-thal + >HbSC Risk factors: TCD >200 cm/sec on 2 exams, low baseline Hgb, high WBC count, prior TIA, frequent/recent acute chest, incr BP, sibling with stroke, dactylitis <age2 (Blood 1998;91(1):288; Blood 2011; Epub PMID:22096242)	Transcranial Doppler screening Chronic transfusion decr stroke risk by 92% in pts with HbSS with repeated TCD >200 (N Engl J Med 1998;339(1):5) Alternative hydroxyurea/ phlebotomy was not inferior at preventing strokes, but did not reduce liver iron content (SWiTCH trial. Blood 2012; Epub PMID:22318199) If untreated, 90% pts with stroke will have recurrence PRBC transfusion volume calculated to raise Hct to 28–33% or Hgb 10g/dL. Repeat q3–6wk Monitor CBC monthly, Hgb E, LFT, ferritin
Acute chest Syndrome	Leading cause of morbidity and mortality in children and adults Infarction, infection, pulmonary fat embolism New infiltrate on CXR with: Tachypnea, fever >101.5°F (38.5°C), chest pain, cough, wheeze, SaO_2 3–5% below baseline Most commonly p/w fever; 50% c/b VOC, VOC involving trunk also causes splinting/decr TV Infections often Chlamydia, mycoplasma, virus Frequent ACS a/w shorter lifespan, severe ACS a/w neuro damage SCD pts tend to have hyperactive airways	Chronic transfusions decr freq of ACS • Work up fever as above • Admit • Correct fluid deficit if dehydrated (but do not fluid overload, consider diuretics if fluid overload or sensitive) • Daily CBC, repeat CXR as needed, viral panel, O_2, incentive spiro, encourage ambulation, chest physio, • Ceftriaxone or Cefuroxime, Azithromycin, Vancomycin for severe • Bronchodilators for wheezing/ RAD • Steroids for RAD or severe resp diff • (may cause rebound VOC, may taper) • Optimize pain control to avoid atelectasis or hypoventilation • Transfuse if SaO_2 <95% or Hct <18 (do not exceed Hct >35)
Pulmonary Hypertension	Found in 30% of children >6 yo with HbSS/Sβ-thal0. But study used tricuspid regurg jet (echo) which has lower PPV for PHN compared to right heart cath. Risk factors: Reticulocytosis, low SaO_2, ↑ plt count (Pediatrics 2008;121;4:777)	Optimal treatment not yet defined.

Priapism	Painful sustained unwanted erection, stuttering (episodic) or prolonged 75–89% prevalence by age 20 Can result in corpus cavernosal fibrosis and ED Increased Hgb F is protective	Home: Increase fluids, urination, oral pain meds, warm baths/soaks Acute mgmt: IV hydration, analgesia, supplemental O_2, pseudoephedrine, CBC diff, retic, UA, catheterization if trouble voiding, urology consult if no relief within 3 hr (for penile aspiration/irrigation with epinephrine) May need percutaneous shunt if no detumescence with medical rx
Osteonecrosis	Dactylitis (hand–foot syndrome) most common initial sx in 40% of children overall, and 50% <age 2. Femoral and humeral heads	
Decreased spleen function	Hyposplenism or functional asplenia due to repeated infarction 2/2 sickling; loss of splenic fxn <12 mo in 86% SCD infants, a/w lower fetal Hgb and higher WBC/retic (Blood 2011;117(9):2614)	
Cardiac	LVH and cardiomegaly may be present in children from chronic incr cardiac demands from anemia and O_2 desat (Blood 2010;116(1):16)	
Renal failure	Painless hematuria from papillary infarcts, proteinuria, renal infarction, papillary necrosis, FSGS, enuresis from hyposthenuria	
Hepatobiliary dysfunction	Hepatic ischemia, benign cholestasis, transfusional iron overload, cholelithiasis (42% by adolescence, pigmented gallstones)	
Retinopathy	Proliferative, retinal artery occlusion, retinal detachment, hemorrhage Risk Hgb SC >Hgb SS	
Leg ulcers	Usually age >10, near medial or lateral malleolus, risk for infection and often recurrent	

Thalassemias (Pediatr Rev 2002;23:75; Pediatr Rev 2007;28:5; Pediatr Clin North Am 2008;55(2):447)

- Nml Hgb (Hgb A) composed of 2 β-chains and 2 α-chains
- Fetal Hgb (Hgb F) composed of 2 γ-chains and 2 α-chains
- Consider dx w/ hypochromic, microcytic anemia, and in pts of appropriate ethnic background
- Other forms: Delta thalassemia (no HbA2); Hgb S/thalassemia (common in Africa/Mediterranean, similar to SCD); Hgb C/thalassemia (β 0 causes mod–severe hemolytic anemia), Hgb E/thalassemia (most common form of severe thalassemia in SE and South Asia, clinically similar to β thal major) (Br J Haematol 2008;141:3)

Beta-thalassemia Trait

- AR, β-chains controlled by two genes on chromosome 11; no Rx needed
- Diminished production of nml β-globin chains → hypochromic, microcytic anemia
- Characterized by mild anemia (hemoglobin 9.5–11) and MCV <80
- Basophilic stippling often seen on blood smear

Beta-thalassemia Major (Cooley Anemia)

- Little to no production of β-chains, and subsequently hemoglobin A (α_2, β_2)
- Usually evident beyond 6 mo of age when fetal hemoglobin production falls
- Severe hypochromic, microcytic anemia requires chronic transfusion
- Enlargement of liver and spleen because of extramedullary hematopoiesis
- Long-term complications those of iron overload; BMT from matched donor curative
- Iron chelator: Deferoxamine (IV), Deferasirox (oral) well tolerated and decr liver iron concentration/serum ferritin (Blood 2011;118:884)

Alpha-thalassemia

- Normal: 4 functional genes for α-chain (on chromosome 16)
- Silent carrier: 3 functional genes
- α-thalassemia trait: 2 functional genes, typically asymptomatic w/ decr Hgb
- Hgb H: 1 functional gene. Hgb H composed of tetrad of β-chains, 2/2 paucity of available α-chains. Characterized by chronic hemolytic anemia w/ splenomegaly
- Bart Hgb: 0 functional genes. Bart Hgb: Tetrad of four γ-chains, leading to catastrophic anemia, hydrops fetalis, and fetal or neonatal loss

PLATELET DISORDERS

Thrombocytopenia (Pediatr Rev 2011;32:135)
- Plt lifespan 7–10 d. Younger plts larger and more hemostatically active → less risk of severe bleeding in destructive thrombocytopenia with brisk production
- **Definition:** Plt count <150,000/μL

Thrombocytopenia and Risk of Bleeding	
Platelet Count (cells/μL)	**Risk**
>100,000	No increased risk
50,000–100,000	Risk with major trauma; can proceed with general surgery
20,000–50,000	Risk with minor trauma or surgery
<20,000	Risk of spontaneous bleeding (less so with immune thrombocytopenic purpura [ITP])
<10,000	Risk of severe, life-threatening bleeding

- **Clinical manifestations:** Petechiae, purpura, gingival bleeding, epistaxis, GI bleed, menorrhagia, hematuria, CNS bleed. Hematomas and muscle hemorrhage rare
- **Etiology**
  - Decreased production: Marrow infiltration or failure (ALL, Fanconi pancytopenia), infection (e.g., EBV, CMV, VZV, Rickettsia, parvo), marrow injury (drugs, toxins), ineffective nutritional deficiencies (folate, B_{12}), cyanotic congenital heart dz, genetic (e.g., Wiskott–Aldrich, thrombocytopenia absent radii, Bernard–Soulier)
  - Increased destruction
    - Immune: Ab/immune complex: ITP; neonatal alloimmune thrombocytopenia (NAIT, maternal allo-Ab against paternal Ag), neonatal autoimmune thrombocytopenia (maternal Ab against maternal and infant plts); infxn; heparin-induced thrombocytopenia (HIT); Evans syndrome (AIHA, ITP), SLE
    - Platelet consumption: Disseminated intravascular coag (DIC); hemolytic-uremic syndrome (HUS), thrombotic thrombocytopenic purpura (TTP), NEC; thrombosis
  - Platelet sequestration: Hypersplenism, Kasabach–Merritt (thrombocytopenia and hemangiomas), chronic liver disease, malaria
  - Platelet loss or dilution: In setting of massive transfusions, pRBC or whole blood
- **Diagnostic evaluation:** H&P: Meds, infxns, PMH, splenomegaly, LAD, bleeding
  - CBC w/ differential: Isolated thrombocytopenia vs. multilineage involvement
  - Peripheral smear:
    - **If ↑ destruction:** Large Plts, schistocytes; **if ↓ production:** Blasts, hyperseg PMNs
  - Additional labs as needed—bone marrow biopsy when indicated
    - Hemolysis: LDH, retic, haptoglobin, bilirubin, Coombs test
    - DIC: Coags, D-dimer, fibrinogen, fibrin degradation products

Immune Thrombocytopenic Purpura (ITP) (Blood 2010;115:168)
- Most common cause of isolated thrombocytopenia in otherwise well children
  - Peak age 2–5 yo
  - 2/2 antiplt Ab binds Plt surface & incr destruction by phagocytosis in spleen & liver
  - 50% cases follow viral infxn (either non-specific or 2/2 EBV, varicella, or HIV), MMR
  - Sudden appearance of bruising or mucocutaneous bleeding in healthy child (epistaxis, gingival bleed, petechiae, purpura, ecchymosis, hematuria)
  - Newly diagnosed, persistent (3–12 mo), chronic (>12 mo)
- **Diagnosis:** Diagnosis of exclusion; patient's Hx (recent URI), meds, diet, travel
  - Isolated thrombocytopenia: Plt count <100 × 10^3/μL, presentation <20 × 10^3/μL
  - Nml WBC, Hgb, MCV, nml smear except thrombocytopenia, nml coags
  - Red flags: Fever, constitutional sx, diet limits, malaria exposure, LAN, splenomegaly, limb defects, hemangiomas, hearing loss
- **Treatment:** Spont resolution in 2/3 within 6 mo
  - Avoidance of aspirin and ibuprofen, avoidance of contact sports; reassurance
  - Platelet transfusions usually ineffective; warranted in life-threatening hemorrhage
  - Medications: No Rx permanently alters natural history of acute ITP
    - Prednisone: 1–2 mg/kg/d for 14 d (Blood 2010;115:168) (oral); up to 75% respond, plt count incr more rapidly with tx (2–7 d) but may decr with taper (caution if active infection esp VZV)
    - IVIG: 0.8–1 g/kg on day 1; blocks FcRs; 80% effective in 1–2 d; side effects are HA, N/V, aseptic meningitis, cataracts, ARF
    - Anti-D Ig: 50–75 μg/kg; for Rh+ patients, coats RBC and overwhelms FcR; 50–77% achieve plt response, >50% in 24 hr; side effects are fever, chills, transient Coombs + hemolytic anemia; contraindicated if Coombs + before

- No data suggesting either IVIG or Anti-D Ig prevents serious bleeding
- Chronic/persistent ITP
  - Splenectomy: 60–70% permanent emission
  - Methylprednisolone or dexamethasone: Decr Ab pdtn, >60% response in 2–7 d
  - Single/combination Cyclosporin A, Azathioprine, Vincristine, Cyclophosphamide, IVIG, Prednisone, Anti-D (70% response over d to mos)
- Rituximab weekly × 4, >30% response within wks, variable duration (Br J Hematol 2009;144(4):552)
- Thrombopoietin receptor agonists Romiplostim (subq), Eltrombopag (PO) (Blood 2011;118(1):28)
- **Complications**
  - Intracranial hemorrhage (ICH): 1 in 200–1,000 cases; risk factors poorly defined: Severe thrombocytopenia + head trauma and/or hematuria (Blood 2009;114:4777)
    - Low threshold for imaging in pts w/ ITP and HA or neurologic symptoms
  - Chronic ITP: ITP >6 mo
    - R/o etiologies: Evan syndrome (ITP w/ AI hemolytic anemia), lupus
    - Generally benign with Plt count from 30–80/μL
    - Prednisone, IVIG, and anti-D Ig raise platelet count but not curative (see above)

Hemolytic-uremic Syndrome (HUS) and Thrombotic Thrombocytopenic Purpura (TTP) (Pediatric Rev 2011;32(4):135; Eur J Pediatr 2010;169(1):7)

- Thrombocytopenia, 2/2 Plt consumption, 2/2 endothelial cell injury, vasculitis, and prothrombotic state (microthrombi confined 1° to kidney in HUS; systemic in TTP)
- **HUS:** Hemolytic anemia, thrombocytopenia, and acute renal failure
  - Classic D(+) HUS: 90% with diarrhea, most often caused by shiga/shiga-like toxin from *E. coli* (O157/H7) or other bacteria (*Shigella, Strep pneumo*), verotoxin inactivates ADAMTS13 → uncleaved vWF multimers initiate plt aggregation
  - Atypical D(–) HUS: No diarrhea, almost all have mutation in complement factor H, factor I or membrane co-factor protein → uncontrolled complement activation (Pediatr Nephrol 2010;25:97)
  - Commonly 9 mo–4 yr in summer & fall; 1° reservoir of bacteria = cattle
  - P/w abd pain, then diarrhea (30–90%); becomes bloody. Avoid abx
  - 2–14 d (mean 6 d) after diarrhea 10–15% develop HUS (40–50% need dialysis)
  - Pts w/ HTN do worse, decr plts w/o signif bleeding, 15–20% w/ neuro sx (szr, coma)
  - Lab: Check CBC, Coombs, smear, BUN/Cr, hemolysis labs, stool culture
  - Treatment supportive, abx controversial, may need dialysis for renal failure
  - Eculizumab is a potential therapy for atypical D(–) HUS: Blocks complement activity of C5 (N Engl J Med 2011;364:2561)
- **TTP:** Primarily in adults; children have autoimmune inhibition of ADAMTS13 or autosomal recessive def → vWF multimers trigger coagulation in multiple organ systems

Disseminated Intravascular Coagulopathy (DIC) (Pediatric Rev 2011;32(4):135)

- Pathologic activation of coagulation → microvascular thrombosis → end-organ ischemia; consumption of plts/coag factors → hemorrhage
- Sepsis, asphyxia, meconium aspiration, ARDS, extensive trauma
- Decr plts, fragmented RBC, prolonged PT/apt, decr fibrinogen, increased FDP. Factor VIII levels differentiate DIC (decr) from liver failure (incr, released during hepatocyte necrosis)
- Treat underlying cause, temporizing plt transfusions for bleeding/severe decr plts and FFP for coag/antithrob factors

COAGULATION

Definition (Pediatr Rev 2008;29:121; Clin Pediatr 2010;49(5):422)

- **1° hemostasis** formation of platelet plug by interaction btw plts and exposed subendothelial layer; plt adhesion via glycoprotein Ib and vWF → plt activation by glycoprotein IIb/IIIa, vWF, and fibrinogen → plt aggregation
- **2° hemostasis** formation of organized fibrin clot for stabilization of platelet plug through activation of the blood coagulation system
- **Physiologic inhibitors** Tissue factor pathway inhibitor, antithrombin, activated protein C and cofactor protein S, fibrinolytic pathway (plasmin)
- **Hemostasis in the newborn:** Need age appropriate assays
  - Immediately postnatally, conc of Vit K dependent coag proteins (FII, FVII, FIX, and FX) and inhibitors protein C and S are ~50% of adult values
  - Concentrations of vWF are incr at birth and for first several postnatal mos

- Factor VIII, V, XIII, and fibrinogen are at/above adult levels
- Inherited severe bleeding disorders present most often in neonatal period or early childhood → may p/w circumcision bleeding, umbilical stump bleeding, cephalohematoma, and subgaleal hemorrhages (as w/ vacuum extractions)

Clinical Manifestations of Bleeding Disorders
- Severe bleeding disorders (hemophilia) usually present at toddler stage, but may present in 1st yr after birth, less severe bleeding disorders, (von Willebrand dz) or platelet fxn abnormality may be clinically silent for yrs
- Easy bruisability; unexpected surgical hemorrhage
- Mucosal bleed (epistaxis, menorrhagia, oral, GU or GI bleed) → think 1° hemostasis
- Deep tissue bleeding into muscles and joints (hemarthrosis) → think 2° hemostasis
- Be sure to always think about child abuse as a cause for bruising
- Family hx, coexisting illness, medication

Diagnostic Studies (Pediatr Rev 2008;29;121)
- CBC, peripheral blood smear
- PT (prothrombin time): Measures extrinsic and common pathways (FVII, FV, FX, prothrombin, fibrinogen); most commonly prolonged w/ Vit K def
- INR (international normalized ratio): Adjust for different reagent sensitivities for PT
- PTT (activated aPTT): Measures contact system (prekallikrein, FXII) as well as intrinsic (FVIII, FIX, FXI) and common pathway; hepzyme prior to further eval
- Mixing study (1:1 pt and normal plasma, PT/aPTT normalizes if missing factor(s) replenished by 50%, PT/aPTT persistent incr suggests presence of inhibitor/antibody
- Fibrinogen, thrombin time (measures fibrin formation, time reqd to form clot on addition of thrombin to plasma), bleeding time (plt interaction with vascular wall, poor predictability, sens, spec), platelet function assay
- Specific factor issues: FXIII not measured by PT/PTT need specific assay, FV only factor not made in liver, FVII shortest 1/2 life of all factors

Abnl PT or aPTT	Abnl PT and aPTT	Abnl CBC or Periph Blood Smear	No Abnl
PTT only prolonged **Hemophilia A or B, Factor XI def, vWD with FVIII dysfxn, Lupus anticoag, Heparin contamination** • *check FVIII, FIX, FXI, lupus anticoag* *PT only prolonged* **early Vit K def, Factor VII deficiency, Warfarin excess** • *check FVII*	*PT & aPTT prolonged, normal platelets* **Liver dz, Vit K def, Common path def (Factor X, V, prothrombin, fibrinogen), dysfibrinogenemia** • *check FV, FX, prothrombin, mixing study, fibrinogen* *PT & aPTT prolonged, low platelets* **DIC, liver disease** • *check fibrinogen*	**von Willebrand dz:-** Check vWF antigen, ristocetin cofactor activity, ristocetin-induced plt aggregation (RIPA), FVIII, vWF multimers analysis **Acute or chronic ITP** • *check platelet count, platelet function assay, meds, systemic disease*	FXIII assay Connective tissue dz Child abuse

Pediatr Rev 2008;29;121; Clin Pediatr (Phila) 2010;49;422

Von Willebrand Dz (Pediatr Rev 2008;29;121; Haemophilia 2008;14;171)
- Most common genetic bleeding disorder, 1% prevalence
- vWF is a large multimeric glycoprotein required for plt adhesion to damaged endothelium and acts as carrier protein for FVIII. High molecular weight multimers have more plt binding sites and adhesive properties
- Note vWF is an acute phase reactant, can incr with stress, exercise, pregnancy, inflamm
- Often asymptomatic, positive FHx, easy bruising, repeat epistaxis, menorrhagia (50% of women), postop bleeding
  - **Type 1:** 70–80% of cases, autosomal dominant partial quantitative decr of vWF and FVIII → decr vWF activity/Ag and FVIII, mild sx
  - **Type 2:** 15–20% of cases, autosomal dominant or recessive, qualitative defect in vWF
    - **2A:** Autosomal dominant, normal–reduced level of FVIIIc/vWF and decr ristocetin cofactor activity due to decr intermediate/high molecular weight vWF multimers
    - **2B:** Autosomal dominant, decr high molecular weight vWF multimers → decr affinity for GPIb complex; intermittent thrombocytopenia
    - **2M:** Decr plt-directed function, decr vWF activity
    - **2N:** Autosomal recessive, decr affinity for FVIII → 5% FVIII levels (appear like hemophilia)

- **Type 3:** Most severe form, autosomal recessive, marked deficiency of vWF and FVIIIc, no vWF on plts/endothelium, no response to DDAVP, severe clinical bleeding
- **Acquired forms** with Wilms tumor, lymphoproliferative d/o, congenital heart dz, antiphospholipid antibody syndrome, aortic valvular stenosis, SLE, angiodysplasia, seizure disorders on Valproic acid, hypothyroid, essential thrombocythemia
- **Treatment** (J Emerg Med 2010;39:158)
  - **Desmopressin (DDAVP) IV, IN, SubQ:** Rx of choice for Type 1 vWD and Types 2A/2M vWD, ineffective in Type 3 and most Type 2B disease (may cause plt drop)
    - Incr endogenous vWF plasma conc 2–4-fold w/ similar rise in FVIII activity
    - Dose for hemostasis ~15× used for DI. Peak values within 1 hr after admin
    - Side effects: facial flushing, HA, tachycardia, HoNa (esp plts <2 yo 2/2 SIADH)
    - For major bleeds, use only if known responder
    - Aminocaproic acid (plasmin inhibitor) is a useful adjunct for mucosal bleed
  - **Transfusional therapy with plasma-derived vWF products**
    - Need for Type 3 and most with Type 2 disease
    - Need plasma concentrates w/ both FVIII and high molecular weight vWF forms (e.g., Humate-P, Alphanate)
    - Cryoprecipitate is not a good choice because it is not virally inactivated

Platelet Function Disorder (w/ exclusion of thrombocytopenia, see earlier)
- **Acquired:** Meds: Antiepileptic meds (valproate) and antidepressants, aspirin, NSAID
  - Systemic: Uremia, liver failure, leukemia
- **Congenital:** Less common, 2/2 inherited defects in receptors needed for Plt adhesion and aggregation, defects in signaling and in Plt metabolism. Variable presentation
  - Bernard–Soulier syndrome: Deficiency in glycoprotein Ib, prevents Plt adhesion
  - Glanzmann's thrombasthenia: Plts lack glycoprotein IIb/IIIa, no Plt aggregation

Hemophilia: X-linked, second most common factor def after vWD
- Hemophilia A: Deficiency/dysfxn in FVIII, 1/5,000 male births, 1/3 no FHx
- Hemophilia B: Deficiency/dysfxn in FIX, 1/30,000 male births
- Hemophilia C: Deficiency in FXI, 10 times less common than hemophilia A, usually mild bleeding tendency, bleeding risk not related to severity of deficiency
- Acquired: Develop FVIII auto-Ab in pts w/o deficiency, idiopathic (age > 50), collagen vasc dz, peripartum, IBD, acute hepatitis B/C, drug reaction (e.g., PCN), autoimmune dz, lymphoproliferative malignancies
- **Presentation:** Weakness/orthostasis from bleeding, spontaneous/excess hemorrhage with trauma/surgery, bleeding sites incl joints, muscles, CNS (2–8% lifetime risk ICH), GI, GU, pulm, cardiovascular, mucosal membranes, circumcision site
  - Hemophilic arthropathy graded in 5 stages (Arnold–Hilgartner classification) synovial cells make high levels tissue factor pathway inhibitor → more FXa inhibition → predisposition to bleed → long-term inflamm, fibrosis, hemosiderin deposition, cartilage damage, subchondral bone-cyst formation
- **Labs:** PTT: Prolonged and PT, platelet count, bleeding time: Normal, vWF: Normal (low value with low FVIII suggests vWF deficiency)

Classification	Severe	Moderate	Mild
FVIII or FIX activity	<1%	1–5%	>5–40%
Frequency	50–70%	10%	30–40%
Cause of bleeding	Spontaneous Hemarthrosis	Minor trauma, rarely spontaneous	Major trauma, surgery
Freq bleeding (w/o prophy)	2–4 times/mo	4–6 times/yr	Uncommon

- **Complications**
  - Inhibitors: 30% hemophilia A pts develop FVIII allo-Ab (IgG), 50% occur by age 10, usually FVIII <1%, a/w certain mutations and purified FVIII products; <5% hemophilia B pts develop FIX inhibitors (J Emerg Med 2010;39(2):158)
  - Inhibitor titer (in Bethesda units <5 BU low titer → pt may respond to higher dose FVIII, >10 BU high titer), bleed severity, responder status determine rx
  - Life expectancy: Now comparable to healthy males
  - ICH is the most common cause of death related to hemorrhage, chronic debilitating joint dz (prevent disability by replacing factors 2–3× weekly)
- **Treatment** (J Emerg Med 2010;39:158)
  - Recombinant-derived FVIII and FIX concentrates, desired FVIII level 30–50% for minor/mod bleed and 80–100% for severe life-threatening bleed
  - Rx for severe bleeds requires loading and maintenance. Each unit FVIII/kg causes 2% rise in FVIII. Each unit FIX/kg causes 0.8–1% rise in FIX

- Episodic ("on demand") or prophylactic infusions of factor concentrates to limit arthropathy (Semin Thromb Hemost 2012;38(1):79)
- Desmopressin IV/IN may be used for mild hemophilia A (baseline FVIII >10%)
- Cryoprecipitate (contains FVIII, vWF) use only when FVIII concentrate not available, diff to achieve hemostatic doses
- FFP (contains FIX) use only when FIX concentrate not available, diff to achieve hemostatic doses due to volume overload
- Recombinant- or plasma-derived FVIII, recombinant activated FVII used against inhibitors

Factor XIII Deficiency
- Factor XIII deficiency: Fibrin stabilizing factor deficiency, rarest form (1 in 5×10^6 births), autosomal recessive, a/w oozing from umbilical stump/circumcision, 25–30% ICH
- FXIII def treated with plasma, cryoppt or FXIII concentrates; desired level >3–5%

Acquired Bleeding Disorders
- Acquired systemic disorders: Liver disease, renal disease w/ uremia
- Acquired Vit K def: In chronically ill, prolonged abx, or w/ malabsorption
- ECMO or DIC

Thrombophilias (Pediatr Rev 2011;32:41; Hematol Oncol Clin N Am 2010;24:151)
- Btw 2001 and 2007, 70% incr in annual rate of VTE in US. 63% pts with at least 1 coexisting chronic medical condition, especially malignancy (Pediatrics 2009;124(4):1001)
- Bimodal distribution of VTE incidence, peak in neonatal period and adolescence
- **Etiology**
  - **Inherited hypercoagulable states** (always ask for FHx)
    - Activated protein C resistance (APCR): Cannot degrade FVa/FVIIIa → 4× incr risk for DVT in lifetime, usually 2/2 FV Leiden mutation (also FV London, FV Toronto)
    - Prothrombin 20210A mutation: 3–5× incr risk for DVT by early lifetime
    - Hyperhomocysteinemia: Can cause either arterial or venous thrombotic disease
    - Heterozygous antithrombin III deficiency
    - Homozygous protein C/S def: Homozygous → purpura fulminans in neonates; heterozygotes have 50% risk of thromboembolism by middle age
    - Elevated lipoprotein (a): 3–4× incr risk venous thrombosis; also arterial
  - **Acquired hypercoagulable states**
    - Virchow triad: Venous stasis, endothelial injury, hypercoagulability
    - 90% VTE in children is risk-associated: Cancer, congenital heart dz, prosthetic heart valves, indwelling vascular access, nephritic syndrome, trauma, recent surgery, infection, autoimmune dz, immobilization, OCP, SCD, smoking, IBD, vasculitis, APLS
    - HIT → suspect if 50% decr in Plt count plus prior heparin exposure (~5–10 d prior), and no other explan +/− Concurrent clot
- **Clinical manifestations**
  - Macrovascular: DVT, pregnancy loss, catheter-related, arterial clot/CVA, pulmonary embolism, antiphospholipid antibody syndrome
  - Microvascular: TTP/HUS, HIT
- **Diagnostic evaluation:** D-dimer, Coags, CBC, Doppler US for DVT or renal vein thrombosis, CT venography, Spiral CT for PE (VQ scan if contrast contraindicated), MRA/V for eval of CVA (sx based), Echo

Laboratory Evaluation of Thrombophilic Conditions	
Factor V Leiden Prothrombin G20210A	PCR
Elevated lipoprotein(a) Protein S deficiency	ELISA
Protein C deficiency Antithrombin deficiency	Chromogenic (functional) assay
Elevated Factor VIII activity	One-stage clotting assay (aPTT based)
Hyperhomocysteinemia	Mass spectrometry
Antiphospholipid syndrome	ELISA for anticardiolipin, anti-β2-glycoprotein IgG/IgM; clotting assay (dilute Russell viper venom time or aPTT based phospholipids neutralization method for lupus anticoagulant
APCR	Clotting assay (aPTT based)

Adapted from Hematol Oncol Clin North Am 2010;24:151

Pediatric Stroke (Stroke 2008;39:2644; Acta Paediatrica 2010;99:1641)
- **Arterial ischemic strokes (AIS)** (Thromb Res 2011;127:6): 2 per 100,000 children per yr, many with cardiac dz (20%) and sickle cell, also previously healthy pts— 80% found to have cervical/cerebral arteriopathy, i.e., dissection, occlusion, stenosis

- **Reported risk factors:** Systemic varicella infection, URI, vasculitis, mitochondrial encephalomyopathies (e.g., MELAS), thrombophilias (Circulation 2010;121:1838), iron def anemia (Arch Dis Child 2011;96:276), dyslipoproteinemias, organic acidurias
- 74% neuro deficit at discharge, 3% death (arteriopathy, b/L ischemia, decr consciousness at presentation a/w worse outcomes (Lancet Neurol 2009;8:1120)
- **Cerebral venous sinus thrombosis (CVST)** (Neurosurg Clin N Am 2010;21:511): 40% occurs in neonatal period, 0.4–0.7 per 100,000 children per yr, tend to have non-focal neurologic signs/sx
  - **Reported risk factors:** Dehydration, infection, HIE, anemia, head injury, post-intracranial surgery, autoimmune d/o, malignancies, cardiac disease, renal disease, drugs, chromosomal d/o, thrombophilias, maternal hx (e.g., chorio, DM, HTN)
- **Hemorrhagic stroke** (Pediatr Neurol 2007;36:73): 2–3 per 100,000 children per yr
  - **Reported risk factors:** AVM, aneurysm, cavernous malformation, plt disorder, coagulation defects
- **Diagnostics:** Cranial Doppler ultrasound; CT and CTA; MRI, MRA, MRV; nuclear medicine, incl SPECT and perfusion techniques and PET; and catheter angiography; TTE/TEE; thrombophilia or bleeding d/o workup; Hgb electrophoresis
- **Management** based on consensus-based guidelines and evidence from adult literature: *Management of Stroke in Infants and Children* (Stroke 2008;39:2644).

Anticoagulation (Pediatr Emerg Care 2011;27:55)

Agent	Mechanism	Pros	Cons	Monitoring
Unfractionated heparin (UFH)	Binds ATIII and incr inhibition of thrombin/FXa	Rapid onset, short half-life, easily reversed with protamine	Continuous infusion, risk of bleeding/ HIT/ osteoporosis	Anti-FXa conc (goal 0.3–0.7) PTT (goal 2–3 × baseline)
LMWH	Inhibits FXa	Long half-life, easy admin (bid subq), minimal monitoring	Subq, incomplete protamine reversal, HIT (lower risk than UFH), osteoporosis	Anti-FXa conc obtained 4 hr after 2nd dose Therapeutic 0.5–1 U/mL Prophylactic 0.1–0.3 U/mL
Warfarin	Inhibit Vit K-dep factors II, VII, IX, X, and protein C and S	Long half-life, oral admin, reverse with Vit K and FFP	Food/med interactions, unpredictable conc, frequent titration	INR goal 2–3 or 2.5–3.5 dependent on indication
Tissue plasminogen activator	Plasminogen → plasmin to promote clot breakdown	Rapid onset, active lytic agent	Higher risk bleed, frequent monitor	Serial imaging of clot, D-dimer incr, fibrinogen decr

Adapted from Pediatr Rev 2011;32:41

- **Heparin:** Loading dose: 75 U/kg IV over 10 min
  - Maintenance <1 yo: 28 U/kg/hr; >1 yo: 20 U/kg/hr; >14 yo: 16 U/kg/hr; adult: 18 U/kg/hr or 1,000 U/hr; need sliding scale (see PE/DVT)
  - Check aPTT every 4 hr, goal 60–85 sec. Anti-FXa may be used in children <1 yo because aPTT less accurate (goal 0.35–0.7 U/mL)
  - When aPTT therapeutic, check CBC/aPTT daily
  - HIT: Type 1 benign self-limited decr plt count within 24–96 hr of exposure. Type 2 severe decr plt count (>50%) 5–14 d after initiation, IgG Ab against plt factor 4 and heparin (ELISA for dx) → stop all forms of heparin rx

aPTT (sec)	Bolus (U/kg)	Stop Infusion (min)	Rate Cange (%)
<50	50	0	+10
50–59	0	0	+10
60–85	0	0	0
86–95	0	0	−10
96–120	0	30	−10
>120	0	60	−15

Adapted from Chest 1998;114:748S

- **Low Molecular Weight Heparin** (LMWH): Lovenox (enoxaparin) or Dalteparin (fragmin) (Chest 1998;114:748S)
  - <3 mo: Treatment 1.5 mg/kg/dose q12h; prophylaxis: 0.75 mg/kg/dose q12h
  - >3 mo: Treatment 1 mg/kg/dose q12h; prophylaxis: 0.5 mg/kg/dose q12h
  - Check antifactor Xa activity after 4 dose, 4 hr after LMWH
    - Anti-FXa activity <0.35; ↑ next dose by 25%; repeat anti-FXa 4 hr after next dose
    - Anti-FXa 0.35–0.49; ↑ next dose by 10%; repeat anti-FXa 4 hr after next dose
    - Anti-FXa 0.5–1; no change; repeat anti-FXa next day, then after 1 wk, then monthly
    - Anti-FXa 1.6–2; Hold dose x 3 hr; ↓ next dose by 20%; repeat anti-FXa before next dose and again 4 hr after next dose
    - Anti-FXa >2; Hold dose till level ≤0.5; ↓ next dose by 40%; repeat anti-FXa before next dose and if not ≤0.5 then again q12h until ≤0.5
- **Warfarin:** Goal INR 2–3 (2.5–3.5 in certain situations, i.e., mechanical valve)
  - Each incr INR 0.5 → incr risk of bleeding 1.4×
  - Overlap w/ heparin. Continue heparin for minimum 5 d and until INR >2 for 2 d
  - Start dose 0.15 mg/kg, max 10 mg (limit 5 mg if liver dysfxn or s/p Fontan proc)

Loading d 2–4	1.1–1.3	Repeat start dose
	1.4–3	Give 50% of start dose
	3.1–3.5	Give 25% of start dose
	>3.5	Hold until INR < 3.5, then restart at 50% start dose
Maintenance	1.1–1.4	Incr 20% dose
	1.4–1.9	Incr 10% dose
	2–3	No change
	3.1–3.5	Decr 10% dose
	>3.5	Hold until INR< 3.5, then restart at 20% less

Adapted from Pediatr Emerg Care 2011;27:55

- Check INR qd for 5–7 d after new dose
- Efficacy affected by Vit K intake; protein bound and affected by other meds
- Reverse effect w/ Vit K (if bleeding; 0.5–2 mg IV + FFP 20 mL/kg IV). If not; Vit K 0.5–2 mg SQ. If reversal wanted but w/ plan to reuse warfarin in near future, do not use Vit K, instead use 10 cc/kg FFP (may need >1 dose)
- **Other agents** (Thromb Res 2011;127:70)
  - **Direct thrombin inhibitors (Argatroban, Lepirudin, Bivalirudin)**
    - Does not require antithrombin, more predictable pharmacokinetics, less bleeding in adult studies, do not cause HIT
    - Used in nephrotic syndrome with proteinuria (where urinary AT III loss)
    - Argatroban: Pediatr Blood Cancer 2011;56:1103, Bivalirudin: Pediatr Blood Cancer 2008;51:798
  - **Fondaparinux** (anti-Xa inhibitor): Selectively binds to ATIII, used in HIT (FondaKIDS. Pediatr Blood Cancer 2011;57:1049)
  - **Thrombolysis:** Can use agents such as TPA (alteplase). Indications/dosing extrapolated from adults. Monitor INR, aPTT, Fibrinogen (goal>1 g/dL), plt (>50–100 × 10⁹/L), D-dimer, FDP. Contraindicated if active bleed, recent surg, HTN, AVM, severe trauma
  - **IVC filter:** Consider if contraindication/failure of anticoagulation

BONE MARROW FAILURE

Definition (Hematology Am Soc Hematol Educ Program 2009:329)
- **Pancytopenia:** Anemia, thrombocytopenia, leukopenia

Diagnostic Evaluation: Exam for signs of anemia &/or thrombocytopenia
- Exam for dysmorphic features (eval for inherited etiologies)
- Labs: CBC, serum aminotransferases, viral serologies (HIV, CMV, EBV, hepatitis, parvo, HSV), folate, B_{12}, Hgb F, BM aspirate and biopsy, marrow cytogenetics, drug screen
- Specific labs: Diepoxybutane for Fanconi anemia; CD 55/59 screen for paroxysmal nocturnal hemoglobinuria, HLA tissue typing

Aplastic Anemia (Lancet 2005;365:1647; Ann Intern Med 2002;136:534)
- Pancytopenia (2 of the following—ANC < 500/μL, retics < 1%, platelets < 20,000), and hypocellular bone marrow; 2/2 injury or loss of hematopoietic stem cells
- Incidence triphasic, w/ 1 peak in childhood (2–5 yr; 2/2 inherited causes), and 2 peaks in adulthood, 20–25 yr and majority pts presenting beyond 55–60 yo

- Complications: Infxns (2/2 neutropenia), bleeding (decr Plts), and findings of anemia, cancer susceptibility (Br J Haematol 2010;150:179)
- Acquired: Idiopathic, chemo/XRT, drugs (gold, NSAIDs, AEDs, sulfa), chemicals (benzene), viral (parvo B$_{19}$, Non-A, B, C hepatitis, HIV, EBV), immune (SLE), misc (pregnancy, thymoma, paroxysmal nocturnal hemoglobinuria)
  - Paroxysmal nocturnal hemoglobinuria: Rare in children, intravascular hemolysis, nocturnal hemoglobinuria, thrombotic events, serious infections, bone marrow failure, a/w GPI-anchor protein deficiency (Br J Haematol 2005;128:571)
- Inherited
  - **Fanconi anemia:** Café-au-lait spots, abn of thumbs, hypogonadism, microcephaly
  - **Dyskeratosis congenita:** Nail dystrophy, early hair graying or loss, leukoplakia, hyperpigmented rash, dysmorphic teeth, enamel hypoplasia, restrictive pulm dz, or pulm vasc dz
  - **Shwachman–Diamond syndrome:** Exocrine pancreatic insufficiency, short stature, skeletal anomalies, transient transaminitis (Hematol Oncol Clin North Am 2009;23:233)
  - **Amegakaryocytic thrombocytopenia:** Isolated thrombocytopenia

Pure RBC Aplasia (Pediatr Rev 2002;23:111) will have reticulocytopenia
- **Diamond–Blackfan** (Consensus conference: Br J Haematol 2008;142:859)
  - Insidious presentation in 1st yr of life (2–3 mo)
  - 25% w/ dysmorphic features (short statues, abnormal facies w/ cleft palate), abnormalities of the thumb, congenital heart disease
  - Increased MCV and red cell adenosine deaminase
  - Rx: Glucocorticoids (initially prednisone 2 mg/kg/d) and check retic response
  - If no response to steroids, will likely need chronic RBC transfusion support
  - If matched sibling, consider BMT
  - Complications of chronic transfusions: Iron overload and need chronic iron chelation therapy. Increased risk of AML
- **Transient erythroblastopenia of childhood (TEC)**
  - Unknown etiology; median age is 2 yr; normal physical exam
  - Resolves spont w/i mo. Recurrence unlikely; can require RBC xfusion
- **Parvovirus:** Significant in prenatal parvo infxn or setting of chronic hemolysis (sickle cell)
  - Has affinity for erythroid precursors; thus in setting of chronic hemolysis and incr reticulocytosis, can lead to severe anemia and aplastic crisis

Bone Marrow Transplant (N Engl J Med 2006;354:1813; Pediatr Clin North Am 2010;57:147)
- **Definitions**
  - Graft vs. host disease (GVHD): Undesirable side effect of allogenic hematopoietic stem cell transplant (HSCT) where donor cells effect the host
  - Graft vs. tumor (GVT) effect: Desired effect of bone marrow transplant, transplanted cells attack host tumor cells
  - Goal is to balance immunosuppression as to minimize the effects of GVHD, while still maintaining an adequate GVT response
- **Indications**
  - Malignancy: Useful in case of refractory dz or non-responsive to usual chemo Rx regimens. Uses GVT effect w/ hopes of eradicating malignancy
  - Non-malignant dzs: Immunodeficiencies, hematologic abn (thalassemia, sickle cell); goal to replace abn lymphohematopoietic system w/ nml donor one
- **Autologous:** Goal is as rescue for pt w/o replacing their lymphohematopoietic sys
  - Allows pts to receive higher than usual doses of chemo w/ rescue in place
  - Often used for neuroblastoma, extraocular retinoblastoma
  - No risk of GVHD, but also no benefit of GVT
- **Allogeneic:** Donor provides host w/ hematopoietic rescue and GVT effect
  - Goal to minimize side effect of GVHD and maximize GVT effect

LYMPHADENOPATHY IN THE PEDIATRIC PATIENT

Definition (Pediatr Rev 2008;29:53)
- Axillary or cervical lymph node >1 cm in size; inguinal lymph node >1.5 cm; epitrochlear lymph node >0.5 cm; supraclavicular—any palpable lymph node
- **Note:** Risk of underlying malignancy increases w/ increasing size, esp >2 cm
- **Localized lymphadenopathy:** Involving one nodal group
- **Generalized lymphadenopathy:** Involving ≥2 nodal groups or sites (i.e., spleen/liver)

Differential Diagnosis of Lymphadenopathy (Pediatr Rev 2008;29:53; Pediatr Rev 2000;21:399)

Infections	Malignancy / Immunologic / Endocrine / Misc

Infections
• **Bacterial:**
  • **Localized:** Lymphadenitis (tender, suppurative node, often unilateral cervical): Staph, GAS, anaerobes (periodontal disease). Cat scratch dz, tularemia, bubonic plague, scrofula (TB), diphtheria, chancroid (inguinal)
  • **Generalized:** Brucellosis, leptospirosis, lymphogranuloma venereum, typhoid
• **Viral:** Adenovirus, influenza, RSV, EBV, CMV, HSV, HIV, HBV, mumps, measles, rubella, dengue fever
• **Fungal:** Coccidiomycosis, cryptococcosis, histoplasmosis
• **Protozoal:** Toxoplasmosis, leishmaniasis
• **Spirochetal:** Lyme disease, syphilis
	Malignancy: Leukemia, lymphoma, metastasis from solid tumor
	Immunologic: Angioimmunoblastic LAD w/ dysproteinemia, autoimmune lymphoproliferative dz, chronic granulomatous dz, dermatomyositis, drug rxn, RA, hemophagocytosis, Langerhans cell histiocytosis, serum sickness, SLE
	Endocrine: Addison disease, hypothyroidism
	Misc: Amyloidosis, Castleman dz, Churg–Strauss, inflammatory pseudotumor Kawasaki dz, Kikuchi dz, lipid storage dz, sarcoidosis

Clinical Manifestations (Pediatr Clin North Am 2002;49:1009)
- Hx: Duration of LAD, assoc sx, recent localized infxn (esp in drainage territory of nodes), skin lesions, trauma, animal scratches/bites, meds, ingestion of unpasteurized milk/undercooked meats, dental problems (cervical LAD), tick bites, travel Hx, sexual Hx
- Exam: Size, location (supraclavicular always concern causing), tender/nontender, mobile/fixed, soft/hard, warm or erythematous, HSM, bruises or petechiae, signs of systemic dz

Diagnostic Evaluation and Management (Pediatr Rev 2008;29:53; Pediatr Clin North Am 2002;49:1009)
- See figure on next page

PEDIATRIC ONCOLOGIC EMERGENCIES

(Principles and Practice Of Pediatric Oncology. 6th ed. Philadelphia, PA: LWW; 2011:1190–1242)

Fever and Neutropenia (Clin Infect Dis 2011;52:e56)
- Definition for purposes of Rx: ANC < 500 & temp 101 (or 100.5–101 × 2 in <24 hr).*
- Background: High risk of bacterial infection w/ overwhelming sepsis. Need to treat empirically with broad-spectrum antibiotics
- Higher-risk pts: ANC < 100, prolonged neutropenia (>1 wk), comorbidities
- Evaluation:
  - Hx: Sx, prior infxns, most recent chemo agents and timing, exposures
  - Exam: Vital signs w/ O_2 sat & attention to oropharynx, lungs, abdomen, skin including nailbeds, central line site & perineal area
  - Dx studies: CBC w/ diff, CMP, blood cx from all lumens CVL (+/– peripheral), blood bank sample, U/A & Ucx. Consider: Coags if toxic, CXR/throat cx/viral panel depending on signs and symptoms
- Rx w/ broad-spectrum IV abx w/i 1 hr of presentation, after blood cx obtained (do not delay rx for other studies such as urine cx)
  - Cefepime is reasonable mono-Rx. Add AG for additional GN coverage for toxic patients, vancomycin empirically after high-dose AraC for α-hemolytic strep or if cellulitis. Consider anti-fungal rx if prolonged F&N >5–7 d
- Usually managed as inpts until afeb with evident neutrophil recovery
- For lower-risk patients consider IV or oral rx and outpatient management

*Do not take rectal temps.

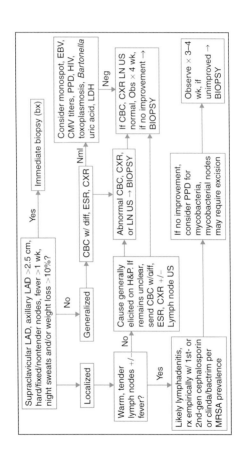

Supraclavicular LAD, axillary LAD >2.5 cm, hard/fixed/nontender nodes, fever >1 wk, night sweats and/or weight loss >10%?

Yes → Immediate biopsy (bx) → Consider monospot, EBV, CMV titers, PPD, HIV, toxoplasmosis, *Bartonella*, uric acid, LDH

No → Localized / Generalized

Localized → Warm, tender lymph nodes +/- fever?

Yes → Likely lymphadenitis, rx empirically w/ 1st- or 2nd-gen cephalosporin or clinda/bactrim per MRSA prevalence → If no improvement, consider PPD for mycobacteria, mycobacterial nodes may require excision

No → Cause generally elicited on H&P. If remains unclear, send CBC w/diff, ESR, CXR +/- Lymph node US

Generalized → CBC w/ diff, ESR, CXR

Nml → Consider monospot, EBV, CMV titers, PPD, HIV, toxoplasmosis, *Bartonella*, uric acid, LDH

Neg → If CBC, CXR LN US normal, Obs × 4 wk, if no improvement → BIOPSY

Abnormal CBC, CXR, or LN US → BIOPSY

Observe × 3–4 wk, if unimproved → BIOPSY

Superior Vena Cava (SVC) Syndrome (Pediatr Clin North Am 1997;44:809)

- **Definition:** Signs and sx from compression &/or obstruction of SVC
- **Etiology:** Often a presenting feature of intrathoracic malignancies
  - Malignancies p/w mediastinal mass most commonly include NHL, T-cell ALL, and Hodgkin dz. Less common: Teratoma, sarcoma, neuroblastoma, thymoma
- **Pathophysiology:** Mediastinal mass compresses SVC causing venous stasis
  - Compression &/or clotting of SVC → ↓ venous return from head, neck, & upper thorax
  - Tracheal compression may also be present, esp with anterior masses
- **Presentation:** Cough, dyspnea, dysphagia, orthopnea, stridor, "wheeze," & hoarseness
  - Later sx of anxiety, confusion, lethargy, HA, Δ vision, and syncope may = CO_2 retention; can also see facial +/− UE swelling, plethora, chest pain, pleural effusions
  - Sx worse when patient is supine; should raise suspicion for mediastinal mass
- **Diagnostic studies:** CXR; typically will show anter mediastinal mass; trach deviation, and narrowing on lateral view. CT neck/chest crucial to assess airway patency
  - CBC, Chem10, LDH, and uric acid; obtain dx tissue sample before Rx if possible
  - Anesthesia may be contraindicated if tracheal compression
- **Treatment:** Depends on underlying malignancy
- If significant CV or resp compromise, emergent XRT and/or IV methylprednisolone/ dexamethasone treatment may be indicated

Tumor Lysis Syndrome (TLS) (Nat Clin Pract Oncol 2006;3:438)

- **Definition:** Metabolic abn 2/2 cell death and subsequent release cell contents into circ
  - Metabolic disturbances can result in severe end-organ impairment, esp renal
- **Etiology/risk factors**
  - Occurs in tumors w/ ↑ growth fraction and large tumor burden/volume
  - Malignancies most commonly assoc w/ TLS include Burkitt lymphoma, ALL (particularly T-cell variant), and lymphoblastic lymphoma; TLS rare in AML
  - Can occur before onset of Rx but typically occurs w/i 12–72 hr of initiation of Rx
  - Risk factors: WBC > 50,000, ↑ LDH, ↑ uric acid on admit, Cr > 1.6 or ↓ GFR
- **Diagnostic studies:** Elevated uric acid (>10) – caused by breakdown of nucleic acids
  - Hyperphosphatemia and secondary hypocalcemia; hyperkalemia
- **Consequences of TLS**
  - Hyperuricemia → precipitation of uric acid in collecting ducts of renal tubules, causing resultant nephropathy and acute renal failure
  - Hyperkalemia → cardiac arrhythmias and sudden death
  - Hypocalcemia → hypotension, EKG changes, tetany, and seizures
  - Hyperphosphatemia → renal precipitation; exacerbate nephropathy and renal failure
- **Management/prevention of TLS:** Electrolyte abn managed acutely as indicated
  - Upon dx of malignancy and before starting Rx, aggressive mgmt to prevent TLS
    - Aggressive hydration (2–4× maintenance) to ↑ GFR and ↑ urinary outflow
    - Urinary alkalization w/ D51/4NS w/NaHCO₃ (40–80 mEq/L) to urine pH ≥ 7 to prevent uric acid precipitation
    - Allopurinol (250–500 mg/m²/d) inhibits xanthine oxidase; ↓ uric acid formation
    - Alternatively, rasburicase (recombinant urate oxidase) in place of allopurinol. More effective & 1st choice in high-risk cases
    - Alkalinization not necessary after uric acid level falls
    - Close observation of electrolytes, Ca, Mg, Ph, LDH, and uric acid (q6–12h upon initiation of Rx) essential to monitor for development of TLS

Spinal Cord Compression (SCC) (Pediatr Clin North Am 1997;44:809)

- **Definition/etiology:** Occurs in 2.7–5% of children w/ cancer
  - Most cases 2/2 epidural compression from extension of paravertebral tumor
  - ↑ risk w/ neuroblastoma, Ewing sarcoma, non-Hodgkin lymphoma, and Hodgkin lymphoma
  - Osteosarcoma and rhabdomyosarcoma typically cause SCC only w/ recurrence
- **Clinical manifestations:** Back pain present in 80% pedi pts w/ cord compression
  - Sx typically present for an avg of 2 wk before dx is made
  - Weakness, sensory loss, and incontinence are later and more concern-causing findings
- **Evaluation/treatment**
  - Detailed neuro exam in any pt p/w suspected malign; rectal exam for sphincter tone
  - Plain radiographs often performed but only show findings in 1/2 of affected patients
  - MRI w/ contrast is study of choice to assess presence and extent of SCC
  - Children w/ neuro findings and/or rapidly progressing spinal cord dysfxn should receive dexamethasone 1 mg/kg IV and have emergent spinal MRI
  - Surgery, XRT, and chemo are other emergent Rx options depending on tumor type

Hyperleukocytosis (Pediatr Clin North Am 1997;44:809)

- **Definition/etiology:** WBC >100,000; presence of high # of circ leukemic blast cells

- Clinically signif hyperleukocytosis >200,000 in AML, >300,000 in ALL and CML
- Occurs in 9–13% of patients with ALL and 5–22% of patients with AML
- **Pathogenesis:** Excessive leukocytes obstruct circulation in brain, lung, and other organs forming aggregates and white thrombi in small veins
  - Excessive leukocytes also compete for oxygen and damage vessel walls
  - Morbidity is directly related to blood viscosity
  - Myeloblasts and monoblasts are larger (AML) and more likely to cause obstruction
- **Clinical manifestations**
  - Pulmonary leukostasis → dyspnea, hypoxia, and right ventricular failure
  - Intracerebral leukostasis → Δ mental status, frontal HA, szr, and papilledema
  - Other possible complications include priapism, renal failure, and dactylitis
  - Major complications of hyperleukocytosis in ALL usually result of TLS
  - Complications of hyperleukocytosis in AML usually are result of intracerebral leukostasis and include stroke and hemorrhage
- **Treatment:** Aggressive hydration, alkalize, & rasburicase or allopurinol (to ↓ risk of TLS)
- Maintain platelet count >20,000 minimize RBC xfusion to prevent further ↑ in viscosity
- Correct coagulopathy w/ FFP and vitamin K as indicated
- Exchange xfusion and leukophoresis also used to help rapidly ↓ leukocyte count
  Prompt initiation of chemotherapy (or ATRA for acute promyelocytic leukemia)

NEUTROPENIA IN THE PEDIATRIC PATIENT

Definition (Pediatr Rev 2008;29:12)
- **Absolute neutrophil count (ANC)** = WBC (cells/μL) × %(PMNs + bands)/100
- Mild neutropenia: ANC 1,000–1,500/μL; moderate neutropenia: ANC 500–1,000/μL; severe neutropenia: ANC < 500/μL. ANC < 500 assoc with significant risk of infections
- **Note:** Lower limit nml ANC = 1,500 for pts >1 yo. For pts 2 wk–6 mo, nml ANC > 1,000. Pts <2 wk nml ANC variable. 3–5% of African-Americans have ANCs < 1,500 normally

Differential Diagnosis (Pediatr Rev 2008;29:12)
- **Acquired causes:**
  - **Infection:**
    - Viral (most common cause neutropenia, 2/2 BM suppression, lasts 3–8 d): EBV, CMV, parvo, RSV, flu A/B, hepatitis, HHV6, VZV, rubella, rubeola, HIV
    - Bacterial: Typhoid fever, *Shigella*, brucellosis, tularemia, TB, malaria, RMSF
  - **Drug induced:** PCNs, sulfonamides, chloramphenicol, phenytoin, ibuprofen, ranitidine, hydralazine, carbamazepine, cimetidine, chlorpromazine, indomethacin, quinidine, propylthiouracil, procainamide, chlorpropamide, phenothiazines
  - **Immune:**
    - Neonatal alloimmune neutropenia (maternal antineutrophil IgG xfer across placenta, dx w/ antineutrophil Ab in infant and maternal serum; self-resolves by 2–3 mo)
    - Primary autoimmune neutropenia (neutropenia may be severe but generally benign clinical course, typically presents btw 5–15 mo, dx by detecting antineutrophil Ab in pt)
    - Secondary autoimmune neutropenia (e.g., SLE, Evans syndrome)
  - **Sequestration** (typically mild neutropenia w/ splenomegaly of any cause)
  - **Nutritional def** (typically p/w anemia, hypersegmented PMNs): B_{12} or folate def
  - **Chronic idiopathic**
- **Inherited causes:**
  - **Severe congenital neutropenia** (early infancy w/ severe neutropenia and infxns, may be AR = Kostmann syndrome (HAX1 gene mut) or AD (ELA2 and GFII mut. High risk of later developing MDS and/or AML)
  - **Cyclic neutropenia** (characterized by 21-d cycles w/ neutropenia lasting 3–6 d in a cycle, sometimes severe. Dx w/ serial CBCs 2–3 × /wk × 4–6 wk, neutrophil elastase)
  - **Shwachman–Diamond syndrome** (mild–mod neutropenia + exocrine pancreatic insuff, short stature, metaphyseal dysplasia. ↑ risk for MDS/AML)
  - **Marrow failure syndromes:** Fanconi anemia (pancytopenia usually in 5–10 yo), dyskeratosis congenita (abn skin pigmentation, dystrophic nails, leukoplakia), Diamond–Blackfan syndrome (anemia, thumb, and craniofacial anom)
- **Syndromes w/ associated immunodeficiencies:**
  - Hyper-IgM syndrome, dys-γ-globulinemia, myelokathexis, Chediak–Higashi (albinism, periph neuropathies), cartilage hair syndrome (fine hair, short limbed, dwarfism, lymphopenia), Wiskott–Aldrich (eczema, neutropenia, thrombocytopenia), selective IgA def, reticular dysgenesis (SCID w/ neutropenia)

- **Hx:** Hx of infxn (esp mouth ulceration), cong anomalies, med exposures, recent illnesses. FHx for neutropenias or serious infxn, hospitalizations, blood dz
- **Exam:** Physical feature c/w immunodeficiency syndrome (see the earlier discussion)
- **Laboratory eval:** CBC w/ diff & retic count. Consider rpt CBC to verify
- **Further eval:** As per suspected cause: Observation (if mild/mod neutropenia and suspected viral cause, rpt CBC 1–2 wk), viral titers/tests, antineutrophil Ab (if AI suspected), serial CBCs (if cyclic suspected), DNA analysis for HAX1, ELA2, GFII (if severe congenital suspected), quant Ig's w/ B- and T-cell subsets (if evidence of immunodef), ANA/anti-dsDNA (if SLE suspected), BM biopsy/aspirate (if multiple lines affected or dx unclear)

ACUTE LYMPHOBLASTIC LEUKEMIA

Definition: Clonal proliferation of either pre-B, mature B- or T-lymphocyte cell lines
Epidemiology (Pediatr Rev 2005;26:96)
- ~2,500–3,500 new pedi cases/yr; most common pedi cancer (25% of all pedi cancer)
- May occur at any age with peak incidence 2–5 yo; males > females, whites > blacks
- Risk factors: Down syndrome, neurofibromatosis type 1, ataxia telangiectasia, Fanconi, other syndromes

Clinical Presentation (Pediatr Rev 2005;26:96)
- Fever (55%), bleeding +/– petechiae/purpura (45%), malaise (40%), bone pain (30%), hepatomegaly (70%), splenomegaly (50%), LAD (50%), abd pain (10%)
- CBC: Leukocytosis or leukopenia and anemia (88%) and/or thrombocytopenia (80%)
- Blasts may be visible on peripheral blood smear, but are not always present

Prognostic Factors and Overall Prognosis (N Engl J Med 2006;354:166)
- **Overall survival:** ~80%
- **Favorable prognostic features:** Age at presentation 1–9 yr, presenting WBC <50,000; favorable cytogenetics include: Hyperdiploidy (>50 chromo) w/ trisomies of 4, 10, and 17, t(12;21)/*TEL-AML1* fusion gene
- **Unfavorable prognostic features:** Age <1 or >9 yr, presenting WBC >50,000; highly unfavorable cytogenetics: Hypoploidy (33–39 chromo) or near haploidy (23–29 chromosomes), t(4;11)/*MLL-AF4* fusion gene in infants (present in 80% of infant ALL), and t(9;22)/BCR-ABL protein/Philadelphia chromosome
- **Other unfavorable features:** Fail to achieve morph remission after induction or >1% blasts detectable by PCR or flow cytometry (min residual dz) at the end of induction

Treatment (Pediatr Clin North Am 2008;55:1; N Engl J Med 2006;354:166)
- Total treatment duration is typically 2–3 yr and consists of 3 phases:
  - Induction (4–6 wk): Prednisone or dexamethasone, vincristine, PEG L-asparaginase +/– anthracycline, also w/ intrathecal Rx
  - Consolidation (4–6 mo): High-dose methotrexate, cyclophosphamide, cytosine arabinoside (AraC), 6-MP, and PEG L-asparaginase
    - Most protocols have delayed intensification or reinduction phase; 4–6 wk pulse intensive Rx similar/identical to Induction during 1st 6 mo of remission
  - Maintenance (2–3 yr): Oral MTX and 6-MP, steroid & vincristine pulses, IT chemo
- **Role of BMT:** Reserved for pts at very high risk; with poor initial response to treatment or with relapse
- **Role of XRT:** Cranial radiation therapy reserved only for very high-risk patients or those with significant CNS leukemic involvement
  - W/ effective risk-adjusted chemo, prophy cranial XRT can be safely omitted from Rx of childhood ALL (N Eng J Med 2009;360:2730)

ACUTE MYELOGENOUS LEUKEMIA

Definition (Pediatr Clin North Am 1997;44:847)
- Clonal proliferation of any of the following (*Parentheses denote French-American British Morphologic Classification*): minimally differentiated myeloid cells (M0), myeloblasts (M1 and M2), promyelocytic (M3), myelomonocytic (M4), monocytic (M5), erythroleukemias (M6), or megakaryoblastic (M7)
- AML distinguished from myelodysplastic syndromes by >20% blasts in BM

Epidemiology (Pediatr Rev 2005;26:96; Pediatr Clin North Am 2008;55:21)
- ~500 new pedi cases/yr in the United States; represents 4% of all childhood cancers
- Males = Females; equal incidence in black and white children
- More common than ALL in neonates; no age peak in childhood (median age = 65 yr)

AML 9-5

- **Environmental:** Exposure to chemo (alkylating agents, topo-2-isomerase inhibitors) or ionizing radiation, exposure to organic solvents, herbicides, pesticides
- **Inherited:** Down syndrome, Fanconi anemia, Kostmann syndrome, Shwachman–Diamond syndrome, Diamond–Blackfan syndrome, neurofibromatosis Type I, Klinefelter syndrome, Bloom syndrome, Li–Fraumeni syndrome

Clinical Presentation (Principles and Practice of Pediatric Oncology. 6th ed. Philadelphia, PA: LWW; 2011:566–587.)

- Fever (30%), bone pain (20%), lymphadenopathy (<20%), leukemia cutis (palpable, nontender nodules; may be colorless or blue) (<10%), gingival hypertrophy (<15%), granulocytic sarcomas/chloromas (solid tumors composed of AML blasts), bleeding (from thrombocytopenia or DIC, esp in APL), leukostasis
- CBC: Anemia (>50%), thrombocytopenia (75%), WBC >100,000 (20%)
- Blasts may be visible in peripheral blood smear

Prognosis (Pediatr Clin North Am 2008;55:21)

- **Overall survival:** ~50%
- **Favorable prognostic features:** Age <50 yr, Down syndrome (special group w/ >80% cure rate) favorable cytogenetics: t(8;21), inv(16), t(15;17), possibly t(9;11)
- **Unfavorable gene prognostic factors:** Black race, WBC >100,000 at dx, monosomy 5 or 7, FLT3 gene mutations. Residual dz after induction either morphologically or by PCR/flow cytometry (minimal residual disease)

Treatment (Pediatr Clin North Am 2008;55:21)

- Generally shorter (<1 yr) and more intensive than ALL treatment
- Induction: Generally w/ cytarabine, anthracycline +/– etoposide given for at least 2 cycles along w/ intrathecal chemotherapy
- Consolidation: 3–4 cycles of high-dose chemotherapy featuring high-dose cytarabine
- AML protocols do not generally include maintenance phase w/ exception of APL Rx, which includes maintenance w/ all-trans retinoic acid (ATRA)
- **Role of BMT:** Major role in AML (most successful curative Rx after remission induced w/ chemo); ~20% children have suitable HLA-identical sibling
- Whether SCT should be performed in 1st remission or reserved until 2nd is under study
  - APL, Down syndrome, or children with t(8;21) or inv(16) should not be transplanted in 1st remission as they have favorable outcomes with chemo rx

HODGKIN LYMPHOMA

Definition (Pediatric Lymphomas. Berlin, Heidelberg: Springer-Verlag; 2007; Pediatr Rev 2003;24:380)

- Histologically, Reed–Sternberg cells or variants. Majority of cases believed to represent proliferation of lymph node germinal center B-cells. Five histologic subtypes
  - **Nodular sclerosing:** Most common (40% younger pts, 70% adolescents). Mediastinal involvement in 80% of cases
  - **Mixed cellularity:** 25% cases. Male predominant (70%). Usually p/w periph LAD of upper body, often at an advanced stage
  - **Lymphocyte depleted:** Rare (<5%). Typically presents late, often w/ BM involvement, retroperitoneal LAD &/or abd organ involv; often w/ constitutional sx
  - **Nodular lymphocyte predominant Hodgkin lymphoma (NLPHL):** Rare (<5%). May not contain classic Reed–Sternberg cells but has lymphocytic and histiocytic cells ("popcorn cells"). Represents monoclonal B-cell neoplasm
  - **Nodular, lymphocyte-rich classic Hodgkin lymphoma (NLRCHL):** Rare

Epidemiology (Pediatr Rev 2003;24:380)

- Lymphoma 3rd most common childhood malignancy, 12% of cancers in kids <15 yo
- 40% are Hodgkin, 60% non-Hodgkin, but Hodgkin is more common in adolescents
- Most common childhood cancer in 15–19 yo
- In developed countries, 50% of cases of Hodgkin lymphoma are EBV positive

Clinical Presentation (Pediatr Rev 2003;24:380)

- Lymphadenopathy (most common, typically cervical, mediastinal, supraclavicular, almost always *above* diaphragm), hepatosplenomegaly, mediastinal mass (w/ or w/o sx of cough, stridor, dysphagia, dyspnea, SVC syndrome)
- B symptoms (fever >38° C × >3 d, >10% wt loss in 6 mo preceding dx, drenching night sweats) present in ~30% of patients, pruritus, alcohol-induced pain
- In contrast to NHL, Hodgkin lymphoma may have indolent (wks to mos) course

Diagnostic Studies (Pediatric Lymphomas. Berlin, Heidelberg: Springer-Verlag; 2007)

- CBC w/ diff, ESR, LDH, CRP, Chem20, alk phos level

- CXR (ratio max diameter mediastinum to max diameter of intrathoracic cavity at dome diaphragm >33% = bulky disease)
- PET-CT of neck, chest, abdomen/pelvis. Bone scan (if ↑ alk phos/bone pain)
- Lymph node biopsy (not needle). BM bx (except for stage IA/IIA)

Staging and Prognosis (Pediatric Lymphomas, Berlin, Heidelberg: Springer-Verlag; 2007)
- **Overall survival:** 90%
- **Prognostic factors:** Ann Arbor stage (most important), presence/absence of bulky mediastinal or other bulk nodal dz (>10 cm), B sx. ↑ age predicts poorer prog
- **Hodgkin lymphoma Ann Arbor staging**
  - Stage I—involves 1 LN region or structure or single extralymphatic site
  - Stage II—≥2 LN regions on same side of diaphragm
  - Stage III—involvement of LN regions on both sides of diaphragm; III-1 includes splenic, hilar, celiac, or mesenteric nodes; III-2 includes involvement of para-aortic, iliac or mesenteric nodes; III-S denotes splenic involvement
  - Stage IV—diffuse or disseminated involvement of ≥1 extranodal organ/tissue w/ or w/o associated LN involvement
  - Additional designations applicable to any stage: A: No B symptoms; B fever >38°, drenching night sweats, ≥10% weight loss in 6 mo; E: Involvement of an single extranodal site continuous/proximal to known nodal site

Treatment (Pediatric Lymphomas, Berlin, Heidelberg: Springer-Verlag; 2007)
- Many Rx regimens for HD, representative examples are given below
- **Low-risk dz (I/IIA w/o B sx or bulky dz):** 2–4 2-wk cycles chemo w/o alkylator, e.g., VAMP (vincristine, doxorubicin, MTX, prednisone), plus low-dose, involved-field XRT
- **Intermediate-risk** (stage I/IIB or bulky dz or IIIA) and **high-risk (IIIB or IVA) disease:** 6–8 cycles of multiagent chemo w/ alkylator, e.g., COPP (cyclophosphamide, vincristine, procarbazine, prednisone), **and/or** ABVD (doxorubicin, bleomycin, vinblastine, dacarbazine) for ~6 mo followed by low-dose, involved-field radiation

NON-HODGKIN LYMPHOMA

(Pediatric Lymphomas, Berlin, Heidelberg: Springer-Verlag; 2007; Ped Rev 2003;24:380)

Definition
- Includes both B- and T-cell neoplasms with Reed–Sternberg cells absent
- Non-Hodgkin lymphomas comprise 10% of all childhood cancers
- In general, vs. Hodgkin lymphoma, sx of NHL more rapid onset and short duration and $^2/_3$ of pts have widespread dz at time of dx
- 4 primary histologic subtypes of pediatric NHL, detailed below
- Presenting signs/sx similar to those for Hodgkin lymphoma above; except as below

Burkitt Lymphoma
- A B-cell lymphoma, most common pedi NHL: ~40–50% of cases
- **Clinical presentation:** Rapidly proliferating tumor often p/w extranodal dz. Intra-abd dz common and may p/w intussusception (acts as lead point in up to 50% of kids >6 yo)
- 95% pts w/ translocation of c-myc oncogene (chromo 8) w/ Ig heavy- or light-chain gene; 80% of time, translocation is t(8:14)
- **Treatment:** No benefit of XRT added to chemo demonstrated
- Generally 2–6 mo chemo w/ many agents, e.g., cyclophosphamide, doxorubicin, vincristine, HD-MTX w/ AraC, ifosamide, etoposide, and intense IT chemo for advanced stage dz
- **Overall survival:** 85–95% depending on stage

Diffuse Large B-cell Lymphoma
- A B-cell lymphoma; represents 20% of pediatric NHLs
- **Clinical presentation:** May occur at single site in nodes or bone. 1° mediastinal presentations in adolescent females and is the type of NHL associated w/ immunodeficiency and post solid organ transplant (PTLD)
- **Treatment:** Same as that for Burkitt lymphoma

Anaplastic Large Cell Lymphoma
- A T-cell lymphoma; 10–15% of pediatric NHLs
- **Clinically:** B sx (~50%) more common than other NHLs. LAD (usually periph) & usually p/w skin or soft tissue sites (skin lesions may wax/wane) 60% pts w/ extranodal involve
- Cells express CD30 and usually have a T-cell phenotype

- **Treatment: Minimal risk for CNS relapse** (minimal intrathecal therapy)
  - Regimens vary; most w/ steroids, vincristine, doxorubicin MTX, +/– alkylating agents

Precursor B- and Precursor T-cell Lymphoblastic Lymphoma
- ~30% of pediatric NHL
- Histologically identical to pre-B/pre-T acute lymphoblastic leukemia, but by definition has <25% involvement of bone marrow
- Clinically: Periph nodal or Waldeyer ring, T-cell lymphoma, may p/w anter mediastin mass
- **Treatment:** Based on high-risk ALL regimens and includes intrathecal chemo

Diagnostic Evaluation of Non-Hodgkin Lymphoma (Pediatr Rev 2003;24:380)
- Same as for Hodgkin lymphoma as previous, plus CSF examination and uric acid level

Staging and Prognosis (Pediatr Rev 2003;24:380)

St Jude/Murphy Staging System for Non-Hodgkin Lymphoma
Stage I: A single tumor (extranodal) or involvement of a single nodal area, excluding mediastinum and abdomen
Stage II: Single tumor (extranodal with regional node involvement) • Two or more nodal areas on the same side of the diaphragm • Two single (extranodal) tumors, w/ or w/o regional node involvement on same side of diaphragm • A primary GI tumor with or without involvement of nodes, which is completely resectable
Stage III: Two single tumors (extranodal) on opposite sides of the diaphragm • Two nodal areas above and below the diaphragm • Any primary intrathoracic tumor (mediastinal, pleural, thymic) • Extensive primary intra-abdominal disease • Any paraspinal or epidural tumor whether or not other sites are involved
Stage IV: Any of the previous findings with initial involvement of the CNS, bone marrow, or both

Overall Survival for Non-Hodgkin Lymphoma
- Stage I/II: ~90–98%; stage III/IV: 70–90%

TRANSFUSIONS

Expected Effect of Transfusions (Lancet 2007;370:415; Lancet 2007;370:427)
- Adult; 1 unit pRBCS → 3% increase in Hct or 1 g/dL increase in Hgb
- Infant/child: 3 cc/kg pRBCs → 3% increase in Hct or 1 g/dL increase in Hgb
- For platelets: 1 U platelets → 5,000 increase in Plt count
- Blood products leuko-filtered to ↓ risk of alloimmunization and prevent febrile xfusion rxn. Products given to children w/ malignancy receiving chemo, to neonates, or pts w/ severely compromised immune fxn are irradiated to prevent xfusion assoc GVHD

Transfusion Risks (Lancet 2007;370:415)

Complication	Estimated Risk	Complication	Estimated Risk
Febrile reaction	1 in 300	HIV1 and HIV2	1 in 2,000,000–3,000,000
Urticaria/cutaneous rxn	1 in 50–100	Hepatitis B	1 in 100,000–200,000
RBC alloimmunization	1 in 100	Hepatitis C	1 in 1,000,000–2,000,000
Mistransfusion	1 in 14,000–19,000	HTLV I and II	1 in 641,000
Hemolytic reaction	1 in 6,000	Bacterial contamination	1 in 5,000,000
Fatal hemolysis	1 in 1,000,000	Malaria	1 in 4,000,000
TRALI (more rare in kids)	1 in 5,000	Anaphylaxis	1 in 20,000–50,000
Immunomodulation	Unknown	GVHD	Uncommon

- Estimated risks in transfusion *per unit* transfused in the United States

- **Acute hemolytic reaction:** Reaction from transfusion of mismatched blood
  - **Symptoms:** Fever, chest pain, back/flank pain, hypotension, flushing, nausea, SOB, anxiety, may progress to DIC and renal failure
  - **Rx:** Stop xfusion IMMEDIATELY, retype pt and donor blood, send UA.
- **Allergic transfusion reaction:** May be IgE-mediated immediate rxn or delayed rxn to proteins present in transfused blood products
  - **Sx:** Immediate or delayed. Sx of allergic resp (anaphylaxis to mild urticaria)
  - **Rx:** Stop xfusion IMMEDIATELY. Give Benadryl. Epi if bronchospasm/anaphylaxis
  - **Note:** Pts w/ Hx of prior allergic rxn should be premedicated w/ Benadryl and Tylenol. No need for premedications in pts w/o Hx of prior rxn
- **Febrile nonhemolytic transfusion reaction (FNHTR):**
  - **Definition:** Recipient immune response to leucocytes and/or cytokines in xfusion
  - **Symptoms:** Flushing, fever, chills
  - **Rx:** Stop xfusion until rxn can be clearly differentiated from allergic or hemolytic rxn. Leukocyte reduced xfusion ↓ risk. May pretreat to prevent sx

Blood Products

Product		Criteria	Dosing	Contraindications
pRBCs	250 cc/U	Hct < 20–25 or w/ sx. Some advocate a xfusion threshold as low as 20 for some PICU pts (N Engl J Med 2007;356: 1609)	10–15 cc/kg given over 3–4 hr	
Platelets (single donor may be required)	5×10^{10} Plts/U	Prophylaxis Plt <10. Bleeding Plt 10–50. If CNS lesion maintain Plt >50,000	2 U infants 2–4 U toddlers 6 U school age 8 U adolesc or pheresis pack (= 5–8 U)	Avoid in TTP, HUS, HIT
FFP	Contains all clotting factors	Bleeding 2/2 clotting factor def, severe liver dz, warfarin or DIC	10–15 cc/kg	
Cryo-precipitate	1 bag: 80–120 U has 80–120 U FVIII, 50 U FXIII, 250 mg fibrinogen 880 U vWF	Fibrinogen deficiency or dysfunction	1 bag/5 kg	Higher-risk product as viral inactivation method not available
rFactor VIIa		Hemophilia w/ inhib, FVII def, liver dz	40 mcg/kg	

PEDIATRIC BRAIN TUMORS

(Principles and Practice of Pediatric Oncology. 6th ed. Philadelphia, PA: LWW; 2011;717)

Overview/Epidemiology
- CNS tumors are 2nd most common cancer of childhood
- CNS tumors have highest mortality rate of all childhood malignancies
- Incidence peaks in the first decade of life
- Supratentorial tumors predominate in 1st 2 yrs of life and again in late adol and adulthood
- Infratentorial tumor predominates from 2nd yr of life through mid-adolescence

Presentation of Pediatric Brain Tumors (Pediatr Clin North Am 2008;55;121)
- Supratentorial tumors may p/w localizing signs and sxs before ICP significantly ↑
  - Include hemiparesis, hemisensory loss, hyperreflexia, szr, or visual complaints
  - Developmental delay/loss of milestones; increased head circumference
  - Rarely, seizures can be the presenting symptom
- W/ tumor growth → ↑ ICP (2/2 mass effect or obstructing CSF outflow) → noncommunicating hydrocephalus, p/w sx ↑ ICP; morning HA, N/V, papilledema
  - Cushing triad: HTN, bradycardia, irregular respirations
- Tumor in pineal region (germinomas, mixed germ cell tumors, pineoblastomas, & lower grade pineocytomas) → compression/destruction of tectal region of brain stem; p/w:
  - Paralysis/paresis of upgaze, nystagmus
  - Pupils that react better to accommodation than to light
  - Lid retraction

Presentation of Posterior Fossa Tumors (Pediatr Clin North Am 2008;55;121)

Tumor (Incidence)	Presentation	Diagnosis	Prognosis
Medulloblastoma (35–40%)	2–3 mo of HA, vomiting, truncal ataxia	Heterog or homogeneously enhancing 4th ventricle mass; +/– disseminated	65–85% survival; depends on stage/type; poorer (20–70%) in infants
Cerebellar astrocytoma (35–40%)	3–6 mo of limb ataxia; 2° HA, vomiting	Cerebellar hemisphere mass, usually w/ cystic and solid (mural nodule) components	90–100% survival in totally resected pilocytic type
Brain stem glioma (10–15%)	1–4 mo of double vision, unsteadiness, weakness, and other CN deficits, facial weakness, swallowing deficits and other deficits	Diffusely expanded, minimally or partially enhancing mass in 80%; 20% more focal tectal or cervicomedullary lesion	Rare survivors except in unusual localized, low-grade tumors
Ependymoma (10–15%)	2–5 mo of unsteadiness, HA, double vision, and facial asymmetry	Usually enhancing, fourth ventricular mass with cerebellopontine predilection	75% + survival in totally resected lesions
Atypical teratoid/ rhabdoid (>5%, 10–15% infantile malign tumors)	As in medulloblast, but 1° in infants; often assoc with facial weakness and strabismus		

Types of Pediatric Brain Tumors

Supratentorial astrocytomas—low grade	15–25%
Cerebellar astrocytoma	10–20%
Medulloblastoma	10–20%
Brain stem glioma	10–20%
Others	12–14%
Supratentorial astrocytomas—high grade	10–15%
Craniopharyngiomas	6–9%
Ependymoma	5–10%
Pineal tumors	0.5–2%

- Most common malignant tumor in childhood; usually in pts <15 yo; ♂ predominance
- Bimodal distribution, peak at 3–4 yo & again btw 8–9 yo; 10–15% dx'd in infancy
- Large cell or anaplastic variant associated with worse outcome
- Amplification of MYCC oncogene assoc w/ the large-cell variant and poor outcome
- Expression of tyrosine kinase receptor ERBB2 in 40% and predictive of poor outcome
- Desmoplastic variant typically more responsive to treatment
- Younger children (<2–3 yr of age) have worse prognosis than older children
- **Presentation:** 80% p/w sx 2/2 obstruction of CSF flow (papilledema, AM HA, N/V); sx usually present for <3 mo; progressive truncal ataxia
  - Infants p/w vomiting, macrocephaly, "sun-setting sign" (unable to look up)
- Staging of medulloblastoma in children >3 yo (Pediatr Clin North Am 2008;55;121)

	Average Risk	High Risk
Tumor extent	Localized	Disseminated
Tumor resection	Total/ near total	Subtotal; biopsy
Histology	Classic; desmoplastic/nodular	Anaplastic/large cell
Biologic parameters	Neurotrophin-3 receptor expression; sonic hedgehog lineage markers	↑ MYCC amplification; ↑ ERBB2 expression; OXT2 amplification

- **Management of medulloblastoma**
  - Initial step is surgical resection: Total/near total resection assoc w/ improved survival
    - Cerebellar mutism syndrome in up to 25% of pts after resected midline cerebellar tumor; ↓/absent speech, hypotonia, & ataxia
    - Pts >3 w/ avg risk of dz Rx'd conventionally w/ craniospinal (2,400 cGy) and local boost XRT (5,580 cGy), supplemented w/ adjuvant chemo
    - Rx of pts <3 yo complicated 2/2 brain immaturity and high likelihood (40%) of disseminated disease at diagnosis
    - 75% desmoplastic variant pts >3 yo respond well to chemotherapy
    - Classical and anaplastic variants Rxd w/ a variety of regimens, including high-intensity chemotherapy w/ peripheral stem cell support
- **Long-term sequelae/outcomes:** High risk of intelligence impairment
  - Many endocrine abnormalities secondary to treatment effects
    - High risk for growth hormone deficiency
    - Decrease in skeletal growth secondary to spinal irradiation
    - Thyroid dysfunction occurs commonly
    - Sex hormone dysfunction (precocious or delayed puberty)
  - Permanent neurologic sequelae, w/ motor difficulties, sensory dysfxn, hearing impairments, and visual abn increasingly recognized in long-term survivors

NEUROBLASTOMA

(Pediatr Clin N Am 2008;55:97; Principles and Practice of Pediatric Oncology. 6th ed. Philadelphia, PA: LWW; 2011:886–922)

Definition: Solid neoplasm of the sympathetic nervous system

Epidemiology

- 650 new cases in the United States per year
- Accounts for 8–10% of childhood cancer and 15% of cancer deaths in children
- Most common non-CNS solid tumor of childhood
- Incidence peaks at 0–4 yrs of age; median age 23 mo

Clinical Presentation

- Depends on location, disease extent, and presence of paraneoplastic syndromes
- Can arise anywhere along sympathetic nervous system; 65% abdomen ($^1/_2$ from adrenal)
- Dz dissemination occurs through lymphatic and hematogenous spread
  - Bone marrow, bone, and liver most common sites of metastasis
  - Periorbital region spread → periorbital swelling and "raccoon eyes" at presentation
- Many well-documented paraneoplastic syndromes
  - Horner syndrome: Unilateral ptosis, miosis, and anhidrosis assoc w/ thoracic or cervical primary tumor (sx not resolved w/ tumor resection)
  - Pepper syndrome: Massive involvement of liver w/ metastatic dz +/– resp distress
  - Opsoclonus myoclonus ataxia syndrome (1–3% of NB cases)
    - Myoclonic jerking and random eye movement with or without ataxia
    - Often assoc w/ favorable and differentiated tumor; may not resolve w/ resection

Diagnostic Testing
- Definitive tissue bx and pathologic diagnosis is required for diagnosis, or positive bone marrow with elevated vanillylmandelic acid (VMA)/homovanillic acid (HVA)
- Urinary testing w/ ↑ HVA or VMA
- Initial dx testing should include CT or MRI; assess tumor site/extent & for metastasis
- Brain imaging only if clinically indicated
- Bilateral bone marrow biopsies to evaluate for bone marrow involvement
- Bone scan and/or MIBG to assess for bone metastasis

Staging
- Stage 1: Localized tumor w/ complete resection; neg lymph nodes (LNs)
- Stage 2A: Localized tumor with incomplete resection; negative LNs
- Stage 2B: Local tumor +/- gross total resxn; + ipsilateral LNs; neg contralateral LNs
- Stage 3: (a) unresectable unilateral tumor infiltrating across midline +/- LN involvement; (b) local unilateral tumor w/ contralateral + LN involvement; (c) midline unresectable tumor w/ bilateral extension or bilateral LN involvement
- Stage 4: Any 1° tumor w/ dissem/extension to LN, bone, BM, liver, skin, other organ
- Stage 4S: Local 1° tumor w/ dissemination to skin, liver, BM (only for infants <1 yo)

Prognostic Features
- Age >1–2 at dx assoc w/ worse prognosis than infants
- N-myc amplified or diploid DNA content assoc w/ worse prognosis
- Pathologic characteristics differentiate into "favorable" and "unfavorable" prognoses
- Treatment based on risk stratification

Treatment/Outcomes
- **Low risk** (Low stage [stage 1, 2A, or 2B], favorable N-myc, ploidy, and histology)
  - Excellent prognosis w/ surgery alone for stage 1 disease
  - 2-yr event-free survival for all low-risk disease 85–100%
  - No chemo w/ incomplete resection for favorable stage 2A/2B dz (survival >95%)
  - If life-/organ-threatening disease at diagnosis or disease progress, chemo effective adjuvant Rx for stage 2A and 2B
  - Stage 4S w/o n-MYC amplification spont regresses w/o Rx or need for resection unless clinical indications to rx (respiratory failure, DIC)
- **Intermediate-risk dz (age <1 yo w/** stage 3 dz (regardless of MYCN status or histology), age >1 yo w/ favorable histologic features, infants w/ stage 4 dz, and a subset of infants w/ 4S dz w/ diploid tumors or unfavorable histology, and no MYCN amplification)
  - Surgical resection and multiagent chemo (cisplatin/carboplatin, doxorubicin, etoposide, cyclophosphamide) are backbone of treatment
  - Survival greater than 95% if favorable histologic and biologic characteristics
  - Long-term survival >90%
- **High-risk disease** (age >1 yr, disseminated dz, or localized dz w/ unfavorable markers such as MYCN amplification)
  - Chemoresponsive but poor long-term prognosis; 40–50% long-term survival
  - Std Rx w/ induction, local control, consolidation, & Rx of min dz w/ biologic agents
    - Great correlation between tumor response at induction and survival
    - Induction includes multiagent chemotherapy
    - Local control w/ aggressive surg resection & external beam XRT to 1° tumor site
    - NB one of most radiosensitive tumors of childhood
    - Consolidation therapy includes myeloablative chemotherapy w/ stem cell rescue
    - Biologic Rx includes cis-retinoic acid & immunorx (monoclonal ab, GM-CSF, IL-2)

OSTEOSARCOMA

(Principles and Practice of Pediatric Oncology. 6th ed. Philadelphia, PA: LWW; 2011;1015–1044; Am Fam Physician 2002;65:1123)

Definition/Epidemiology
- Most common malignant bone tumor of childhood
- Primary malignant bone tumor, derived from bone-forming mesenchyme
- Production of immature bone tissue or immature bone by malignant spindle cell stroma
- ~400 new diagnoses in U.S. per yr; higher incidence in males than females
- Peak incidence in 2nd decade of life (during growth spurt)
- 80% in extremity; predilection for rapid growing bones (distal femur, proximal tibia, proximal humerus)
- 15–20% present with metastases to lung and/or bone

Pathology
- Histologic diagnosis depends on the presence of frankly malignant sarcomatous stroma associated w/ production of tumor osteoid and bone
- Great variability in histologic patterns often require extensive review of path material

Clinical Presentation/Evaluation
- **Sx:** Pain, soft tissue mass, occasionally pathologic fx; rarely constitutional sx. Avg duration of symptoms is 3 mo
- **Exam:** Tender soft tissue mass, limited range of motion
- **Labs:** May have increased LDH (30%) or alk phos (40%)
- **Imaging:** Plain radiograph, MRI of primary lesion, CT chest, bone scan
- **Biopsy:** Usually needle or incisional; carefully to allow for future complete resection

Treatment
- **Surgery:** Aggressive gross total resection w/ wide margins required to prevent local recurrence (either amputation or limb salvage procedures). Often preceded by two cycles of chemo and followed by multiple cycles of chemo
- **XRT:** Highly radioresistant. XRT rarely included as part of treatment plan
- **Chemo:** Current regimens include doxorubicin, cisplatin, and high-dose methotrexate. Ifosamide is also incorporated into a number of treatment plans
- **Treatment of metastases:** Frequent CT surveillance makes individual resection of pulmonary nodules possible by thoracotomy

OTHER CHILDHOOD TUMORS

Wilms Tumor (*Principles and Practice of Pediatric Oncology*. 6th ed. Philadelphia, PA: LWW; 2011;861–885)
- **Overview/Epidemiology**
  - Malignant tumor of kidney arising in nephrogenic rests; 500 new U/S cases annually
  - 2nd most common abdominal tumor in childhood; occurs early (mean age 3.5 yr)
  - Usually sporadic but ↑ risk in several genetic d/o 2/2 involvement of WT1 tumor suppressor gene (Beckwith–Wiedemann, Denys–Drash, WAGR, hemihypertrophy, aniridia)
  - May be bilateral (especially if genetic predisposition)
  - Classic histology: Triphasic ("favorable")
  - Histologic variants: Focal or diffuse anaplasia (more aggressive)
- **Clinical presentation/Evaluation**
  - Most common is asymptomatic abdominal mass
  - Also: Hematuria, fever, hypertension, abd pain, anemia from intratumoral hemorrhage
  - Metastasizes to regional lymph nodes, lung, liver
  - Imaging: CXR, abdominal CT or MRI, U/S to assess for IVC thrombus, chest CT
- **Treatment/Outcome**
  - Surgery is crucial: Nephrectomy up-front unless bilateral or unresectable
  - Radiation post-operatively for stage III and IV disease
  - Chemotherapy with 2 drugs (stage I/II) or 3 drugs (stage III/IV): Vincristine, actinomycin D, +/– doxorubicin
- **Prognosis** generally excellent for all stages unless more aggressive histology

Rhabdomyosarcoma (*Principles and Practice of Pediatric Oncology*. 6th ed. Philadelphia, PA: LWW; 2011;923–953)
- **Overview/Epidemiology**
  - Most common soft tissue sarcoma (STS) in children; $1/2$ of STS, 3% of childhood CA
  - Malignant tumor arising from muscle (primitive mesenchymal cell) occurs anywhere
  - 350 new cases in the United States per year; 2/3 of cases under 6 yr of age
- **Clinical presentation/Evaluation**
  - Symptoms depend on site involved
  - Most common sites: Head & neck, esp orbit, GU, trunk, extremities
  - 2 major histologies: Embryonal (favorable), alveolar
  - Metastasizes to lung, bone, bone marrow
  - Imaging: CT or MRI primary site, chest CT, bone scan and/or PET
- **Treatment/Outcome**
  - Multi-modality with chemotherapy (most common regimen is VAC: Vincristine, actinomycin D, cyclophosphamide) plus local control with surgery and/or radiation
- **Prognosis** related to age (infants and teens higher risk), histology, site, stage

Ewing Sarcoma (*Principles and Practice of Pediatric Oncology*. 6th ed. Philadelphia, PA: LWW; 2011;987–1014)
- **Overview/Epidemiology**
  - 2nd most common primary malignant bone tumor

- Family of tumors thought to be of neural crest origin. Includes Ewing sarcoma of the bone, soft tissue, Askin tumor of thoracic wall, and primitive neuroectodermal tumor
- 200 new cases in the United States per year; >50% occur in 2nd decade (mean age = 15 yr)
- More common in Caucasians; very rare in African-Americans
- Pathology: Small, round, blue-cell tumor, 85% with translocation EWSR1/FLI1 t(11;22)
- **Clinical presentation/evaluation:** Pain, swelling, tenderness over involved bone or soft tissue. Can affect any bone, but most commonly pelvis and femur. If more advanced/metastatic may have systemic sxs (fever, weight loss, etc)
  - Imaging: X-ray may show osteolysis, detachment of the periosteum from the bone (Codman triangle) given an "onion-skinning" appearance of the affected bone. MRI of primary site, chest CT, bone scan +/− PET scan
- **Treatment/Outcome**
  - Multi-modality w/ chemo (most common regimen; vincristine, doxorubicin, cyclophosphamide, ifosfamide, and etoposide) plus local control with surgery and/or radiation
- **Prognosis:** Better prognosis in pts w/o mets, tumor size <200 mL, good response to chemo, extremity lesions vs. axial), younger children, type I transcript (EWSR1/FLI1)

CHEMO-ASSOCIATED NAUSEA/VOMITING

(Adapted from *Principles and Practice of Pediatric Oncology.* 6th ed. Philadelphia, PA: LWW; 2011;1262–1280)

- Easier to prevent n/v than to treat
- **Antiemetic regimens used at MGHfC**

For highly emetogenic regimens: (cisplatin, actinomycin, ifosfamide/doxorubicin, cyclophosphamide, carboplatin >300 mg/m²):
• Give on a scheduled basis: Dexamethasone daily for ≥3 d, ondansetron, aprepitant for 3 d; additional agents on prn basis (see below)

Moderately emetogenic regimens (cytarabine, ifosfamide/etoposide, lower-dose cyclophosphamide and carboplatin):
• Give on a scheduled basis: Dexamethasone on chemo days, ondansetron
• Additional agents on prn basis

Agents	Characteristics	Toxicities
5-TH3 receptor antagonists (ondansetron, granisetron, palonosetron)	Most important frontline agent, wide therapeutic index, threshold effect w/ little or no dose response, min toxicity Efficacy enhanced by steroids and human substance P/ neurokinin antagonists	QTc prolongation, headache, LFT elevations, constipation
Steroids (dexamethasone)	Effective adjunct to 5-TH3 receptor antagonists	Facial flushing, hyperglycemia, HTN, behavioral changes
Substance P/ neurokinin recept antagonist (aprepitant, fosaprepitant)	Effective adjunct to 5-TH3 receptor antagonists for highly emetogenic regimens. High cost	Fatigue, constipation, nausea, hiccups infusion reactions with IV formulation

PRN Agents

Agent	Characteristics	Toxicities
Benzodiazepines (lorazepam, diazepam)	Anxiolytic, useful for anticipatory n/v	High doses can cause perception disturbance, sedation, dizziness
Scopolamine	Dermal patch	Sedation, dry mouth, cannot be used in small children because of fixed dosing
Antihistamines (diphenhydramine, hydroxyzine)	Mild antiemetic properties. Can be used in combo with other antiemetics	Drowsiness, behavioral changes (sometimes paradoxical hyperactivity)
Cannabinoid (marinol)	Active ingredient of marijuana. Relief of nausea w/o sedation. Only available in oral formulation	Drowsiness, dysphoria, or euphoria

CHEMOTHERAPY ADVERSE EFFECTS

Agent	Toxicities	Things to Follow
Actinomycin D (dactinomycin)	Myelosuppression (nadir 7–20 d), hepatotoxicity, tissue necrosis if extravasates, mucositis, nausea/vomiting, radiation recall	LFTs pre and post, CBC pre and post
Anthracyclines (adriamycin, doxorubicin, daunomycin, daunorubicin, mitoxantrone)	Myelosuppression (nadir 7–10 d, recovery 14–21 d), cardiomyopathy (acute/chronic), red urine, alopecia, N/V, mucositis, hepatotoxicity, vesicant, radiation recall	Echo pre and post, CBC and LFTs pre and post, mucositis
AraC (cytosine arabinoside)	Myelosuppression (nadir 10–14 d, recovery 21–28 d), N/V, fever, ataxia, nystagmus, alopecia, rash, diarrhea, conjunctivitis w/ high dose, hepatotoxicity. Can see high fever w/ infusion; R/o infxn	Eye drops w/ high dose. Neuro exam before each dose. Renal function and LFTs pre. CBC pre and post
Asparaginase	Hypersensitivity reaction, hypoalbuminemia, pancreatitis, azotemia hypercholesterolemia, hypercoagulable w/ inc risk of thrombosis (DVT/PE/ cerebral) or cerebral bleed	Check glucose, amylase, lipase, LFTs pre and post
Nitrosureas (BCNU, CCNU, nitrogen mustard)	Myelosuppression (nadir 4–6 wk, recovery 6–8 wk), N/V, pulmonary fibrosis, nephropathy, cellulitis if extravasates	LFTs, BUN, Cr pre and post
Bleomycin	Mucositis, alopecia, rash, pulm fibrosis, hyperpigment, hypersens	Test dose first. PFTs prior to every other dose
Carboplatin	Delayed myelosuppression, less nephrotoxic and neuropathy than cisplatin, potentiates toxicity of aminoglycosides, mild hepatotoxicity, hypersensitivity	Audiogram pre 1st dose. LFTs, BUN, Cr
Cisplatin	Myelosuppression, renal tubular nephropathy with Mg wasting, high-frequency hearing loss, N/V, peripheral neuropathy	Audiogram pre-each dose. Mg, K—renal function prior. Watch I/ Os closely
Cyclophosphamide (cytoxan)	Myelosuppression (nadir 8–14 d, recovery 18–25 d), N/V, hemorrhagic cystitis (↓d by MESNA), SIADH, alopecia, myocardial necrosis with very high (BMT) doses, immunosuppression	Urine SG < 1.010 to start. Follow lytes, urine output, hematuria. CBC and LFTs prior
Dacarbazine (DTIC)	N/V, myelosuppression, hepatotoxicity, pain at IV site. Phenobarb and dilantin may change metabolism	CBC and LFTs prior
Etoposide (VP-16)	Myelosuppression (nadir 7–14 d), hypotension with rapid infusion, N/V, secondary AML	Monitor BP closely, CBC and LFTs pre and post

CAE 9-15

CAE 9-16

Ifosfamide	Hemorrhagic cystitis (must be given with MESNA), altered mental status, SIADH, CNS effects, myelosuppression, renal (glomerular and tubular)	CBC and renal function pre and post. Monitor urine output, check U/As, Fanconi's syndrome, hematuria.
Mercaptopurine, Thioguanine (6-MP, 6TG)	Hepatotoxicity, myelosuppression, N/V, mucositis, 6-TG has mild GI effects	CBC and LFTs prior
Methotrexate	N/V, myelosuppression (nadir 7–14 d, recovery 14–21 d), hepatotoxicity, nephrotoxicity, osteoporosis, pneumonitis, alopecia, mucositis, CNS effects with intrathecal	Renal fxn & LFTs pre high dose. Follow MTX levels per protocol. Keep Urine pH >6.5 w/ high/intermed dose. Mucositis.
Prednisone	HTN, osteoporosis, immunosuppression, gastritis, pancreatitis, mental status changes, adrenal suppression, hyperglycemia	Follow glucose and BP
Procarbazine	Myelosuppression (nadir 25–36 d, recovery 30–50 d), N/V, peripheral neuropathy, hypertension (drug interaction), confusion	Avoid MAOs
Taxol (paclitaxel)	Acute hypersensitivity, bradycardia, HoTN, myelosuppression (nadir 10 d, recovery 18 d), mucositis, myalgias, alopecia, N/V	CBC and LFTs prior. Test dose
Topotecan	Dose limiting leukopenia (nadir 10–12 d, recovery 15–21 d), prolonged thrombocytopenia, N/V/D, alopecia, HA, fever, fatigue	LFTs prior
Vincristine (oncovin)	Alopecia, constipation, peripheral neuropathy, tissue necrosis if extravasates, SIADH, jaw pain	Neuro exam pre each dose. LFTs pre dose. Constipation, neuropathies
Vinblastine (velban)	Myelosuppression (nadir 7–9 d, recovery 14–21 d), peripheral neuropathy (rare), cellulitis if extravasates, N/V, myalgias	CBC, LFTs prior
Irinotecan (CPT-11)	Diarrhea, N/V, abdo cramps, diaphoresis; use atropine for early onset diarrhea, loperamide for late diarrhea, oral abx to prevent diarrhea	CBC prior
Temozolomide (temodar)	Myelosuppression, N/V, diarrhea, fatigue	CBC prior
Vinorelbine (navelbine)	Neuropathy, paresthesias, N/V, constipation, fatigue. CBC, LFTs prior	Neuro exam pre each dose
Gemcitabine (gemzar)	Myelosuppression, N/V, fatigue, fever, edema, radiation recall	CBC prior

FEVER OF UNKNOWN ORIGIN

Definition
- Fever >101°F ≥8 d w/o clear etiology after H&P and basic lab eval; definitions vary

Etiology (Feigen et al. *Textbook of Pediatric Infectious Disease*, 4th ed. p. 820)
- Most often uncommon presentation of a common disease (Pediatrics 1975;55:468)

Infectious	Malignancy	Autoimmune	Other
• **Viral:** EBV (mono), CMV, HIV, hepatitis, parvovirus, arbovirus • **Bacterial:** Cat scratch dz (*B. henselae*) URIs (mastoiditis/sinusitis/OM, etc.), tuberculosis, bacterial endocarditis, osteomyelitis, urinary tract infection, intra-abdominal abscess, (liver, perinephric, pelvic), Lyme disease, *mycoplasma*, brucellosis, leptospirosis, tularemia, occult infections • **Rickettsial:** Rocky Mountain spotted fever, ehrlichia, anaplasma, Q-fever • **Parasitic:** Malaria, babesia, toxoplasmosis • **Fungal:** Histoplasmosis, blastomycosis, coccidioidomycosis	• Leukemia • Hodgkin's disease • Non-Hodgkin lymphoma • Neuro-blastoma	• Juvenile idiopathic arthritis/Still's dz • Systemic lupus erythematosus • Polyarteritis nodosa	• Drug fever • Kawasaki disease • IBD • Thyrotoxicosis • CNS dysfunction • Diabetes insipidus • Periodic fever syndromes and other auto-inflammatory conditions (e.g., TRAPS) • Factitious fever/ MBP • Sarcoidosis

Arch Pediatr 1999;6:330; Acta Paediatr 2006;95:463; Clin Infect Dis 1998;26:80.

Diagnostic Studies
- Hx (fever pattern, assoc sx, ethnicity, ingestion, travel, animal and insect exposure, meds, FHx); complete exam (including accessible LNs, HSM, scalp and skin, MSK, and GU); review meds
- Labs: CMP, U/A, ESR and CRP, CBC w/ diff and periph smear, PPD (purified protein derivative) +/– IGRA (interferon-gamma release assays) (especially in children older than 5 s/p BCG immunization), HIV, Bld and U cx
- Additional testing (based on H&P, sx): stool cx and O and P, viral serologies, ANA, immunoglobulin levels (if h/o recurrent infections), toxoplasmosis serologies, Lyme serologies, ehrlichia/anaplasma serologies, or PCR
- Imaging: CXR, abd CT (if ↑ inflammatory markers or other concern for IBD), consider chest CT, CT sinuses, cardiac echo

Management
- Generally avoid empiric Abx or corticosteroids until potential dx available
- Empiric broad-spectrum antibiotics may decrease diagnostic yield

Complications
- Mortality previously reported at <10%; less in more recent cohorts (Pediatrics 1975;55:468; Acta Paediatr 2006;95:463)

INFECTIOUS MENINGITIS

Etiology
- Inflammation of meninges, covering brain and spinal cord 2/2 infection
- Peak incidence in 6–12 mo (infants = perinatal exposure and relatively immunocompromised); though 2/2 vaccinations, bulk of disease shifted to adulthood
- Incidence: 2,500 cases in US annually; *S. pneumo* 7.5/1/0.2 per 100,000 in >2 yr/2–4 yr/ 5–17 yr. (Pediatrics 2006;118:e979; JAMA 2001;285:1729)

Neonate	1–3 mo	3 mo–3 yr	3–12 yr	12 yr–adult
GBS (early onset) E. coli/Gm-neg rods Listeria monocytogenes	GBS; late-onset = ↓ severe S. pneumoniae Listeria and Hib (rare) N. meningitidis, Salmonella	S. meningitidis N. meningitidis H. influenzae • rare 2/2 immunity	S. meningitidis N. meningitidis H. influenzae • rare 2/2 immunity	N. meningitidis S. pneumoniae

- Aseptic meningitis: Enterovirus (Coxsackie B and echoviruses, ~85–95% of all viral meningitis), HSV, EBV, CMV, VZV, human parechoviruses, arbovirus (EEE, West Nile), influenza A/B, mycoplasma, Lyme (Semin Neurol 2000;20:277)

Risk Factors
- Functional/anatomic asplenia, sickle cell disease, nephrotic syndrome, IgG deficiency → ↑ risk encapsulated organism infections (S. pneumo, Hib, N. meningitidis)
- Late complement deficiency (C5–C8) → N. meningitidis
- Anatomic defects/CSF leak → S. pneumo, S. epi, S. aur, Strep spp., Corynebact
- VP shunt for hydrocephalus → Staph. epidermidis (coagulase-negative staph)
- Galactosemia → E. coli; HIV → C. neoformans; Endemic area → Lyme

Clinical Manifestations
- Bacterial meningitis tends to present acutely (<24 hr)
- Infant (non-specific): Fever, irritable, lethargy, ↓feeding, abn tone, bulging fontanel, szr's, vomiting, Δ body temperature; e/o sepsis (hypotension, respiratory distress, jaundice)
- Older children: Fever, headache, vomiting, neck stiffness, photophobia
- Skin: Widespread petechiae/purpuric rash (esp associated with meningococcemia)

Diagnostic Studies (Pediatr Infect Dis J 1996;15:298)
- Hx: Neck stiffness or pain, progressive petechial/purpuric rash, seizure, vaccine Hx; recent infxns (sinusitis, otitis media); exposure of pts w/ meningitis; travel; h/o head trauma/craniotomy; VP shunt; immunodeficiency; Hx of recent Abx use
- Neurologic exam; assess risk of ↑ ICP/herniation → follow neurologic exam during Rx
- Meningeal signs: Nuchal rigidity; in >2 yr: Kernig (straighten flexed leg at knee → neck/back pain) and Brudzinski (passive neck elevation → hip flexion). Tripod sign; Pt sitting w/ legs flexed and arms outstretched at the elbow
- ↑ ICP: Bulging fontanel in infants, ↑ head circum, papilledema in older, CN palsies
- Labs: CBC w/ diff, blood culture × 2; chem. 10, LP (if suspect bacterial, do not delay)
  - LP most important dx test; low threshold in infants (↑ risk of untreated meningitis)
  - Contraindicated if e/o intracranial mass/↑ ICP/abscess (focal neuro deficit/papilledema) → herniation risk check CT/MRI
  - Safe to perform LP on infants with bulging fontanel if (–) focal neurologic signs
  - Herniation unlikely if (–) focal neurologic signs or comatose
  - LP: Cell count, diff, gluc, prot, GS (↑ yield w/ cytocentrifug), cx/PCR/latex agglutination (latex agglut testing useful in partially rx'd meningitis)
    - Consider enterovirus PCR, very low risk of bacterial meningitis if positive, (Clin Infect Dis 2010;51(10):1221–1222), HSV PCR, Lyme abs, Parechoviruses PCR, viral encephalitis panel

Bacterial Meningitis CSF	Viral Meningitis CSF
1° neutrophils	1° lymphocytes (may show neutrophils early)
↑ protein	Mildly ↑ protein
↓ glucose	NL glucose
↑ opening pressure (20–75+ cm water)	NL or slightly ↑ opening pressure
Opalescent to purulent CSF appearance	Clear unless ↑ cell count

- Normal CSF findings
  - Neonate (<1 mo): WBC < 15–20; 60% PMNs; protein < 90; glucose 70–80
  - Infant (>1 mo): WBC < 10; 0% PMNs; prot < 40; gluc 50–60 (↑ BBB maturity)
- CSF GS (+) 90% S. pneumo and 80% N. mening; Bcx (+) 90% Hib and 80% S. pneumo
- Repeat LP in 24–36 hr if: Possible resistant organism (e.g., PCN-resist S. pneumo); s/p dexamethasone; poor Rx response; GNR (after 2–3 d of Rx)

Management (Cochrane Database Syst Rev 2007:CD004405; AAP Red Book 2009)
- Empiric Abx after LP: 3rd gen. cephalosporin (ceftriaxone, cefotaxime) + vancomycin (+ ampicillin if <3 mo for Listeria coverage)→ Δ when cx/sensitivities available

- Acyclovir prophylactically while HSV PCR on CSF pending if HSV suspected
- Rx duration: 7 d *N. mening*; 10 d *S. pneumo/H. influenzae*; 14–21 d for others
- Consider early dexamethasone w/ 1st Abx doses to ↓ risk hearing loss in *H. influenza*
- Most studies w/ no mortality difference w/ steroid Rx; limit to 2 d to dec side effects
- AAP rec's steroids for Hib meningitis only; eval risk/benefit for *S. pneumo* in >6 wk old
- Acyclovir (21 d) for HSV meningoencephalitis; supportive care for other viral etiologies

Complications: (Pediatr Infect Dis J 1993;12:389)
- Hypovolemia, HypoNa (2/2 SIADH), hypoglycemia, acidosis, septicemia, seizures, DIC, metastatic infection, cerebral edema, ↑ ICP/herniation, stroke
  - Mortality ~100% in untreated meningitis vs. 0–15% mortality in treated pts >1 yr
  - Sig morbidity even w/ appr Rx (15–30% permanent neuro sequelae)
    - Sensorineural hearing loss most common, 5–10% w/ Hib
    - Seizures: Up to 30%; neonates > older; recurrent focal sz suggests focal lesion; Rx early w/ phenobarbital vs. phenytoin (less sedating than phenobarb)
    - Subdural effusions: Up to 50% w/ Hib; noted on CT, no Rx unless ↑ ICP; consider aspiration/drainage if persistent fever
    - Cerebral edema: Steroids, mannitol, diuretics, hypervent; consider pressure monit

Prevention (MMWR 2005;54:893; Eur J Clin Microbiol Infect Dis 2006;25:90)
- Pneumococcal vaccine (PCV-13) → has replaced PCV-7, children 14–59 mo who have received PCV-7 series should receive one dose of PCV-13
- MCV-4 conjugate vaccine (covers A, C, Y, W-135 strains (no B); ~3–5 yr efficacy)
  - AAP recommends routine primary vaccination at 11–12 yr with booster at 16 yr; for details see AAP policy statement (Pediatrics 2011;128:1213)
- Hib vaccine → 75+ % decrease in Hib meningitis rates
- Close contact chemoprophy in *N. meningitidis* (rifampin, Cipro, CTX) and Hib (rifampin)

PERIORBITAL (PRESEPTAL) AND ORBITAL CELLULITIS

Definition
- Infxn's of eyelids, orbit, & surrounding structures. Separated by orbital septum
- Periorbital cellulitis is a simple skin infxn and involves structures anterior to septum. Orbital cellulitis is posterior to septum; involves infxn of soft tissues w/i the orbit

Pathophysiology (Pediatr Infect Dis J 2002;12:1157)
- Periorbital infxn 2/2 direct inoculation of bacteria (trauma, insect bite) or via bacteremia
  - Etiology if 2/2 trauma usually skin flora (*S. aureus*, GAS); if bacteremia, *S. pneumo*
- Orbital infxn generally sinusitis complication w/ infxn extension, rarely 2/2 trauma
- Periorbital cellulitis does not spread and become orbital cellulitis (Pediatr Infect Dis J 2002;12:1157)
  - Ethmoid sinus most common source; separated from orbit by thin lamina papyracea
  - Bacteria same as sinusitis (*S. pneumo*, nontyp *H. influ*, *M. catar*, GAS, *S. aureus*, anaerobes)

Clinical Manifestations (Pediatr Infect Dis J 2002;12:1157)
- Essential to differentiate the 2 entities; can be challenging as symptoms overlap
- **Periorbital cellulitis** p/w erythema, induration, tenderness, and warmth of eyelid and periorbital tissue. No limitations or pain w/ eye mvmt. Systemic sx infrequently present
- **Orbital cellulitis** w/ same superficial inflamm, but w/ vision Δs, pain w/ and limitation of eye mvmt, chemosis (edema of bulbar conjunctiva), or proptosis (Pediatr Rev 2004; 25:312)
  - Eye pain can precede signif swelling; impaired ocular mvmt usually w/ upward gaze

Differential (Pediatr Rev 2004;25:312)
- Noninfectious causes of periorbital swelling
  - Blunt trauma (black eye), p/w ecchymosis/swelling; ↑ first 48 hr then slowly resolves
  - Tumor usually more gradual onset, w/ proptosis but usually no inflammation
    - Hemangioma of the lid; stereotypical vascular appearance
    - Ocular tumors (retinoblastoma, choroidal melanomas)
    - Orbital neoplasms (neuroblastoma, rhabdomyosarcoma)
  - Allergy w/ either hypersensitivity (more itchy than painful) or angioedema
  - Local edema 2/2 over hydration, CHF, or hypoproteinemia, usually w/o tenderness
- Infections that can be mistaken for periorbital cellulitis
  - Dacryoadenitis: Infxn of lacrimal gland w/ sudden and max at onset inflamm at outer upper eyelid (viral [EBV, mumps, CMV, Coxsackie, echo, VZV] or bacterial)

- Dacryocystitis: Bacterial infxn of lacrimal sac as complication of URI w/ inflamm most prominent at medial corner of the eye
- Hordeolum: Infxn of sebaceous glands at eyelashes base; meibomian gland abscess

Diagnostic Studies
- No imaging needed with periorbital cellulitis
- CT of orbits/sinuses for orbital cellulitis, esp if persistence or worsening sx on appt Rx

Treatment (Pediatr Rev 2004;25:312)
- For periorbital cellulitis, Rx PO if >1 yo and full vac w/o systemic sx to cover Gram+'s (cephalexin, dicloxacillin, clinda). Good outpt f/u. Duration of Rx: 7–10 d
- For orbital cellulitis, Rx w/ IV Abx against potential pathogens
  - Amp/sulbactam ≥200 mg/kg/d divided q6h. Add vancomycin if MRSA suspected. Duration of Rx depends on clinical picture; usually 3 wk (1st 5–7 d parenterally)
  - Pts w/ large, well-defined abscess, ophthalmoplegia and/or visual impairment, or those w/o clinical improvement w/ 24–48 hr of IV Abx usually require surgical drainage of abscess and involved sinuses (J Fam Pract 2007;56:662)

ACUTE OTITIS MEDIA

Definition (Pediatrics 2004;113:1451)
- AAP guidelines require Hx acute onset of signs/sx, presence of middle ear effusion (MEE) on exam, and signs/sx of middle ear inflammation for diagnosis

Epidemiology (Pediatr Rev 2004;25:187)
- Accounts for ~20% of pedi clinic visits and for most outpt Abx prescriptions
- 50% of pediatric patients will have 1st episode of AOM before 6 mo, 90% by 2 yr
- Risk factors: Atopic dz, low socioeconomic status, immune def, craniofacial abn (cleft palate), genetic syndr (Downs), day care, siblings, smoke exposure, pacifier use, bottle feeding, 1st AOM before 6 mo

Pathophysiology
- Middle ear connected to nasopharynx by Eustachian tubes, drain middle ear secretions and protect middle ear from nasopharyngeal secretions
- Eustachian tube obstruction and drainage impairment more common in children; more horizontal, less stiff, and surrounded by lymphoid follicles (inflamed w/ URI)
  - W/ obstruction, nasopharyngeal secretions reflux into middle ear → infection
  - E. tube dysfunction → negative pressure → sterile MEE
  - Micro: S. pneumo (25–50% cases, 50% resistant, 20% resolve spont), H. influ (25% cases, 40% w/ β-lactamase activity, 50% resolve spont), and M. cat (12.5% cases, 100% w/ β-lactamase, 80% resolve spont) (Pediatr Rev 2004;25:187)

Differential Diagnosis
- Distinguished from simple otitis media w/ effusion (OME); fluid in middle ear space but no acute inflamm (otalgia or erythema of the TM)
- **Otitis externa** (swimmer's ear) bacterial infxn involving inflamm and skin breakdown of external ear canal (Pediatr Rev 2007;28:77)
  - Peak btw 7–12 yo and most common agents are P. aeruginosa and S. aureus
  - Exam w/ pain on pushing tragus or pulling pinna, edema in canal w/ secretions
  - Rx focuses on pain control and topical Abx (fluoroquinolones are Rx of choice)

Clinical Manifestations and Physical Exam (Pediatrics 2004;113:1451)
- Rapid onset signs and sx; otalgia, otorrhea, and/or fever; may be irritability in infant
  - Prospective studies show sx present in 90% of children w/ AOM, but also in 72% of those w/o (Pediatr Rev 2004;25:187)
- MEE via otoscopy; w/ bulging tympanic membrane (TM), ↓ mobility TM, TM air fluid level, or otorrhea. Can be benign finding w/ URI
  - Bulging TM has the highest predictive value for presence of MEE
- For MEE to indicate AOM, need middle ear inflamm (erythema of TM or otalgia)

Dx Studies
- Generally none. Definitive dx via tympanocentesis (rarely) (Pediatr Rev 2004;25:187)

Treatment (Pediatrics 2004;113:1451)
- Pain; Rx w/ Tylenol/ibuprofen and/or topical agents in pts >5 yo (Auralgan)
- Observe w/o Abx (Abx at 1st visit course 1 d in 5–14% vs. Abx adverse rxn in 5–10%)
  - Applies in pts 6 mo–2 yo where dx uncertain and sx nonsevere, pts >2 yo where dx uncertain, and pts >2 yo where dx certain but nonsevere

- Antibiotics: In all pts <6 mo; pts 6 mo–2 yo w/ certain dx or w/ uncertain dx & severe dz; or failure to improve after 24–72 hr obs w/o Abx. In children 6–23 mo w/ dx of AOM based on sx + MEE + either mod TM bulging or slight TM bulging w/ otalgia or marked erythema, Rx w/ 10 d Augmentin reduced overall sx burden & rate of persistent signs of AOM on otoscopic exam (N Engl J Med 2011;364:105–115)
- Choice of Abx
  - At dx or clinical failure following obs w/o Abx: Amoxicillin at 80–90 mg/kg/d
    - Amox/clav (90 mg/kg/d amox) in severe dz (temp >39°C and mod/sev otalgia)
  - At clinical failure after 48–72 hr of initial Abx Rx: Amox/clav (90 mg/kg/d amox)
    - Ceftriaxone × 3 d, in severe disease (temp >39°C and mod/sev otalgia)

Complications (Pediatr Rev 2004;25:187)
- TM perforation is most common complication, seen in 5% of patients
  - Antibiotic drops are suggested if perforation is present, but no clear data for this
  - Persistent drainage or prolonged perforation is an indication for ENT referral
- MEE (OME) persists following AOM normally, if it persists it can increase the risk for language delay due to partial hearing loss
  - If effusion persists >3 mo, if child has >4 episodes of AOM in 6 mo or >5 in 12 mo, then formal hearing evaluation is recommended
  - Consensus for tympanostomy tubes for children w/ persistent effusion bilaterally, >3 mo, >4 episodes AOM in 6 mo or >5 in 12 mo; no data supports this
- Mastoiditis rare but is most common serious complication of AOM; p/w fever, mastoid tenderness, displacement of the ear anteriorly
- Other much less common complications include bacteremia, meningitis, and abscess

LYMPHADENITIS

Definition
Enlarged, inflamed, lymph node(s); also see Oncology section for more details

Clinical Manifestations (Pediatr Rev 2000;21:399)
- **Hx:** Duration, laterality, location, exposures (TB, kittens, uncooked meat), dental problems, vaccination Hx, B sx (F/C/S, weight loss), recent illness, travel, & sexual Hx

Etiology (N Engl J Med 1963;268:1329)

Infectious Cervical Lymphadenitis in Children	
Position and Time Course	**Etiologies**
Unilateral – acute	**S. aureus** or **Group A strep** (up to 80%), GBS (infants), tularemia, anaerobes
Unilateral – subacute/chronic	Mycobacteria (TB vs. atypical), Bartonella henselae (CSD), toxoplasmosis
Bilateral – acute	Viral URI, Group A strep, enterovirus, adenovirus, influenza, EBV, CMV, Mycoplasma pneumoniae
Bilateral – subacute/chronic	EBV, CMV, HIV, toxoplasmosis

- Noninfectious causes: Neoplasms, Kawasaki, PFAPA (**P**eriodic **F**ever, **A**phthous stomatitis, **P**haryngitis, **A**denitis), connective tissue disease, Kikuchi dz, branchial cleft cyst, cystic hygroma, medications

Diagnostic Studies
- Unilateral (acute) → if mod sx, FNA for Cx. If severe → U/S/CT, I&D, Bcx
- Bilateral (acute) → usually no w/u aside from throat swab for group A strep; likely viral
- Unilateral/bilateral (subacute/chronic) → consider CBC/diff, ESR, PPD (or IGRA for pts >5 yo), serologies for EBV/CMV/Bartonella/Tularemia/Toxoplasma, HIV, excisional biopsy

Management
- Unilateral (acute) → Abx cover for staph, GAS, +/– oral flora; if mild sx → cephalexin, clinda, amox/clav, TMP–SMX (if CA-MRSA prevalence high, but need additional agent if want to cover GAS). If mod/severe sx, consider IV cefazolin, nafcillin, ampicillin/sulbactam, clindamycin, or vancomycin

LYME DISEASE

(Clin Infect Dis 2006;43:1089)

Epidemiology
- Most common vector born dz in U S, ↑ trend; peak incidence in summer, incubation period (for early localized disease) 2–31 d, mean 11
- Endemic areas include Northeast, Great Lakes, mid-Atlantic regions, usually in rural, wooded areas (for local prevalences: American Lyme disease foundation: http://www.aldf.com/usmap.shtml)
- Most prevalent in children 2–15 yo (Pediatrics 1998;102:905)

Microbiology
- Spirochete *Borrelia burgdorferi* spread by tick (*Ixodes scapularis*) on deer and mice
- Coinfection w/ *Babesia*, and other rickettsial species not uncommon (up to 10%), may contribute to prolonged sx despite Rx for Lyme
- Infection usually requires tick attachment >36 hr

Clinical Manifestations

System	Stage 1 (Early Localized – wk)	Stage 2 (Early Disseminated – mo)	Stage 3 (Late Chronic – yr)
Cardiac	N/A	**AV block;** myopericarditis, pancarditis	N/A
Constitutional	Flu-like sx	Malaise; fatigue	Fatigue
Lymphatic	Regional LAD	Regional or generalized LAD	N/A
MSK	Myalgia	Migratory arthralgias, myalgias, oligoarthritis	Prolonged/recurrent arthritis, synovitis
Neurologic	Headache	**Meningitis,** CN7 palsy, cranial neuritis, mononeuritis multiplex, transverse myelitis	Encephalopathy, polyneuropathy, leukoencephalitis
Cutaneous	**Erythema migrans** (~80%), macular lesions with central clearing, 6–40 cm	Multiple annular lesions	Lymphocytoma; acrodermatitis chronica atrophicans, panniculitis

From: N Engl J Med 2001;345:115; Lancet 2003;362:1639; Ann Intern Med 2002;136:421.

Diagnostic Studies
- Clinical dx during early stages (erythema migrans), Ab against *B. burgdorferi* not detectable w/i first few wks after infection
- In early disseminated or later dz, dx based on clinical findings and serologic tests
  - 2-step approach: 1st, screening test for serum Ab's (IFA or EIA)
  - If +, then standardized Western blot (False +'s 2/2 EBV, other spirochete, HIV, SLE)
  - Early dz, IgG and IgM; late dz, IgG (if IgM false +)
  - A + IgM test needs 2 of 3 bands (Ab's). A + IgG test requires 5 of 10 bands
- Note: Rx'd individuals early in course of infection might not develop Ab's
- Consider PCR in joint fluid, and serologies in CSF. Culture is not recommended

Treatment
- Prophylaxis: RCT (>12 yr) w/ efficacy doxycycline 200 mg × 1 w/i 72 hr of tick bite (must have seen and removed tick) to prevent Lyme dz (N Engl J Med 2001;345:79)
- Recommended treatment of Lyme disease in children (Lyme Disease. Red Book 2009)

Disease Category	Drug(s) and Doses[a]
Early localized disease[a]	
>8 yo	Doxycycline 100 mg PO bid × 14–21 d[b]
All ages	Amoxicillin 50 mg/kg/d PO divided tid (max 1.5 g/d) for 14–21 d **-OR-** Cefuroxime 30 mg/kg/d PO divided bid (max 1 g/d) for 14–21 d

Early disseminated and late disease	
Multiple erythema migrans	Same oral regimen as for early localized dz but for 21 d
Isolated facial palsy	Same oral regimen as for early localized dz but for 21–28 d[c,d]
Arthritis	Same oral regimen as for early localized dz but for 28 d[c,d]
Persistent or recurrent arthritis[e]	Ceftriaxone 75–100 mg/kg IV or IM qd (max 2 g/d) for 14–28 d **-OR-** Penicillin 300,000 U/kg/d IV, divided q4h (max 20 million U/d) for 14–28 d **-OR-** Same oral regimen as for early disease
Carditis	Ceftriaxone or penicillin: See persistent or recurrent arthritis
Meningitis/ encephalitis	Ceftriaxone or penicillin: See persistent or recurrent arthritis for 14–28 d

[a]For pts who are allergic to PCN, cefuroxime, and erythromycin are alternative drugs.
[b]Tetracyclines contraindicated in pregnancy.
[c]Corticosteroids should not be given.
[d]Rx has no effect on the resolution of facial nerve palsy; its purpose is to prevent late disease.
[e]Arthritis not considered persistent or recurrent unless objective evidence of synovitis exists at least 2 mo after Rx initiated. Some experts administer 2nd course of oral agent before using IV antimicrobial agent.

UTI/PYELONEPHRITIS

Etiology
- Most 2/2 ascending infxns; only ~4% children w/ UTI/pyelonephritis are bacteremic

Microbiology
- 80% of infections 2/2 *E. coli*
- Gram-neg rods (*Klebsiella, Proteus, Enterobacter, Citrobacter*) = 2nd most common group
- Gram-pos cocci (*Enterococcus, Staph. saprophyticus* [mostly adol], *Staph. aureus* [rare])
- ↑ rates bacterial resistance in community acquired strains; risk for resistant infection inc w/prolonged or recent hospitalization, instrumentation, indwelling Foley
- Mediated by interaction of bacterial adhesins and receptors on host cells (e.g., *E. coli* pili – virulence factor → adhere to uroepithelium and ascend)

Risk Factors (Arch Dis Child 2006;91:845; Pediatrics 1998;102:e16)
- Age: Females <4 yo and males <1 yo
- FHx: Patients w/ 1° relatives w/ h/o childhood UTI more likely to have UTI (↑ adherence)
- Female (2/2 shorter urethra, possible ↑ adherence to female periurethral mucosa)
- Uncircumcised (mucosal foreskin vs. keratinized glans; partial phimosis → mild obstruction)
- Voiding dysfunction (frequent/infrequent voiding; urinary/stool incontinence; withholding); ~15% prevalence in school-aged children
  - Dx of exclusion after H&P/U/A/bladder U/S; often overlooked UTI risk-factor
  - ~40% school-aged pts w/ 1st UTI & 80% w/ recurrent UTI have sx c/w voiding dysfxn
  - Risk factor for persistent vesicoureteral reflux (VUR) and renal scarring
- VUR; 2/2 short intravesical ureter > posterior urethral valves
  - ~1% prevalence in childhood; ~40% of children w/ febrile UTIs; less common in AAs
  - Grades I–V, depending on prox vs. distal reflux and presence/severity of ureteral dilatation; ~95% of VUR is Grades I–III
  - Equivocal studies about link between VUR and pyelonephritis/renal scarring
  - Most w/ recurrent pyelo or scarring do *not* have VUR
  - Most VUR resolves w/i 5 yr
- Obstruction (anatomic [post urethral valves, UPJ obstruction, constipation] ~1–4%; neurologic bladder; functional withholding)
- Sexual activity (strong correlation in sexually active adolescent and young adult females)

Clinical Manifestations
- Fever, abd or back pain, dysuria, ↑ urinary frequency, urgency or incontinence, hematuria, suprapubic tenderness (JAMA 2007;298:2895)

Diagnostic Studies (Pediatrics 2011;128:e749; Pediatr Infect Dis J 2002;21:1)
- Samples for UA and cx: Midstream clean catch if possible. Otherwise, cath or suprapubic

Test	Sensitivity (%)	Specificity (%)
Leukocyte esterase (LE)	84	78
Nitrite (several hr req'd in bladder for +)	50	98
Nitrite *or* leukocyte esterase	88	93
Nitrite *and* leukocyte esterase	72	96
>10 WBC/cc – all ages (uncentrifuged)	77	89
>10 WBC/cc – under 2 yr	90	95
Bacteriuria (Gram stained)	93	95
Pyuria *or* bacteriuria	95	89

- "Enhanced U/A"; uncentrifuged U/A + GS + quantitative WBC/cc; most accurate screening test
- Difficult to distinguish cystitis from pyelonephritis via clinical criteria (some show pyelo on DMSA) → treat febrile UTI like pyelo in children <2 yo = 14 d Abx course
- **Urine culture very important to guide management**
  - Cath urine cx significant if >1,000–50,000 CFU/mL especially if UA suggestive of an UTI if single pathogenic organism and consistent clinical picture
  - Urine cx >50,000 CFU/mL indicator of significant bacteriuria if single pathogen present
  - Clean-catch urine cx significant if >100,000 CFU/mL
  - Up to 85% of +cx's from bag urine specimens represent false-+ results
  - Suprapubic bladder tap cx significant if *any* pathogenic bacteria present
- Blood cultures not routinely recommended in children >2 mo
- Need LP in children <1 mo, since 1% w/ UTI may have concurrent bacterial meningitis; LP for older infants is not absolutely indicated
- ↑ WBC, CRP not good predictors for UTI
- Pyuria present in UTI but not asymptomatic bacteriuria
- Consider checking serum creatinine if suspect acute renal failure 2/2 pyelonephritis
- Imaging: Renal U/S on all 1st UTIs (eval hydronephrosis) or pts w/ worsening dz (r/o abscess). Optimal imaging strategies controversial (Curr Opin Pediatr 2007;19:705)
  - VCUG now only recommended if hydronephrosis, scarring, or anatomical abnormality found on renal ultrasound (Pediatrics 2011;128:e749)
  - VCUG can be done as soon as cx negative (eval reflux, bladder anatomy, obstruction and voiding patterns) (Isr Med Assoc J 2008;10:453)
  - Large prospective trial (RIVUR) study underway to evaluate role of antibiotic prophylaxis in children with VUR
  - Antibiotic prophylaxis currently only recommended for patients with higher grade VUR (III–V), structural abnormalities, or urinary/bowel dysfunction

Management (Pediatrics 2011;128:e749; Pediatrics 2011;128:595; Pediatr Nephrol 2011;26:1967; N Engl J Med 2011;365:239; Pediatrics 2006;117:626; Pediatrics 2006;117:919; Arch Dis Child 2002;87:118)

- Base Rx on Ucx results & sensitivities or w/o these then local abx resistance patterns
- Initial antibiotic choice and route should be based on age of pt, clinical status, comorbidities, and associated problems (e.g., bacteremia)
- Empiric Rx in newborns & young infants: Amp + gent; to treat *E.coli* and *E. faecilis*
- Empiric Rx in ill appearing children: 3rd-gen cephalosporin (ceftriaxone, cefotaxime) and/or gentamicin (if possible bacteremia): Add amp if enterococcus suspected
- Most pts (infants >3 mo and children) are outpt Rx candidates (based on resistance): Amoxicillin; amoxicillin/clavulanate; TMP/SMX; cefixime; quinolones (effective, though safety concerns in younger children, now w/ FDA warning, risk of arthopathy)
- IV therapy for neonates/infants and children w/ urinary tract abnormalities/toxic/ unable to PO/concern for noncompliance w/ treatment and follow-up
- Rx duration: For younger children typically 10–14 d w/ pyelonephritis (IV and PO) and 7 d for cystitis; 3 d for uncomplicated 1st UTI in older adolescents, males w/ UTI typically considered complicated (10–14 d Rx)
- Patients and families should be instructed to seek medical care with any recurrence of UTI symptoms after initial UTI diagnosis to prevent subsequent scarring

CELLULITIS

Definition
- Infection of superficial, deep dermis, subcutaneous fat, and lymphatic system in the absence of an underlying suppurative focus

Microbiology
- Skin flora: *Strep/staph* (increasingly, CA-MRSA)
- Dog/cat bites: *Pasteurella multocida, bacteroides, Fusobacterium, Erysipelothrix*
- Human bites: *Eikenella*
- Fresh water exposure: *Vibrio vulnificus*
- Puncture wounds/piercings: *Pseudomonas*

Clinical Manifestations
- Pain, warmth, swelling, erythema, tender LAD of draining LN, may or may not have assoc abscess, lymphangitis. Less commonly systemic sx → fevers, chills, myalgias
- Red flags (see Ddx below): Pain out of proportion to clinical findings, rapidly progressive erythema, paresthesias, crepitus, bullae, or signs of systemic toxicity

Differential Diagnosis
- Distinguished from other potentially fatal infxn's, including necrotizing fasciitis and clostridial myonecrosis. Eval for underlying process, such as collection, septic arthritis, or osteomyelitis
- Erythema migrans, foreign body reactions, folliculitis, drug reactions, insect stings, contact dermatitis, lymphedema, DVT

Diagnostic Studies (N Engl J Med 2004;350:904)
- Virtually always a clinical dx as blood cultures have low yield (~2%)
- Radiographs not necessary for routine evaluation of patients w/ cellulitis
- U/S if collections suspected
- Cx's of drainage, pus, bullae. Cx's of intact skin are generally not helpful

Treatment
- Incision and drainage of any large collection of fluid within the pustule or abscess
- Warm compresses and soaks to facilitate spontaneous drainage
- Elevation of limb to decrease edema
- For CA-MRSA infections, effectiveness of decolonization uncertain (Lancet Infect Dis 2011;11:952)
- **Antibiotic Rx**
  - Outpt → cephalexin, dicloxacillin. If CA-MRSA rates ↑, known colonization or previous infection w/ CA-MRSA and other MRSA risk factors, consider empiric TMP–SMX or clindamycin. However, the utility of antibiotics in uncomplicated superficial infections is uncertain (Pediatrics 2011;127:e573; J Pediatr 2011;158:861–862. commentary)
  - Inpt → IV nafcillin, cefazolin, clindamycin. If concern for MRSA, unresponsive or severe disease → IV vancomycin first line; alternative: Linezolid

SEPTIC ARTHRITIS AND OSTEOMYELITIS

Etiology
- **Septic arthritis:** Most cases in kids <3 yo; typically 2/2 bacteremia → seeds joint space
  - Spread from adj osteomyelitis (most common in <18 mo, esp prox femur and prox humerus (prox metaphysis = intracapsular))
- **Osteomyelitis:** Starts in spongy/medullary bone → spreads to compact/cortical bone
  - Hematogenous (bacteremia) > direct invasion (e.g., nail, open fracture, puncture wound, pressure ulcers, sinusitis, mastoiditis, dental abscess) > vascular insuff
  - 50% of cases in children <5 yr, 25% < 2 yr
  - Symptoms: Fever (including FUO), fatigue, local symptoms over the involved bone including pain, edema, and erythema

Etiology (Pediatr Clin North Am 2005;52:779; Pediatr Infect Dis J 2010;29:639)

Age	Bacterial Etiology
Neonates	• *Staph. aureus* • Group B Strep (*Strep. agalactiae*) • Enteric GNR Septic arthritis: *Neisseria gonorrhoeae, Candida* (risk factors include CVL, broad-spectrum Abx)
<5 yr	• *Staph. aureus* = #1 (70–90% overall; 85% of hematogenous) • MRSA (~50% CA-MRSA) ↑ common • *Strep. pyogenes* (GAS; 10% of hematogenous, peak 3–6 yr) • Often recent h/o varicella infxn • *Strep. pneumoniae* (PCV-7 benefit)

	• *Kingella kingae* (day care, 2/2 URI and stomatitis) • *Kingella* replaced Hib as #1 GNR arthritis in 2 mo–5 yr (inoculate aspirates directly into blood cx bottles to ↑ yield) • *H. influenzae* B (unvaccinated, typically <5 yo); some nontypeable dz
>5 yr	• Staph. aureus, Strep. pyogenes (GAS)
Adolescents	• Neisseria gonorrhoeae (arthritis-dermatitis 2/2 hematogenous)
Other	• Salmonella (e.g., sickle cell disease) • Borrelia burgdorferi – Lyme arthritis (cause of septic arthritis in children and adolescents, initial arthralgia → pauciarticular arthritis, 1° knee) • Pseudomonas/mixed (e.g., shoe puncture) • Anaerobes (sinusitis, mastoiditis, dental abscess) • Aspergillus, S. aureus, Serratia (chronic granulomatous disease)

Evaluation (Am Fam Physician 2011;84:1027)
- **Septic arthritis:** Prompt eval needed, degradation of articular cartilage w/i 8 hr
  - Untreated hip septic arthritis can → ischemic necrosis of femoral head
    - Hip and knee joints most commonly affected
  - Joint fluid and blood cx's; inoculate joint fluid directly into blood cx bottles to ↑ yield
    - Cell count: >50 K WBC w/ PMN predom suggests septic arthritis > rheum dz
  - WBC, ESR, CRP, Lyme serology/Western blot, as well as Lyme PCR for joint fluid
  - Fever, nonweight bearing, ESR > 20–40, CRP > 1, WBC > 11–12 K, hip joint space >2 mm suggest septic arthritis (vs. transient synovitis) (Krocher criteria)
  - Also cx pharynx, skin lesions, cervix, urethra, vagina, and rectum if suspect *N. gonorrhoeae*; PCR of urine, urethral, cervical cx
  - ASLO, anti-DNaseB if suspect acute rheumatic fever 2/2 GAS; throat cx if pharyngitis
- **Osteomyelitis**
  - Infants: Nonspecific, +/– pseudoparalysis of limb, often no leukocytosis
    - Location: Long bones, multifocal ↑ likely in NICU pts or w/ CA-MRSA
  - Older pts: More dramatic; refusal to bear weight; ~30% h/o prior trauma, ↑ WBC
    - Local: Around knee most common in 7–10 yo; >50% femur, tibia
    - ↑ ESR (80–90%, often >50, peaks in 3–5 d → ↑ for 3–4 wk even on approp Rx)
    - ↑ CRP (98% of cases, peaks in 48 hr → nml after 7–10 d Rx)
  - Patients w/ MRSA osteomyelitis more likely to have HCT <34%, CRP >13, Temp >38, and WBC >12,000 compared to pts w/ MSSA osteomyelitis (J Bone Joint Surg Am 2011;93:1693)
  - Bone aspirate: Gram stain and culture most useful in guiding treatment
    - Can hold off antibiotics in stable patient if aspiration is imminent
    - Bacterial diagnosis made in 50–80% of cases if blood and bone cultures taken
    - Bone bx if cx-neg osteo not responding to Rx → cx for bacteria/mycobacteria/fungi
  - Blood cultures often positive (associated w/ ↑ fever, antecedent trauma)
- **Imaging** (J Pediatr Surg 2007;42:553)
  - **Septic arthritis:** Plain film to evaluate for trauma, malignancy, osteomyelitis; U/S to evaluate if hip joint effusion adequate for aspiration, +/– bone scan, +/– MRI
  - **Osteomyelitis**
    - X-ray: Nonspecific soft tissue swelling (w/i days) → then periosteal elevation w/ new bone formation and lytic changes late (10–21 d); may not be seen if prompt dx and Rx. However, X-ray remains a useful initial modality to help rule out other causes of local pain and swelling
    - Demineralization of bone 2/2 infxn spread down medullary canal = ischemic dead bone fragments (sequestra)
    - MRI: Most sensitive in early osteo; best for dx of pelvic or vertebral (>8 yo) osteo; ↑ resolution than bone scan (for surgical/IR planning)
      - Good eval of adjacent soft tissues: Gadolinium eval for soft tissue abscesses, marrow edema, bony destruction; vertebral osteo, diskitis (<5 yo)
      - Sedation required in younger children, ↑ expense, only evaluates limited area
    - Bone scan: 80–100% sensitive (+ w/i 48–72 hr of sx onset) but nonspecific
      - Can see "cold" scans if compromised blood flow to infected bone; false (+) in malignancy, trauma, cellulitis, postop, arthritis
      - Less expensive than MRI, no sedation, useful if exact locale of osteo unclear

Treatment (Pediatr Infect Dis J 1998;17:1021; Infect Dis Clin North Am 2005;19:787; AAP Redbook 2009; Pediatr Infect Dis J 2008;27:765)

- Prompt decompression of joint in septic arthritis; hip/shoulder often need prompt drainage

Empiric Septic Arthritis/Osteo Treatment	
Neonate (0–2 mo)	**Nafcillin** (or **Vancomycin** if >5–10% MRSA) + **cefotaxime** (or gentamicin)
Children <5 yr	**Cephalosporin** (Kingella) + **Vancomycin** (MRSA) (Pediatr Infect Dis J 2008;8:765)
Children >5 yr	**Vancomycin** (if MRSA suspect). **Ceftriaxone** if suspect *N. gonorrhoeae* or Gram negative on Gram stain, Ceftazidime if following foot puncture (*Pseudomonas*)

- Surgical debridement needed for osteomyelitis complicated by collections, pseudomonal osteomyelitis, and chronic osteomyelitis
- Continue empiric Rx if cx-neg and patient improving; bone bx/reimaging if not improving
- Patients often managed w/ sequential therapy with IV transitioning to PO
  - Post-debridement treatment with 2–4 d IV antibiotics followed by 6–8 d PO supported by an RCT for septic arthritis vs. 30 d Rx (Clin Infect Dis 2009;48:1201)
  - No difference in complications in retrospective analysis of patients receiving prolonged IV or PO treatment for osteomyelitis (Pediatrics 2009;123:636) even with MRSA (Pediatr Infect Dis J 2012;5:436)
  - Longer durations (4 wk) with Kingella (Arch Pediatr 2000;9:927), PsA, Salmonella

Complications (Pediatr Infect Dis J 2002;21:431)
- **Septic arthritis**
  - 10–25% complications; abn bone growth, limp, unstable joint, ↓ range of motion
  - Risk factors: Delay in diagnosis >4–5 d; infant; *S. aureus* or GNR
- **Osteomyelitis**
  - Loss of bone structure & growth abn if significant delay in Rx (e.g., 7–10 d)
    - Pelvic osteo 1–11% hematog osteo (1° ilium/ischium); often delayed dx
  - Recurrent osteo ~5% after appropriate Rx (delay in dx, Rx <3 wk, young age)
  - Chronic osteo <5%; ↑ in contiguous osteo → bone necrosis/fibrosis; Rx with month + Abx +/– surgery
  - 5–60% neonate sequelae: Subnormal bone growth, limb-length discrep, arthritis, abnormal gait, pathologic fracture
  - Similar MRSA/MSSA outcomes; MRSA typically longer duration fever; PVL-1 MRSA → DVT/complications
  - Chronic recurrent multifocal osteo: 1° female, multiple symmetric lesions in long bones/clavicles; assoc w/ psoriasis and palmopustular pustulosis
  - Reactive arthritis at other joints 2/2 inflamm from 1° septic arthritis

SEXUALLY TRANSMITTED INFECTIONS

(CDC STD Treatment Guidelines, 2010)

Disease	Sx/Signs	Investigations	Treatment	Notes
Urethritis/Cervicitis/Epididymitis				
	Urethritis: Mucopurulent discharge, dysuria, pruritus, urgency, nocturia, frequency	Urethral Gram stain with ≥5 WBC (if GNID then *NG*), UA leukocyte esterase(+) Urethral/urine NAAT for *CT/NG* (urine preferred)	Empiric Rx for *CT/NG* if high risk (≤25 yo, new/multiple partners, unprotected sex, poor follow-up) see below If recurrent or persistent consider other organisms (*Ureaplasma urealyticum, Mycoplasma genitalium, T. vaginalis*, HSV, HPV, adenovirus) trial: Metronidazole 2 g OR tinidazole 2 g + azithromycin if not used initially	Abstinence for 7 d post-Rx + no sx + partner treated If sx >3 mo, consider chronic prostatitis, chronic pelvic pain syndrome Retest ♀ 3 mo. post-rx (both ♂ and ♀ if gonococcal)

	Signs/Symptoms	Diagnosis	Treatment	Comments
	Cervicitis: Mucopurulent endocervical exudate, dyspareunia, postcoital bleeding, signs of PID	Cervical/urine NAAT for CT/NG, wet prep, *T. vaginalis* cx/Ag (swab preferred, urine okay) Leukorrhea by microscopy GNID on endocervical fluid Gram stain		
C. trachomatis (CT aka NGU)	**Annual screening of all females <25 yr, and males and females at high risk Complications: Epididymitis, prostatitis, Reiter syndrome, PID, ectopic, infertility		Azithro 1 g PO × 1 OR doxy 100 mg PO bid × 7 d. Consider treating for NG as well and pt-delivered therapy to heterosexual partner	
N. gonorrhoeae (NG)	Often no sx in ♀. Complications: PID, ectopic, infertility Disseminated: Petechial, pustular acral lesions, septic arthritis, perihepatitis, endocarditis, meningitis	NAAT, cx (esp for nongenital sites: Rectum, pharynx), nucleic acid hybridization	CTX 125 mg IM × 1 OR cefixime 400 mg PO × 1 PLUS CT Rx if not ruled out. Disseminated: CTX IM/IV q24h + hospitalization Recommended for pharyngeal infection	Quinolones no longer recommended due to resistance Consider patient-delivered therapy + CT Rx to heterosexual partner
Pelvic Inflammatory Disease				
Mostly C. trachomatis and N. gonorrhoeae Though often polymicrobial	CMT, uterine/adnexal tenderness, fever, discharge, endometritis, salpingitis, TOA, pelvic peritonitis	Abundant WBC on wet prep, ESR, CRP, microbiology Most specific: Endometrial hx, transvaginal U/S, laparoscopy	Inpatient (severe): Cefotetan 2 g IV q12h OR cefoxitin 2 g IV q12h PLUS doxy 100 mg PO or IV q12h After 24 hr of parenteral Abx, continue doxy × 14 d. Add metronidazole or clindamycin if +TOA Outpatient (mild–moderate): CTX 250 mg IM × 1 PLUS doxy 100 mg PO bid × 14 d +/− metronidazole 500 mg bid × 14 d	Empiric Abx prevents long-term sequelae Consider oral quinolone regimen + metronidazole if mild disease and no quinolone resistant Neisseria gonorrhoeae
Vaginal Discharge				
Bacterial vaginosis (*Gardnerella*, other anaerobes)	Homogenous, thin-white, malodorous discharge; pruritic	Clue cells, pH >4.5, +Whiff test, Gram stain – gold standard, cx is nonspecific	Metronidazole 500 mg PO bid × 7 d OR Metronidazole gel 5 mg intravag qd × 5 d OR clinda 2% cream 5 g intravag QHS × 7 d	Complications: Endometritis, PID, postprocedure cellulitis Rx ♂ partners does not reduce recurrence

Trichomoniasis (T. vaginalis)	Malodorous, yellow-green discharge, vulvar irritation, or no sx	Nucleic acid probe, SN >83%, SP > 97% Wet prep 60–70% SN Cx most SN/SP	Metronidazole 2 g × 1 or 500 mg bid × 7 d Tinidazole 2 g PO single dose (longer half-life and higher tissue penetration)	Consider re-screening ♀ at 3 mo; low level metronidazole resistance in 2–5%; consider patient-delivered therapy to rx partner
Vulvovaginal candidiasis (VVC) (C. albicans or other species)	Pruritus, soreness, dyspareunia, external dysuria, abnormal/ curdy discharge Vulvar edema, fissures, excoriations	Saline, 10% KOH wet prep or Gram stain with yeast or pseudohyphae Cx for yeast species (for negative wet mounts)	*Immunocompetent/ sporadic:* Short course topicals (single dose and regimens of 1–3 d) or fluconazole 150 mg PO × 1 *Suppressive therapy for recurrent:* Longer courses i.e., fluconazole 150 mg PO weekly for 6 mo	75% of ♀ will have one episode, 40–45% ≥2, 10–20% will have VVC oil-based creams may weaken condoms Topical azoles more effective than nystatin

Ulcerative Disease (HIV testing should be performed on all individuals with genital ulcers)

| Syphilis (T. pallidum) | 1° ulcer/ chancre 2°: Rash, mucocutaneous lesions, LAD 3°: Cardiac/ ophthalmic, auditory, gumma Neurosyphilis Latent: (early latent vs. late latent) no sx | *Definitive:* Darkfield exam/DFA of lesion *Presumptive* • Nontreponemal (VDRL, RPR) correlate w/ dz activity/Rx response confirm with • Treponemal (FTA-ABS, TP-PA) If neurologic sx (necessary to exam CSF in all infants with suspected or proven syphilis) • CSF:VDRL is SP, FTA-ABS is SN, serologies, CSF cell count/protein • Ocular slit-lamp exam | 1°/2°/early latent (infection within 1 yr): Benzathine PCN G 2.4 million U IM × 1 (50,000 U/kg up to adult dose in kids) 3°, late latent: PCN G 2.4 million U × 3 doses at 1 wk interval Neurosyphilis: Aqueous crystalline PCN G 18–24 million U/d (100,000–150,000 U/kg/d infants) (q4h or continuous) × 14 d Presumptive Rx for sex partners w/i 90 d | Jarisch–Herxheimer rxn: Acute febrile rxn with HA, myalgia within 24 hr of Rx F/u evaluation at 6 and 12 mo (and 24 mo for latent, and q6mo for neurosyphilis) RPR+ gets reflex treponemal test; if RPR-but strongly suspected request treponemal test through micro |
| Chancroid (H. ducreyi) | Painful genital ulcer, tender suppurative inguinal LAD | Dx w/ following criteria • Painful genital ulcer(s) • No syphilis • Ulcer exudates HSV (–) | Azithro 1 g × 1 or CTX 250 mg IM × 1 OR Cipro 500 mg PO bid × 3 d OR Erythro 500 mg PO tid × 7 d | Re-exam in 3–7 d for improvement. 10% coinfected with T. pallidum or HSV Cofactor for HIV transmission |

entity STI's 10-14 marker on side.

Genital HSV • HSV-2 > HSV-1 • First-episode likely HSV-1 • Recurrence likely HSV-2	Most w/ no sx Small, painful, grouped vesicles on an erythematous base/shallow ulcers Erythema multiforme, neuro sequelae, dissemination	DFA and cx, HSV DNA PCR and neg virologic test does not rule out infection due to intermittent shedding Type-specific serum Ab	Valacyclovir (1 g PO bid) OR famciclovir (250 mg PO tid) both have good oral bioavailability, OR acyclovir (400 mg PO tid OR 200 mg PO fid). Duration 7–10 d. *Severe* (complications, hospitalization, CNS): IV acyclovir *Acyclovir-resistant:* ID consult, consider foscarnet/	Treat patients with initial genital herpes Consider 2° prevention suppressive Rx (>5 episodes/yr, HIV coinfection, etc.) CDC STD Rx guidelines for details Episodic Rx (start on 1st day of onset of recurrent ulcer to shorten duration of outbreak [does not clear latent virus]) Counsel re: pregnancy
Granuloma inguinale; Donovanosis (*Calymmatobacterium granulomatis*)	Painless, progressive, beefy-red, vascular ulcerative lesions, no LAD	Visualization of dark-staining Donovan bodies on tissue crush preparation/biopsy	Doxy/bactrim/fluoroquinolones	Rx halts lesion progression
Lymphogranuloma venereum (*C. trachoms* L1, L2, L3)	Unilateral, tender inguinal/femoral LAD, self-limited ulcer/papule often gone, proctocolitis if anal exposure	Nucleic acid probe Urine, genital, and/or LN specimens for cx, direct immunofluorescence	Doxy 100 mg PO bid × 3 wk Buboes require aspiration	Rx cures infection and prevents ongoing tissue damage
Genital Warts (HPV)				
HPV types 6 and 11 common	Flat, papular, or pedunculated growths on genital mucosa Generally asymp, can be painful, friable, or pruritic	3–5% acetic acid turns infected genital mucosa white, but little evidence Bx only if dx uncertain, no response to Rx, or patient immunocomp	*Primary Prevention:* HPV vaccines offer 3-vaccine series starting at 11–12 yo, bivalent (Cervarix HPV types 16 & 18) OR quadrivalent vaccine (Gardasil HPV types 6, 11, 16, & 18 better for genital wart protection) *External:* No definitive treatment Podofilox 0.5% bid. × 3 d, then 4 d no therapy, repeat prn ≤4 cycles (total area ≤10 cm²) Imiquimod 5% cream QHS, TIW ≤16 wk Cryotherapy (various forms) Podophyllin resin 10–25% OR trichloroacetic acid OR bichloroacetic acid	Rx may reduce, does not eliminate infxn, unclear impact on transmission *Genital warts* not indication for HPV testing, change in freq of Pap, or colpo *Cervical:* Exclude high grade SIL before Rx, consult specialist *Vaginal:* Liquid nitrogen, Trichloroacetic acid/Bichloroacetic acid (TCA/BCA)

		Surgical removal, laser therapy, intralesional interferon	*Urethral meatus:* Liquid nitrogen or podophyllin *Anal:* Cryotherapy, TCA/BCA, surgical removal
Ectoparasitic Infections			
Pediculosis pubis (pubic lice)	Lice or nits on pubic hair	Recommended: Permethrin 1% cream or Permethrin with piperonyl butoxide Alternative: Malathion 0.5% lotion or ivermectin 250 μg/kg repeated in 2 wk	Resistance to pediculicides inc Use malathion when Rx failure believed 2/2 resistance Rx sex partners w/i previous mo
Scabies (*Sarcoptes scabiei*)	Classic burrowing rash, pruritus may persist for ≤2 wk	Recommended: Permethrin cream 5% to all areas of the body from neck down, wash off after 8–14 hr Ivermectin 200 mcg/kg PO, repeated in 2 wk Alternative: Lindane 1% total body, neck down (toxicity: Aplastic anemia, seizure) Decontaminate bedding/clothing	Sensitization to *Sarcoptes scabiei* occurs before pruritus. With 1st infection takes ≤ several wks to develop, may occur ≤24 hr of reinfection In adults usually sexually acquired, but not in children Norwegian scabies (i.e., crusted scabies): Aggressive infestation occurs in immune-deficient, debilitated, or malnourished persons

STI's 10-15

cx, culture; SN, sensitivity; SP, specificity; CT, C. trachomatis; NG, N. gonorrhoeae; Rx, treatment; **NAAT**, nucleic acid amplification test; **GNID**, Gram neg intracellular diplococci.

Evaluation and Management of High-risk Exposure (Red Book 2009; 2010 Guidelines on HIV PEP beyond the perinatal period)
- Eval & Rx for sexual assault should be managed by a multidisciplinary team that is experienced in the care of children or adolescents who have been sexually assaulted
- **Diagnostic testing (within 72 hr of exposure and repeated at 2 wk)**
  - CT and GC urine NAAT or cervical culture; swab of throat and rectum if relevant to exposure
  - HIV ELISA
  - Wet prep for trichomonas and bacterial vaginosis if cervical exam performed
  - Hepatitis B surface antibody if status of vaccination unknown
- **Prophylaxis** (recommended in all postpubertal ♀, discuss w/ ID & sexual assault specialist & family in prebuteral children, typically only Rx for Sx, always after consent from appt care givers)
  - Ceftriaxone 125 mg IM × 1 if <45 kg; 250 mg IM × 1 if >45 kg for Gonorrhea
  - Metronidazole 2 g PO × 1 for trichomonas
  - Azithro 1 gm PO × 1 for >45 kg; 20 mg/kg × 1 PO for <45 kg for Chlamydia

- **Hep B:** Immunoprophylaxis depends on type of exposure & immune status of exposed individual. Not all immunized patients respond to the vaccine at protective levels. Please consult the Red Book (HBV section) for details
- **HIV:** Risk of transmission after exposure is <0.3% from puncture wound from a needle in the community, 0.1% from receptive vaginal intercourse, and 0.5% after penile–anal sex exposure
- **HIV:** <36 hr since high-risk exposure and source is HIV-positive or unknown start Kaletra & Truvada (http://aidsinfo.nih.gov – National HIV consultation center 24 hr hotline: 1-888-448-4911)

TUBERCULOSIS

Epidemiology
Worldwide incidence 9 million cases and 1.4 million TB-related deaths annually
- In US, btw 1985–1994 ↑ TB incidence in children by 33%
- Main risk factors: +TB contacts, +immigration from high prevalence country, +HIV, other immunodeficiencies, malnutrition, low SES

Pathophysiology
Mycobacterium tuberculosis bacillus is usually inhaled in droplets
- Early infxn → localized alveolitis, regional LAD, and either spont resolution (latent TB), or spread via hematolymphatics → disseminated TB (military or meningitis)
- Risk of progression: Infants and young children (<4 yo), immunocompromise (HIV, immunosuppressive drugs, Hodgkin disease, lymphoma, diabetes mellitus, chronic renal failure, and malnutrition)
- Reactivation TB is much less common in children than in adults

Screening (Arch Dis Child Educ Pract Ed 2007;92:27, AAP Red Book 2012)
- Technique: PPD, 0.1 mL, intradermal wheal on forearm, Eval btw 48–72 hr, determine diameter of induration, *not* erythema
  - TST relatively nonspecific & insensitive in invasive Tb
- Serum IGRA measure ex vivo interferon-gamma production from T cells in resp to stim specific for *M. tuberculosis* complex
  - Similar sensitivity to Mantoux skin test, higher specificity
  - Recs for use: Immune-competent children ≥ 5 yo; to confirm active case or LTBI and likely will yield fewer false-positive test results (i.e., BCG-vaccinated children)
- Generally, interpretation of TST results in BCG recipients is the same as for people who have not received BCG vaccine
- Who should be screened: Known TB contact, immigration from high prevalence country, HIV (yearly), incarceration, radiographic findings suggestive of TB

Size of Induration	Persons Considered to be +
>5 mm	HIV+; close contact of suspected TB; child with suspected TB (e.g., positive CXR); receiving immunosuppressive therapy
>10 mm	↑ risk of dissemination: <4 yo; malnutrition; immigration from high-risk area; living in high-risk environment (shelter, prison, etc.) recent travel to high-risk area; h/o chronic diseases; latent TB in family
>15 mm	>4 yo w/o risk factors

Clinical Manifestations (Arch Dis Child 2000;83:342)
- Cough, constitutional sx (fever, night sweats, weight loss), FTT, lymphadenopathy
- Extrapulmonary dz more common in kids, esp <5 yo; up to $^1/_3$
  - Scrofula → TB adenitis, bony involv →TB osteomyelitis (in spine = Pott dz), pericarditis, meningitis, hepatitis, adrenal dz, cutaneous dz
- HIV coinfection is major risk factor for active TB and predicts more severe course

Diagnostic Studies
- More difficult to dx than in adults because children often have paucibacillary disease
- Induced sputum in younger children, and AM gastric aspirates in children <5 yo
- Acid fast bacillus (AFB) smear: Rapid diagnosis, but not sensitive
- Culture: Takes weeks, allows for drug sensitivity testing (DST)
- PCR: More sensitive than smear
- CXR: Look for consolidation, pleural effusion, LAD, cavitary lesions, "millet seed" opacities in disseminated or "miliary" TB
- If your suspicion is high, then no diagnostic test will definitively rule out TB

- R/o active dz w/ CXR in all pts w/ +PPD, and further w/u in pts who have any sx
- If CXR neg, and no sx, preventive Rx w/ INH (isoniazid) can ↓ chances of reactivation
- INH + Vit B6 (pyridoxine) ×6–9 mo (should monitor carefully for hepatitis); >12 yr and not on HAART: INH and Rifapentine × 3 mo; INH-resistance: Rifampin QD × 6 mo

Treatment of Active TB

- AFB+, culture+, or high level of suspicion
- Isolate pt (test family and close contacts/prophylaxes as needed)
- 1st-line regimen is 4 drug Rx (usually HREZ – see later) ×2 mo, then HR ×4 mo
- *Do not* give fewer than 3 drugs to prevent resistance
- If TB meningitis: HRZ (+/– ethionamide 20 mg/kg/d) × 2 mo and prednisone 1–2 mg/kg/d taper over 3 wk, then HR ×9–10 mo
- In developing countries, WHO recommends directly observed therapy (DOT) to increase compliance/cure and decrease resistance
- Multidrug-resistant (MDR) TB: Worldwide prevalence in 2007 ~5%, definition → resistant to at least HR → refer to ID for Rx; also XDR-TB (extremely resistant)

Pediatric Dosing of Antituberculosis Medications (non-MDR)		
Drug	Dosing[a] (daily, mg/kg)	Common Side Effects
Isoniazid (H)	5 (4–6)	Hepatitis, peripheral neuropathy, GI upset
Rifampin (R)	10 (8–12)	Orange urine, elevated LFTs, GI upset
Ethambutol (E)	20 (15–25)	Arthralgia, GI upset, HA, malaise
Pyrazinamide (Z)	25 (20–30)	Hepatitis, arthropathy, hyperuricemia
Streptomycin (S)	15 (12–18)	Ototoxicity, nephrotoxicity

[a]Might utilize higher doses in invasive disease and meningitis. In some cases, serum drug level testing might be appropriate.
Adapted from WHO "Hospital Care for Children" 2005: 352.

HIV

Etiology (AAP Redbook 2009)

- HIV-1 most common in US, HIV-2 more common in West Africa
- Retrovirus infection, which infects and depletes CD4 cells over time, leading to severe immunocompromise (AIDS) and opportunistic infections (OIs)

Epidemiology

- Preadolescent infections: 100–200 infant infections/year in US
- Adolescent infections on the rise: In 2005, ~14% of newly diagnosed HIV-1 infections in US were among 13–24 yo, most asymptomatic and unaware of HIV status (RF: Minority, MSM)

Transmission (JAMA 2000;283:1175)

- Vertical transmission: In utero (↑ risk w/ ↑ maternal viral load): 5–10% transmission
  - During delivery (↑ risk w/ vaginal delivery): 10–20% transmission
  - Breast-feeding (↑ risk w/ mixed formula + breast milk): 5–20% transmission
- Horizontal transmission: Sexual contact, injection drug use, blood transfusions

Clinical Manifestations (AAP Redbook 2009)

- Early manifestations: Unexplained fevers, generalized LAD, HSM, FTT, persistent/recurrent oral & diaper candidiasis, recurrent diarrhea, parotitis, hepatitis, central nervous system (CNS) disease, recurrent invasive bacterial infections, and other opportunistic infections (e.g., viral and fungal)
- Median age until sx after perinatal infxn is 12–18 mo, some asymptomatic >5 yr
- Historically, 15–20% mortality in perinatally infected pts by 4 yo if no Rx available
- Newly HIV-infected adolescents and adults may be asymp for yrs (latent infxn) until they progress to severe immunocompromise

Diagnostic Studies (N Engl J Med 1988;319:961; MMWR 1990;39:380)

- HIV ELISA: 1st-line screening test (99+% sensitivity and specificity)
- Western blot: Confirmatory test (99+% sensitivity and specificity)
- HIV-1 PCR: (99% sensitivity, 98% specificity)
  - Used to dx acute HIV before HIV ELISA turns + (usually w/i 3 mo)

- CD4 absolute count predicts risk for opportunistic infections
  - CD4% more reliable in young children (less variability between tests)
- Indications to initiate antiretroviral therapy (www.aidsinfo.nih.gov); initiation of therapy depends on a combination of factors including the age of the child, and virologic, immunologic, and clinical criteria

Infants (<1 yo)	Children (1–4 yo)	Older Children and Adolescents (>5 yo)
Treat HIV-infected children under 12 mo age, regardless of CD4 or viral load	AIDS, significant HIV-related sx (CDC clinical category B or C) or CD4 <25%	AIDS, significant HIV-related symptoms (CDC clinical category B or C) or CD4 <350
	Consider Rx for VL >100,000 even w/o sx	Consider therapy for VL >100,000 even without symptoms

Management

Nucleoside RT Inhibitors	Nonnucleoside RT Inhibitors	Protease Inhibitors
Class-wide NRTI toxicity: Myelosuppression including anemia, peripheral neuropathy **Zidovudine (AZT, ZDV)** • tox: Anemia, marrow suppress **Lamivudine (3TC)** • tox: GI intolerance **Tenofovir (TDF)** • tox: Acute renal failure **Emtricitabine (FTC)** • tox: Hyperpigmentation **Abacavir (ABC)** • tox: Potentially-fatal hypersensitivity rxn in 7% **Stavudine (d4T)** • tox: Lactic acidosis, peripheral neuropathy **Didanosine (ddI)** • tox: Pancreatitis, lactic acidosis, periph neuropathy	**Efavirenz (EFV)** • tox: Teratogenic (esp early), vivid dreams, psychosis (esp in patients with preexisting psychiatric disease) **Nevirapine (NVP)** • tox: Hepatotoxicity (women <250, men <400), Stevens–Johnson syndrome	**Class-wide PI toxicity:** High pill burden, GI intolerance, lipodystrophy, hyperlipidemia, hyperglycemia, neuropathy **Lopinavir/ritonavir** Do not use in neonates <42 W, or 14 d **Atazanavir** • tox: Hyperbilirubinemia, mild–mod rash **Nelfinavir** • tox: Nephrolithiasis **Saquinavir** **Fosamprenavir** • tox: Mild–moderate rash, Stevens–Johnson **Indinavir** • tox: Nephrolithiasis

- Typical ARV treatment regimens (www.aidsinfo.nih.gov)
  - In general, combinations of at least 3 drugs are recommended
  - 1st-line Rx: 2 NRTIs PLUS 1 PI or NNRT (≥42 wk & postnatal ≥14 d of age: Lopinavir/ritonavir; ≥6 yr: Atazanavir/ritonavir)
  - 2nd-line Rx: 2 NRTIs and 1 NNRTI
  - Not generally recommended: 3 NRTIs (AZT, 3TC, abacavir)
  - Goal to suppress viral load to undetectable levels and allow restoration CD4
  - Recommend to screen all Rx-naïve pts or pts failing ARV Rx for viral resistance
  - All std vaccinations recommended (including MMR), except varicella 2/2 risk of systemic disease (MMWR Recomm Rep 2006;55:Q1 PMID: 17136024)

Opportunistic infections & prophy (USPS/IDSA Guidelines for OI Prevention 2002)

Etiology	Threshold to Prophylax	Prophylaxis
Pneumocystis jiroveci (PCP)	CD4 < 200 or CD4% < 14% Oropharyngeal candidiasis	TMP/SMX daily or 3×/wk Alternatives: Dapsone, pentamidine, atovaquone
Toxoplasmosis	CD4 < 100 and toxo IgG-positive	1° ppx: TMP/SMX daily or 3×/wk 2° ppx: Sulfadiazine + pyrimethamine Alternatives: Dapsone, atovaquone
Mycobacterium tuberculosis	Positive PPD (>5 mm) or exposure to active TB case	Rule out active TB disease → Isoniazid for 9 mo

Mycobacterium avium complex	CD4 < 50	Azithromycin weekly or clarithromycin twice daily
Influenza		Influenza vaccine annually
Pneumococcus		Pneumococcal 23-valent vaccine
Cryptococcal meningitis	Documented cryptococcal disease	1° ppx not routinely recommended 2° ppx: Fluconazole or itraconazole
CMV	Documented end-organ disease	Ganciclovir or foscarnet
Herpes simplex virus	Recurrent HSV disease	Consider valacyclovir or acyclovir

Care of Infants Born to HIV Positive Mothers (http://AIDSinfo.nih.gov)

Age	Labs	Prophylaxis/Comment
Birth	CBC diff, electrolytes, BUN, Cr, SGOT, alk phos HIV DNA PCR (R/o in utero transmission, which accounts for ~30% of cases of perinatal HIV infection) The sensitivity of a single HIV DNA PCR test performed <48 hr of age is <40%	**Zidovudine** (ZDV) syrup (50 mg/5 cc) **2 mg/kg/dose** (If IV, use 1.5 mg/kg/dose) FIRST DOSE OF AZT SHOULD BE GIVEN @ <12 HR OF LIFE **Dosing intervals:** Term newborn: q6h Preterm newborn: q12h initially • If EGA ≥ 30 wk, change to q8h dosing at 2 wk of age • If EGA < 30 wk, change to q8h dosing at 4 wk of age Consider giving nevirapine (2 mg/kg) (NVP) in addition to ZDV if the mother received no antepartum treatment (regardless of whether intrapartum ZDV was given) • Give *at birth* if mother did not receive NVP during labor and delivery • Give at 2–3 d of age if mother did receive NVP during labor and delivery
2 wk	CBC diff HIV DNA PCR	Continue zidovudine – make sure family has enough to last 6 wk, check dose, adjust for weight if necessary
1–2 mo of age	CBC diff HIV DNA PCR	Instruct the family to stop zidovudine prophylaxis at 6 wk of age if HIV infection is presumptively excluded HIV infection may be *presumptively* excluded if HIV DNA PCRs done after both 14 d and 1 mo of age are negative Start PCP prophylaxis with trimethoprim–sulfamethoxazole prophylaxis if HIV infection is *NOT* presumptively excluded
4–6 mo of age	DNA HIV PCR	HIV infection can be *definitively* excluded if HIV DNA PCRs done after both 1 and 4 mo of age are negative
≥9 mo of age	HIV screen (ELISA) – optional to document sero-reversion	No further PCR testing is necessary, assuming the infant has had negative PCRs after both 1 and 4 mo of age

- Any +HIV, RNA, PCR, or HIV ELISA should be repeated promptly and ID notified
- HIV-infected patients should be immunized with age-appropriate inactivated vaccines as well as annual influenza vaccine
- Unless severely immunosuppressed, MMR is appropriate for children >1 yo. Infants with HIV should not receive MMR

PEDIATRIC PNEUMONIA

(N Engl J Med 2002;346:429; AAP Red Book 2009, IDSA/PIDS guidelines: Clin Infect Dis 2011;53(7):e25–76)

Definition
- Pulm infxn beyond terminal bronchioles, including alveoli; whereas bronchitis involves proximal to distal bronchioles

Clinical Manifestations
- Fever, cough, dyspnea, &/or hypoxia

- Viral PNA often preceded by URI sx; diffuse bilaterally abnormal lung exam; interstitial infiltrates
- Bacterial PNA suggested by leukocytosis, chills, may show signs of sepsis
- Atypical PNA often w/ gradually worse cough ("walking PNA"), interstitial infiltrates, malaise, myalgia, headache
- Nonspecific in younger children: Fever, irritability, poor feeding, restless
- Abn lung exam (rhonchi, ↓ breath sounds, dullness to percussion, ↑ tactile fremitus)
  - Rhonchi (low-pitched coarse) more common in broncho PNA (larger airways involved)
  - Inspiratory rales more common in lobar PNA and bronchiolitis (alveoli involved)
  - Diminished or bronchial breath sounds in consolidation
  - Expiratory wheezes in bronchiolitis and viral interstitial pneumonitis

Etiologies

Neonates (<1 mo)	Infants (<1 yr)	Younger Children <5 yr	Older Children 5–15 yr

Early onset
 • Group B streptococcus
 • Gram-negative rods
 • Listeria
  • Rx – **amp + gent**
 • Viral (transplacental)
 • TB (transplacental)
 Late onset
 • *Staph. aureus*
 • *Group A Strep*
 • *Strep. pneumoniae*
 • GNR (often nosocomial)
  • tx – **vanc + AGs**
 • *Chlamydophila trach.*
  • 2 wk–4 mo of age
 • Viral
  • RSV, adeno, paraflu, enterov
	Viruses (most common)
	 Afebrile pneumonia
	 • *Chlamydophila trachomatis*
	 • CMV; *Mycoplasma h.*, Ureaplasma
	 Bacterial
	 • S. pneumoniae – #1
	 • *Bordetella pertussis*
		Viruses: RSV = #1
		 • Influenza/paraflu
		 • Adenovirus
		 • Human metapneumovirus
		 • Rhinovirus, coronavirus
		 • Measles (developing co.)
		 Bacterial:
		 S. pneumo – #1
		 • H. influenzae, Moraxella
		 • S. aureus, inc. CA-MRSA
		 • –c/b necrosis, empyema
		 • Often after 1° influenza
		 PNA: GAS
		 • Often after 1° varicella PNA
		 Atypical bacteria (↑ freq)
		 • *Mycoplasma pneumoniae*
		 • *Chlamydophila pneumoniae*
		 Mycobacterium tuberculosis
			Atypical bacteria
			 • *Mycoplasma pneum* (#1 overall)
			 • *Chlamydophila pneum*
			 Bacterial
			 • *S. pneumoniae* = #1
			 • *H. influenzae*, Moraxella
			 • *Staph. aureus*, inc. CA-MRSA
			 • GAS
			 Aspiration pneumonia
			 • Anaerob strepto
			 • *Fusobacterium*
			 • *Bacteroides*
			 • *Prevotella*
			 Nosocomial pneumonia
			 • Gram-negative rods
			 • Staph. aureus
			 • risk: Vent, broad Abx

Diagnostic Studies

- CBC diff (leukocytosis w/ left-shift, occ leucopenia); consider ESR/CRP, blood cultures in moderate to severe infections
- Sputum GS and culture (if productive cough)
- CXR (preferably PA/lateral; lateral decubitus if suspect pleural effusion)
  - Not necessary for dx of simple outpatient CAP, recommended for: Hypoxemia or significant respiratory distress. Routine CXR for follow-up *not* recommended
  - Lobar PNA (single lobe or lobar segmental) classic for pneumococcal PNA
    - Pleural effusion, cavitation/pneumatoceles, sepsis, ↑ WBC, chills suggest bact PNA
  - BronchoPNA (1° airways & surrounding parenchyma): Group A strep & *Staph. aureus*
  - Necrotizing pneumonia: Aspiration pneumonia, *S. pneumoniae*, *Staph. aureus*
  - Interstitial: Suggests viral or atypical etiology
  - Interstitial w/ 2° parenchymal infil: Classic for viral PNA → c/b bacterial PNA
  - Rare to have complete lobar consolidation in infants
  - CXR improvement typically lags behind clinical improvement (up to 1 mo)
- Mycoplasma IgM/IgG complement; fixation or PCR (cold agglutinins not clinically useful); pertussis culture/antibody/antigen PCR

Admission Criteria

- Hypoxia (sat <90% consistently), dehydration, respiratory distress (infant RR >60, children RR >40, grunting, retractions), toxic appearance (↑ common in bacterial PNA), serious underlying disease (e.g., cardiopulmonary), empyema/effusion – requires further evaluation/treatment, failed outpatient therapy (24–72 hr)

	Bacterial	Atypical[a]	Aspiration Nosocomial	Suspected Influenza
Outpt	• Amoxicillin (high-dose = 80–100 mg/kg/d) • *or (if PCN-allergic)-* • Clindamycin • Macrolides (up to 50% macrolide-resistant *S. pneumo*) • IM ceftriaxone → PO Abx • Quinolones[b] (adol)	• Macrolides • Doxycycline (>8 yo) • Quinolones* (adol)	Aspiration • Amoxicillin– clavulanate • Clindamycin	• Oseltamivir Dosage depends on age and weight of patient Duration: 5 d
Inpt	• Ampicillin • Consider Ceftriaxone (50–100 mg/kg/d)/ Cefotaxime/ Cefuroxime; all have better β-lactamase coverage than ampicillin • Continue IV tx until afebrile × 24–48 hr and tolerating PO • If complicated (effusion/abscess) or severe, consider adding • Vancomycin (MRSA) • Nafcillin (MSSA) • Clindamycin • Linezolid (MRSA; resistant *S. pneumo*)	• Macrolides • Doxycycline (>8 yo) • Quinolones* (adol)	Aspiration • Ampicillin– sulbactam • Clindamycin Nosocomial (anti-pseudomonal) • Piperacillin– Tazobactam • Ticarcillin– clavulanate • Meropenem • Quinolones[b]	• Oseltamivir Dosage depends on age and weight of patient Duration: 5 d

[a]Send diagnostic studies for Mycoplasma when results available in clinically-relevant time-frame.
[b]Fluoroquinolone associated with arthropathy, use w/ caution in the pediatric population.

• For *C. trachomatis* or *B. pertussis* Rx w/ macrolides
• PCP (*Pneumocystis j.*): Seen in immunocompromised; Rx w/ TMP/SMX and add corticosteroids if hypoxic/or ↑ A-a gradient

Complications
• Rpt CXR 2–3 wk after d/c for complicated comm.-acquired PNA or if persistent sx
• Parapneumonic effusion (initially sterile) → empyema (pus); U/S is excellent screening
  • Broaden antibiotic coverage and thoracentesis to determine effusion etiology (evid of pus, (+)GS, pH < 7, ↑↑ LDH, ↓ glucose suggest empyema)
  • Chest tube if empyema or for severe effusion → VATS if no improvement after 48 hr of chest tube (remove loculations/adhesions); alt fibrinolytics
• Lung abscess: Aspiration/IR drainage if no improv after 72 hr Rx; lobectomy only after >3 wk appropriate Abx therapy

INBORN ERRORS OF METABOLISM

Definition
- Inherited enzyme mutation alters metabolism → excess or lack of certain metabolites

Incidence
- 1:1,400–200,000 live births; NBS screens for many of the disorders

Neonatal Presentation (Pediatr Rev 2009;30:131; Pediatrics 1998;102:E69; Vademecum Metabolicum 2004:3)
- Sx at 24–72 hr of life; prior, mother's metabolism eliminates metabolic intermediates
- Ill infant w/ nonspecific sx: Lethargy, diff feeding, vomiting, abn resp, hypotonia and szrs, see the acute presentation differential table below
- Abnormal body or urinary odor
  - MSUD: Urine smells of maple syrup or burnt sugar
  - Isovaleric acidemia and glutaric acidemia type II → pungent, "sweaty feet" odor

Late Presentation (Crit Care Clin 2005;21:S9; Vademecum metabolicum 2004:3)
- >28 d of life; recurrent vomiting, lethargy, or fasting → coma with nonfocal neuro exam, liver dysfxn + mental status changes: Consider urea cycle disorders (UCD)

Adolescent/Adults Presentation (J Inherit Metab Dis 2007;30:631)
- Psychiatric d/o, often w/ additional recurrent rhabdo, myoglobinuria, cardiomyopathy
- Acute cyclic confusion → urea cycle defect, porphyria, homocysteine remethylation defect
- Chronic psych sx → homocystinuria, Wilson dz, adrenoleukodystrophy, lysosomal d/os
- Mild mental retardation & personality Δ → homocystinuria, nonketotic hyperglycemia

Specific Triggers of Decompensation (Vademecum Metabolicum 2004:3)
- Vomiting, fasting, infection, fever, vaccinations, surgery, accident or injury, changes in diet → protein or carbohydrate metabolism disorders
- High-protein diet and/or catabolic state → aminoacidopathies, organic acidemia, UCD
- Fruit, sugar (sucrose), liquid medicines → fructose intolerance
- Lactose → galactosemia
- High fat → fatty acid oxidation disorders
- Drugs → porphyria, glucose-6-phosphate-dehydrogenase deficiency
- Extensive exercise → disorders of fatty acid oxidation, glycolysis, respiratory chain

Differential Diagnosis based on Initial Presentation

Presenting Findings w/ Encephalopathy		
Primary	**Secondary**	**Potential Disorder**
Acidosis	+/– Hypoglyc, +/– LA, +/– keto, +/– ↑NH₃, ↑AG	Various organic acid disorders
	Significant LA, normoglycemia	Mito d/o, pyruvate dehydrogenase def, α-ketoglutarate dehydrogenase, pyruvate carboxylase def
	Significant LA, Hypoglyc	Glycogen storage type I, Fructose-1,6-bisphosphatase def
	Nml AG, lactate, no ketosis	RTA
Hyperammonemia	Alkalosis/nml pH, nml lactate	Urea cycle disorders
	Hypoglycemia, ↑LFT, nml ketones	Fatty acid oxidation defects
	Acidosis w/ ↑AG +/– LA, +/– keto, +/– Hypoglyc	Various organic acid disorders
Hypoglycemia	Acidosis w/ ↑AG +/– keto, +/– LA, +/– w/ ↑NH₃	Various organic acid disorders
	Hepatomegaly, +/– LA	Glycogen storage disorder
	No ketosis or acidosis, nml LA	Hyperinsulinemia Fatty acid oxidation defects
	HypoNa, HoTn	Adrenal insufficiency
	Signs liver failure	Tyrosinemia, glycogen storage dz type IV, galactosemia, Niemann–Pick type C

LA, lactic acidosis; AG, anion gap; Hypoglyc, hypoglycemia; HypoNa,: hyponatremia; HoTn, hypotension; dz, disease. *Adapted from Pediatr Rev 2009;31:131*

EMERGENCIES

Critical Labs (Pediatrics 1998;102:E69; Vademecum Metabolicum 2004:4)
- Stat D-stick, CBC w/diff, chem 7, blood gas, NH₃, lactate, plasma and urine amino acids, U/A, urine reducing substances, urine ketones, urine organic acids, ESR
- CRP, CK, ALT, AST, coagulation studies
- Store plasma samples for amino acids, acylcarnitine and filter paper ("Guthrie" card)
- If LP done → freeze CSF for further studies
- Consider ECG, echo, head imaging

Emergent Treatment (Pediatrics 1998;102:E69; Vademecum Metabolicum 2004:5)
- Obtain critical sample as above
- Start Rx before confirmed dx; stop protein, fat, galactose, and fructose intake
- Consult metabolic specialist
- 1st goal: Remove metabolites (organic acid intermediates or ammonia)
  - Hyperammonemia: Immediate HD for coma, vent dependency, or cerebral edema
  - Urea cycle defects: 6 cc/kg of 10% arginine HCL IV over 90 min
  - Organic acidemia: Vit B₁₂ (1 mg) IM for B₁₂-responsive form of methylmalonic acidemia. Biotin (10 mg) PO or NGT for biotin-responsive carboxylase deficiency
  - Acidosis: Give bicarb with frequent ABGs; severely acidotic: HD
- 2nd goal: Prevent catabolism
  - IV glucose (calories & substitute for gluconeogenesis) → D10, 150 cc/kg/d w/ lytes
  - Stop protein as above, IV lipids for urea cycle defects
  - If unclear diagnosis: Continue glucose drip, review history
  - Follow lytes, glucose, lactate, ABG, keep Na >135 to avoid cerebral edema
  - http://newenglandconsortium.org/for-professionals/acute-illness-protocols

HYPOGLYCEMIA

Definition (Pediatrics 1998;192:E69; Vademecum Metabolicum 2004:6)
- Glucose <2.6 mmol/L (45 mg/dL) at all ages

History and Clinical Manifestations
- Determine time since last meal, drugs
- Check for hepatomegaly, liver failure signs (palmar erythema, spider angiomata, gynecomastia, jaundice), small genitals, hyperpigmentation, short stature

Ddx
- Disorders of protein intolerance, carbohydrate metabolism, or fatty acid oxidation
- Hepatic glycogen storage dz (except Pompe); no glycogenolysis (worse with fasting)
- In neonate: Need to rule out sepsis, SGA, maternal diabetes; may show slow adaptation
- Persistent neonatal hypoglycemia → hyperinsulinemia or hypopituitarism

Labs While Hypoglycemic
- As above + insulin, cortisol, lactate, free fatty acids, 3-hydroxybutyrate, Ketostix (urine)
- Acylcarnitine (dried blood spots or plasma); for fatty acid ox d/o + organic acidurias, C-peptide level
- Spare tube for additional labs
- Organic acids in the urine

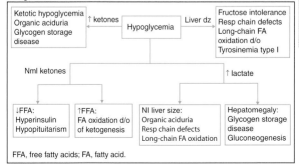

FFA, free fatty acids; FA, fatty acid.

Treatment
- IV glucose at 7–10 mg/kg/min, for calories and to replace normal liver glucose production → D10% glucose, 110–150 cc/kg/d with electrolytes
- Keep FS >100; if glucose needs >10 mg/kg/min → likely hyperinsulinism

HYPERAMMONEMIA

Definition (Pediatrics 1998;192:E69; Vademecum Metabolicum 2004:8)
- Suspect metabolic dz in neonate if NH_3 >200 μmol/L; all other ages NH_3 >100 μmol/L

Ddx: Always consider medication effect
- Urea cycle defects (no acidosis) and organic acidemias (+ metabolic acidosis), liver failure
- Neonates can have transient hyperammonemia of the newborn → sx w/i 24 hr of birth; large premature infants with pulm dz. Usually no recurrent hyperammonemia

Labs
Labs as above; must have uncuffed venous or arterial sample, on ice, sent stat
- AA in plasma and urine, organic acids and orotic acid in urine
- Acylcarnitine in dried blood spots

Treatment
- *Must* contact metabolic team immediately
- NH_3 >500 → central line, art line, HD
- 1st infusion: 12 cc/kg D10 over 2 hr with lytes
  - Arginine hydrochloride 360 mg/kg
  - Na-benzoate 250 mg/kg (alternate pathway for nitrogen excretion)
  - Carnitine 100 mg/kg
  - Ondansetron 0.15 mg/kg IV bolus in noncomatose (to prevent N/V)
- Follow glucose, add insulin if needed, check ammonia after 2 hr
- Ref: Neonate: http://newenglandconsortium.org/for-professionals/acute-illness-protocols/urea-cycle-disorders/neonate-with-hyperammonemia/
- Infant/child: http://newenglandconsortium.org/for-professionals/acute-illness-protocols/urea-cycle-disorders/infantchild-with-hyperammonemia/

ABNORMAL NEWBORN SCREEN

Newborn Screen (Vademecum Metabolicum 2004:53)
http://newenglandconsortium.org/for-professionals/acute-illness-protocols
- Started in the 1960s for PKU → broadened to many d/os w/ regional variations

GALACTOSEMIA

Definition (J Inherit Metab Dis 2006;29:516; Pediatrics 1998;102:E69; Pediatrics 2006;118:E934; Vademecum Metabolicum 2004:3)
- Lactose is broken down into glucose and galactose for absorption
- AR deficiency in enzymes → accumulation of glactose-1-phosphate and galactitol

Incidence
- "Classic galactosemia": Most common with galactose-1-phosphate uridyltransferase (GALT) deficiency → 1:23,000–44,000 newborns
- Galactokinase (GALK) def → 1:1,000,000; galactose-4'-epimerase (GALE) def → rare

Presentation
- Progressive jaundice & liver dysfunction, HSM, food intolerance, hypoglycemia
- First 2 wk of life → V/D, poor weight gain, cataracts, indirect hyperbili from hemolysis
- Most states screen for it on NBS, if picked up <5 do can avoid acute morbidity/mortality
  - Galactose (total) 20–30 mg/dL; no Rx. Outpatient review
    - Repeat screening of dried blood spot, galactose, GALT activity
  - Galactose (total) 30–40 mg/dL; repeat as above
    - Start lactose-free milk, outpt review, follow-up repeat labs
  - Galactose (total) >40 mg/dL; hospitalization, lactose-free diet
    - Check liver and kidney function, coagulation, and ultrasound
    - Check galactose, galactose-1-phosphate, GALT activity

Treatment

- Galactose-free formula
- If ill: Supportive care, Vit K, FFP, Abx for presumed gram-negative sepsis and phototherapy for hyperbilirubinemia
- Usually improves w/ removal of galactose; check meds after dx (many contain galactose)

Prognosis

- Despite dietary therapy, pts develop mental retardation, verbal dyspraxia, motor abnormalities, & hypergonadotrophic hypogonadism
- Many die of *E. coli* sepsis

PHENYLKETONURIA/PHENYLALANINEMIA

Definition (Genet Med 2011;13:697; Pediatrics 2006;118:E934)

- Autosomal recessive d/o: W/ abnormal increase in amino acid phenylalanine in blood
- Deficiency of phenylalanine hydroxylase → impairs neurotransmitter production
- If >20 mg/dL accumulation of phenyl ketones → phenylketonuria (PKU) & musty body odor
- Spectrum of severity depending on degree of residual enzyme function; in most if untreated → severe brain damage, MR, seizures, spasticity

Incidence

- ~1:15,000 for PKU (most common in Turkish (1/2,600) and Irish populations (1/4,500))

Treatment

- Early Rx important → admit to the hospital, inverse relationship btw time to Rx and IQ
- Positive NBS → check quantitative level of phenylalanine and tyrosine concentration
- Provide w/ protein sources low in phenylalanine; titrate to [Phe] 1–6 mg/dL for 1st 10 yr of life
- Follow phenylalanine levels; despite Rx pts w/ ↑ neuropsych complications

MANAGEMENT OF KNOWN INBORN ERRORS OF METABOLISM

Urea Cycle Disorders

Definition (Vademecum Metabolicum 2004; Pediatr Rev 2009;30:e22)

- Inherited enzyme and transport protein def w/ ↓ removal of excess NH_3 from protein metabolism; 6 disorders known

Incidence

- Most common inborn errors of metabolism; 1:8,000
- Usually presents after newborn period, at all ages

Presentation

- Neonates → lethargy, poor feeding, emesis, tachypnea, seizures, encephalopathy
- Infants/children → FTT, feeding problems, vomiting, neuro sx, lethargy, ataxia, szrs
- Teens/adults → Chronic neuro or psych sx, behav probs, lethargy, psychosis
- Of note, arginase deficiency w/o hyperammonemia, p/w progressive neuro deterioration

Diagnosis

- Check NH_3, Dx based on abn plasma & urine amino acid levels, routine labs often nml

Ornithine Transcarbamylase Deficiency (OTC)

- Most common; 1:14,000; X-linked, many w/ residual enzyme activity; ↑ orotic acid level
- Can present between 1 mo of age to childhood with significant illness; inc urine orotic acid

Treatment

- Acute therapy → see the previous discussion
- Long-term management: Metabolic team to assess diet, low-protein diets, good fluid intake, vaccinations, and treating infections early

Aminoacidopathies

Definition (Vademecum Metabolicum 2004:57; Pediatr Rev 2009;30:e22)

- Def of enzymes for AA metab → toxic substances accumulate in brain, liver, and kidneys
- If known disorder of AA metabolism and ill → call metabolic team; often p/w acidosis
- Labs as above and emergency Rx glucose as above, stop protein intake, keep Na >140 to prevent cerebral edema, Abx, detox prn w/ diuresis or HD, Vits and carnitine depending on dz

Tyrosinemia (Am J Med Genet C Semin Med Genet 2006;142C:121; Vademecum Metabolicum 2004:72)

- Accumulation of tyrosine in fluids and tissue
- Type I is the most severe → liver failure, neurologic crises, rickets, hepatocarcinoma
  - 1:100,000 newborns; deficiency of fumarylacetoacetate hydrolase (FAH)
  - Untreated → death before 2 yo
- Type II: Deficiency of tyrosine aminotransferase (TAT)
  - Presents with hyperkeratotic plaques on the hands and soles of the feet and photophobia secondary to tyrosine crystals within the cornea
- Type III: Extremely rare 2/2 deficiency of 4-hydroxyphenylpyruvate dioxygenase
- Treatment → urgent therapy with nitisinone (blocks accumulation of toxic metabolites)
- Long term → phenylalanine and tyrosine restricted diets

Maple syrup urine disease (Pediatrics 2006;118:e934; Vademecum Metabolicum 2004:70)

- Deficiency in activity of branched-chain α-oxoacid dehydrogenase complex → accumulation of leucine, isoleucine, and valine
- AR with 1:185,000. More common in the Mennonite population
- Best outcomes when treated within first 2 wk of life
- Encephalopathy at 4–7 d w/ lethargy, feeding probs, somnolence, cerebral edema, coma
- Urine w/ maple syrup/burnt sugar smell. If breast fed, see in 2nd wk (↓ protein intake)
- Intermittent dz may go undx'd until 5 mo–2 yr of age → dx'd during a mild illness
- Intermediate dz → progressive neurologic probs w/ MR & dx'd btw 5 mo & 7 yr
- Dx → ↑ valine, leucine (plasma > 4 mg/dL) and isoleucine in plasma. Urine w/ branched-chain oxo-/hydroxyacids
- Rx → glucose and insulin infusion, avoid deficiency of isoleucine and valine
- Long term → follow these AAs in the plasma and adjust diet
- Must have low level of these AAs for growth and development
- Trial of thiamine supplementation 50–300 mg/d × 3 wk is recommended

Organic Acidurias

Definition (Pediatrics 1998;102:e69; Vademecum Metabolicum 2004:65)

- D/o of intermediary metabolism w/ accumulation of acids in urine
- Presents with systemic illness ± cerebral abnormalities
- Neonatal → metabolic encephalopathy, lethargy, feeding problems, truncal hypotonia, limb hypertonia, myoclonic jerks, cerebral edema, coma, multiorgan failure
- Chronic intermittent → present up to adulthood, recurring ketoacidotic coma, lethargy, focal neurologic signs
- Chronic progressive form → FTT, chronic vomiting, anorexia, osteoporosis, hypotonia, psychomotor retardation, recurrent infections

Presentation

- Ketosis/ketoacidosis, ↑ lactate, ↑ NH₃, hypo- or hyperglycemia, neutropenia, thrombocytopenia, pancytopenia, hypocalcemia

Diagnosis

- Abnormal organic acids in the urine

Treatment

- As above with glucose, eliminate protein, supplement with carnitine
- Propionic OA →↓ isoleucine, valine, methionine, threonine in diet. Give L-carnitine 50–100 mg/kg/d
- Methylmalonic OA → as for propionic + vitamin B₁₂
- Isovaleric OA → L-carnitine 50–100 mg/kg/d ± L-glycine 150–250 mg/kg/d. Low leucine diet, low protein

Fatty Acid Oxidation Defects

Definition (Pediatrics 2006;118:E934; Pediatr Rev 2009;30:e22)

- Unable to use stored fat during fasting
- P/w hypoketotic hypoglycemia & metabolic acidosis, ↑ transaminases & hyperammonemia ± hepatomegaly

Medium-chain Acyl-CoA Dehydrogenase Deficiency (MCAD)

Definition (Pediatrics 2006;118:E934)

- Most common d/o of fatty acid oxidation; AR, 1:6,500–46,000
- Defect in mito β-oxidation → affects liver (unable to Δ fats to ketones → hypoglycemia)

Clinical Manifestations
- Vomiting and lethargy after fasting in a 3–15 mo child
- Most diagnosed <4 yo, undiagnosed mortality = 20–25%
- Hypoketotic hypoglycemia provoked by fasting (do not present in nonfasting conditions) → may develop coma (from hypoglycemia + toxicity of fatty acids and metabolites)
- Muscle weakness worsens with increased delay in diagnosis

Diagnosis
- Detected on NBS
- Confirm dx with plasma acylcarnitine analysis and urinary organic acids
- May need skin bx for enzyme eval of fibroblasts to narrow down actual enzymatic defect

Management
- Avoid fasting or decreased dietary fat intake
- Supplement with L-carnitine (especially during illnesses)
- Treat aggressively even during mild illnesses with IV glucose and carnitine

POSTMORTEM LABS

(Pediatrics 1998;102:e69; Urea Cycle Disorders, Vademecum Metabolicum; 2004:25)
- Serum and plasma: Centrifuge several ccs immediately and store frozen
- Dried blood spot on filter paper card
- Urine: Freeze immediately
- Bile: Spot on filter paper and store, if available
- 3–10 cc EDTA whole blood for DNA analysis
- Skin bx: Up to 24 hr postmortem, stored at room temp or 37°C in tissue cx med or sterile saline
- Consider CSF and vitreous fluid; both should be frozen
- Autopsy is encouraged

TRISOMY 13

Definition (Am J Med Genet A 2006;140:1749; Nelson Textbook of Pediatrics, 17th ed.)
- Patau syndrome
- 0.85:10,000 live births, large percentage terminated before birth
- Death frequently in 1st mo of life
- Clinical manifestations: Cleft lip, polydactyly, low-set ears, holoprosencephaly, microphthalmia, cardiac defects, absent ribs, visceral and genital anomalies

TRISOMY 18

Definition (Am J Med Genet A 2006;140:1749; Nelson Textbook of Pediatrics, 17th ed.)
- Edwards syndrome
- 1.29:10,000 live births, large percentage terminated before birth
- Death frequently in 1st mo of life, 5% survival to 1st birthday
- Clinical findings: Closed fists w/ index finger overlapping 3rd digit and 5th digit overlapping 4th digit, rocker-bottom feet, microcephaly, micrognathia, cardiac/renal malform

TRISOMY 21

Definition (Lancet 2003;361:1281; Am Fam Physician 1999;59:381)
- Down's syndrome; most common genetic syndrome. 1:800–1,000 live births
- Congenital heart disease, myelodysplasia in newborn and duodenal atresia highly specific for Trisomy 21
- 95% 2/2 nondisjunction (nonsegregation) chromo 21 in oocyte or spermatocyte

- 4–5% caused by translocation of one chromosome 21 to another
- 1% of cases are mosaics (nondisjunction occurring after conception)

Diagnosis
- At birth: Constellation of features and confirmation by karyotype
- Prenatal: Quad screen: Maternal α-fetoprotein & Estriol lower than nml and β-HCG & Inhibin A higher (70–84% sensitivity)
- Fetal US w/ nuchal translucency, short femurs, cardiac anomalies, and duodenal atresia
- Women >35 yo w/increased risk. Chorionic villus sampling can be done btw 9 and 11 wk gestation, amnio btw 16 and 18 wk. Fetal cells examined for chromosomal abn
- Physical attributes: Hypotonia, flat face, upward/slanted palpebral fissures, epicanthic folds, Brushfield spots, mental retardation, cardiac malformations, simian crease

Complications
- Congenital heart disease: 40–60% of infants → ECG and TTE
  - Complete AV canal defects (60% of heart defects); VSD (32%); TOF (6%)
- GI defects: Esophageal atresia, TEF, pyloric stenosis, duodenal atresia, Meckel, Hirschsprung, imperforate anus, and GERD; 5–15% w/ Celiac dz
- ENT: Midfacial malformations interfere with nml drainage of Eustachian tube and sinuses
  - Recurrent otitis media, sinusitis, and pharyngitis
- Orthopedic:
  - Atlanto-occipital instability, hyperflexibility, scoliosis
  - Atlantoaxial instability: 13% asymp & need monitoring. No contact sports
  - Late hip dislocation (>2 yo), SCFE, patellar subluxation or dislocation, foot deformities
- Thyroid dz followed by yearly TSH. GH def and gonadal dysfunction may also be present
- Congenital cataracts and other eye disease
- Transient myeloproliferative disorder (leukemoid reaction) in 10% of newborns (rare in non-Down's infants). Increased risk of ALL
- Seizure disorder in 5–10%
- Dental problems and feeding difficulties
- Refer for early intervention to help with development

TURNER SYNDROME

Definition (Am Fam Physician 2007;76:405; Clin Pediatr (Phila) 2006;45:301)
- Partial or complete absence of X chromosome, 45 X karyotype
- 50 per 100,000 live female births

Diagnosis (Nat Clin Pract Endocrinol Metab 2005;1:41)
- Consider in girls with short stature (2 SD below mean height for age), primary amenorrhea, lack of breast development, delayed puberty
- Consider in fetus w/ hydrops, ↑ nuchal translucency, cystic hygroma, or lymphedema
- Dx made with karyotyping → chromosomal analysis of 30 peripheral lymphocytes
- 50% w/ missing X chromosome in all cells studied, others w/ 45, X/46, XX mosaic

Clinical Manifestations
- Risk of congenital heart defects → 75% with either coarctation of the aorta or bicuspid aortic valve. Risk of progressive aortic root dilation or dissection
- Risk of cong lymphedema, renal malform, hearing loss, osteoporosis, obesity, and diabetes
- Normal IQ, although may have difficulty w/ nonverbal, social, and psychomotor skills
- Physical exam: Misshapen or rotated ears, low posterior hairline, webbed neck, broad chest with widely spaced nipples and cubitus valgus, shortened 4th metacarpal
- Almost all are infertile

Management (Endocrine 2011 PMID 22147393)
Treat short stature with GH therapy through bone age of 14 yo.
- Estrogen in adolescence for pubertal development and prevention of osteoporosis with Ca + Vit D. Continue throughout life
- Hearing tests, pediatric optho for hyperopia and strabismus, regular dental visits
- Echocardiogram to r/o congenital heart defects, 4 ext BPs to follow for coarctation
- Renal ultrasound for renal malformations
- >4 yo r/o celiac with tissue transglutaminase immunoglobulin A & rpt q2–4yr

TURNER SYN 11-7

- Annual TFTs, LFTs, fasting lipids, and glucose
- If Y chromosome is present, 12% risk of gonadoblastoma; must refer for removal

Complications

Strabismus, hearing loss, recurrent otitis media, tooth anomalies, renal malform, autoimmune thyroiditis, celiac dz, congenital hip dysplasia, and scoliosis. ↑ risk colon, breast, and endometrial Ca (from estrogen use). Aortic dissection or rupture especially w/ pregnancy.

FRAGILE X

Definition (Curr Genomics 2011;12:216; Clin Pediatr (Phila) 2005;44:371)
- X-linked dominant w/ ↓ penetrance. 2/2 abn complement of trinucleotide repeats
- Full mutation usually w/ phenotype. Mosaicism common
- Full mutation has >200 CGG repeats → absence of FMR-1 protein, which is responsible for the symptoms. The greater the repeats, the more severe the disease
- Occurs in both males and females
- Most common inherited cause of mental retardation
- Prevalence rate of 1:4,000 males, 1:8,000–9,000 females

Diagnosis
- Classic triad: Macro-orchidism, large or prominent ears, and a long narrow face
- Suspect dx in any infant or toddler w/ developmental delays (esp speech) or maternal FHx of MR, developmental disabilities or learning disabilities
- Males w/ full mutation: Global dev delays and MR, may have autistic spectrum disorder
- Physical exam: Look for macrocephaly, prominent forehead, hyperextensible joints, stretchy skin, MVP, and large testicles
- Females w/full mutation → mildly affected with normal development to MR
- *FMR-1* gene is located on X chromosome

Medical Complications
- Have normal life expectancy; recent studies demonstrate stat sign increase in rate of obesity (31% compared to 18% in age-matched controls; associated w/ Prader–Willi phenotype)
- Recurrent otitis media and sinusitis
- MVP develops in adolescence or adulthood
- Hypotonia is common, may have seizures
- Macro-orchidism
- ♂s tend to exhibit social avoidance. May have ADHD; benefit from early intervention

KLINEFELTER

Definition (Am Fam Physician 2005;72:2259)
- Usually 47, XXY karyotype. Can include extra X chromosomes or Y chromosomes
- Nondisjunction during meiosis with origin from either parent
- 1:1,000 boys; mosaicism in 15% of men

Diagnosis (Int J Endocrinol 2012; PMID 22291701)
- Males present w/ infertility or gynecomastia as teens or adults
- 50% <18 yo w/ mild neurodevelopmental disorders
- Late or incomplete puberty should prompt a workup
- FSH and LH nml in pre-pubertal pts, then high from mid-puberty w/ low testosterone
- Karyotype to count sex chromosomes in 50 cells (in case of mosaicism)

Clinical Manifestations
- Almost all men are infertile (3% of all male infertility)
- Testosterone def, small testes, ↓ facial hair, gynecomastia, ↓ pubic hair, and small penis
- Tall and slender with long legs and short torso
- May develop osteoporosis

Management
- Neurodevelopmental evaluation at diagnosis
- Hormone therapy for low testosterone levels or if hypergonadotropism is present
- Gynecomastia predisposes men to breast cancer; frequency 20–50×s > in normal men

VACTERL

Definition (Orphanet J Rare Dis 2011;6:56; J Med Genet 2006;43:545)
- Association of 3 of the following: Vertebral defects, anal atresia cardiac defects, tracheo-esophageal fistula, renal malformations and limb defects; incidence 1:10,000–1:40,000, ↑ risk in infants of mothers w/ DM

Assessment
- Infants with esophageal atresia or TEF should be assessed for VACTERL
- Hx of teratogen exposure (especially methimazole), maternal DM, FHx of similar issues
- TTE, limb or vertebral x-rays, renal ultrasound, upper & lower GI evals
- Karyotype for exclusion of Trisomy 18, 21, FISH for 22q11 deletion. Array-CGH if karyotype and FISH studies are nml to assess for chromosomal abnormality.
- Multidisciplinary management for abnormalities

LYSOSOMAL STORAGE DISEASES

Gaucher Disease

Definition (Eur J Pediatr 2004;163:58; Curr Opin Pediatr 2005;17:519)
- Defective glucocerebrosidase activity → accumulation of glucocerebroside in macrophage lysosome
- Autosomal recessive. 1:75,000 births
- Glucocerebroside accumulation → hepatosplenomegaly, anemia, thrombocytopenia, growth retardation, skeletal disease

Non-neuronopathic (Type 1)
- Visceral, hematologic, and skeletal involvement
- Develops in childhood/adulthood; 1:40,000–60,000 (predilection for Ashkenazi Jews)
- Survival 6–80 yr; early dx and Rx with enzyme replacement → better prognosis

Acute Neuronopathic (Type 2)
- Visceral + heme involvement with a neurodegenerative course
- Develops in infancy; <1:100,000; survival <2 yr
- Strabismus, saccadic initiating defects, opisthotonic posturing (decerebrate w/neck and back arched posteriorly), bulbar palsy/paresis within the first 6 mo of life
- No data to support enzyme replacement

Subacute Neuronopathic (Type 3)
- Develops in childhood; <1:100,000; survival 20–40 yr
- Saccadic initiation defects 1st 3 mo of life but little progression of CNS dz until later yrs
- No data to support enzyme replacement

Fabry Disease

Definition (J Inherit Metab Dis 2012;35:227; Genet Med 2006;8:539; J Pediatr 2004;144:S20)
- Deficiency of α-galactosidase A, which breaks down glycosphingolipids → accumulates in vascular endothelium → ischemia/infarction
- Average age of diagnosis is 29 yo, with a life span of 50 yr
- 1:40,000–60,000 males, X-linked recessive. Female carriers may develop mild manifestations
- Not associated with MR or physical abnormalities
- Angiokeratomas, hypohidrosis, and acroparesthesia (burning/tingling pain in extremities)

Clinical Manifestations (4–16 yo)
- Neuropathic pain (burning/tingling) that usually begins in hands and feet
- May have fever + elevated ESR, diarrhea, abd pain, N/V, FTT
- Triggered by stress, heat, fatigue, or exercise (cannot sweat) Angiokeratomas (purplish/red nonblanching telangiectases); ↑ in size and # w/ age
- Eyes with whorled corneal opacity

Clinical Manifestations (Teens → Adulthood)
- Renal complications → uremia + HTN → ESRD
- May have MI, valve abnormality, arrhythmias, LVH, early strokes, and dyspnea

Diagnosis
- Deficient or absent α-galactosidase A activity
- Can be dx'd prenatally with chorionic villi or cultured amniocyte

Treatment
- α-galactosidase A replacement (J Inherit Metab Dis 2012;35:227)
- Avoid pain triggers such as heat, cold, stress, or exertion
- Some benefit from carbamazepine, gabapentin, diphenylhydantoin, NSAIDs
- GI symptoms are helped with pancrelipase or metoclopramide
- Check baseline renal, heart, and brain MRI before enzyme Rx to follow disease

Follow-up
- CBC, chemistries, U/A, creatinine: Albumin ratio, CrCl
- In adolescents: Every other yr echo and ECG to monitor for cardiac abnormality

Pompe Disease

Definition (J Pediatr 2004;144:S35)
- Glycogen storage type II disease or acid maltase deficiency; lysosomal storage disorder
- Considered a neuromuscular, metabolic myopathy, & glycogen storage disease
- Muscle d/o caused by deficiency of acid α-glucosidase → lysosomal glycogen accumulation in cardiac, skeletal, and smooth muscle cells

Infantile Onset
- Death within 1st yr of life; present in 1st few mo → floppy baby
- Hypotonia, muscle weakness, HCM → death from cardiopulmonary failure

Juvenile and Adult Onset
- Less severe cardiac issue; presents at any age; survival: Early childhood to late adults
- Progressive skeletal muscle dysfunction, calf muscle pseudohypertrophy
- Gower sign → using hands and arms to stand up from a lying position
- Require wheelchairs and eventual artificial ventilation → respiratory failure

Diagnosis
- Clinical syndrome and muscle bx → check acid α-glucosidase activity in skin/muscle fibroblasts
- Other family members should be tested; genetic counseling recommended

Treatment
- Supportive care

Mucopolysaccharide Disorders (MPS)

Definition (Pediatr Rev 2009;30:e22; J Pediatr 2004;144:S27)
- Def of enzyme for degradation of glycosaminoglycans (previously mucopolysaccharides)
- Accumulation of glycosaminoglycans in lysosomes → cell, tissue, organ dysfunction
- Incidence: ~1:22,500; AR except type II (Hunter syndrome), which is X-linked recessive

Presentation
- Nml at birth → chronic progressive course w/ multisys involv, abn facies, organomegaly
- Loss of developmental skills, frequent pneumonias, cardiomyopathy

Diagnosis
- Specific enzyme assays for each type
- 7 types: I–IV, VI, VII, IX; III and IV having subtypes
- Recommend genetic counseling

Hurler Syndrome
- Most severe form (MPS I)
- Deficiency of α-L-iduronidase → dermatan sulfate and heparan sulfate stored
- Usually normal at birth; death before 10 yo
- Presents in early infancy or childhood w/ severe somatic & neurologic dz, progressive MR
- Bone marrow transplantation is helpful; enzyme replacement also available

Hunter Syndrome (MPS II)
- Severe MPS II disease, X-linked, seen in males
- Deficiency of iduronate sulfatase → dermatan sulfate and heparan sulfate stored
- Supportive therapy

MITOCHONDRIAL DEFECTS

Definition (Am J Med Genet 2001;106:4; Pediatr Rev 2009;30: e22)
- Enzyme or enzyme complex disorder involved in ATP production via oxidative phos
- Enzymes involved include pyruvate dehydrogenase complex, tricarboxylic acid cycle, the respiratory chain and ATP synthase
- Affects high-energy–requiring organs → brain, skeletal muscle, heart, kidney, & retina
- Inheritance can be recessive, dominant, X-linked, or maternal with variable penetrance

Clinical Presentation
- Suspected in the following: Combo of neuromuscular and/or non-neuromuscular sx
  - Progressive course; unrelated organs or tissues involved in disease process
- Neurologic presentation:
  - Central and/or peripheral sx, seizures, hypotonia, abn movements, resp distress, encephalopathy, coma, poor head control as an infant, cerebellar ataxia, MR, poor psychomotor development, or loss of skills
- Muscular presentation
  - Can range from fatal infantile myopathy → progressive muscle weakness
  - Generalized weakness, resp distress, lactic acidosis, exercise intolerance and rhabdo
  - Fatal form results in death before 1 yo
- Multisystem disease
  - Anemia, FTT, liver dysfunction, diarrhea, short stature, DM, cardiomyopathy, FSGS, retinopathy, hearing loss, feeding difficulties

Diagnosis
- Full assessment of muscle function, CK, EMG, neuro exam with EEG
- Lactic acid, CSF lactate, urine organic acids, plasma and CSF amino acids, CSF protein
- MRI, consider NMR spectroscopy
- Surgical muscle bx in mitochondrial center → EM for quant mitochondria and morphology, enzyme histo, immunohisto, genetic studies, enzyme studies, and light microscopy

Treatment
- Fluids, electrolytes, restrict glucose, and avoid drugs that affect the respiratory chain (valproate, tetracyclines, chloramphenicol)
- Treat acidosis; consider cofactors: Coenzyme q10, biotin, creatine

EHLERS–DANLOS SYNDROME

Definition (Clin Genet 2012 PMID: 22353005; Adv Neonatal Care 2005;5:301)
- Heterogeneous connective tissue disorders involving skin, organs, and joints
- Autosomal dominant, recessive, or X-linked inheritance
- Villefranche classification w/ 6 subtypes; many rare, uncommon forms

Epidemiology
- Overall prevalence 1:5,000; Classic type 1:10,000–20,000
- Affects males and females of all racial and ethnic backgrounds

Diagnosis
- Based on family history and clinical exam

Prognosis
- Based on type; sudden death from vascular rupture or perforation is not uncommon
- Children with CVA should be evaluated for EDS

Classic EDS
- Affects 20,000–40,000 people
- AD mutations of collagen type 1 α 1 (COL1A1), COL1A2, COL5A1, COL5A2
- Dx confirmed by FHx and clinical features
- Clinical features: Skin hyperextensibility, IUGR, premature birth, joint hypermobility, redundant skin folds, joint scarring, congenital diverticula of the bladder and inguinal hernias (in males), muscle hypotonia, delayed gross motor development
- MVP and regurgitation

Hypermobility
- AD, most common type: 1:10,000–15,000
- No known genes and diagnosis is by clinical exam and confirmed by FHx
- Clinical features: Smooth, velvety skin; easy bruising, joint hypermobility with unusual ROM, inguinal hernias (males), recurrent joint dislocation, chronic joint/limb pain
- MVP and regurgitation

Vascular
- 1:100,000–200,000
- AD mutations of COL3A1 with over 320 mutation variations. Responsible for procollagen, which provides strength in connective tissue
- Dx is confirmed by skin biopsy

- Clinical features: Thin translucent skin over chest and abdomen, acrogeria (loss of subcutaneous fat and collagen of hands and feet), lobeless ears, short stature, extensive bruising, hypermobility of small joints

Clinical Management
- Classical and hypermobile types may develop aortic root dilatation (up to 28%) → root should be measured at 5 yr of age then q5yr
- Less strenuous activities recommended in order to avoid joint strain and damage

MARFAN DISEASE

Definition (Heart 2011 Aug;97:1206; Eur J Hum Genet 2007;15:724)
- Connective tissue d/o secondary to fibrillin mutation (FBN 1) affecting CV, eyes, & bones
- Variable autosomal dominance, fibrillin-1 on chromosome 15 in up to 91% of cases
- Transforming growth factor β-receptor 1 and 2 genes may also be factors
- Adult diagnosis is made with new Ghent criteria although it is found to be unreliable in children

Epidemiology
- 1:9,800 births; 27% are from a new mutation

Diagnosis (J Med Genet 2010;47:476)
- Suspect if tall, thin, long limbs, arachnodactyly, pectus deformity, and/or scoliosis
- Family history of aortic aneurysm or familial thoracic aortic aneurysms
- Original Ghent criteria replaced by new Ghent criteria (see J Med Genet 2010;47:476)
- CV: TTE eval of aortic diameter; use pediatric nomogram (Am J Cardiol 1989;64:507)
- Ophthalmology: Myopia and lens subluxation
- Skeletal: Pectus, wrist and thumb signs, scoliosis, arm span:height >1.05

Complications
- Progressive aortic dilation, usually at sinus of Valsalva → AV incompetence → aortic dissection and rupture; ↑ risk of aortic dissection in pregnant women
- LV dilatation → cardiac failure
- Mitral valve prolapse → regurgitation
- Lens dislocation, myopia, and retinal detachment
- Scoliosis in approximately 60%
- Joint hypermobility in 85% <18 yo and 56% of adults
- Arthralgias, myalgias, and ligamentous injuries
- Spontaneous pneumothorax in 4–11% of patients
- Most common cause of death → aortic dissection

Clinical Management (N Engl J Med 2008;358:2787)
- β-blockers if aorta is dilated; ARBs/ACEI can slow dilation
- Follow aortic diameter w/ biannual/annual TTE, and consider surgery when >5 cm
- Surgery usually involves replacing the valve and aorta (Bentall procedure)
- Should avoid high-intensity activity

FEBRILE SEIZURES

Definition (Pediatrics 2008;121:1281; Pediatr Rev 2007;28:363)
- **Simple febrile seizure:** Brief (<15 min), generalized (nonfocal) occurring once in a 24-hr period in a febrile child. Usually limited and no further workup required.
- **Complex febrile seizure:** Prolonged (>15 min), focal component, and/or >1 episode within 24-hr period. Often requires ancillary workup/neuroimaging to r/o focal etiology.

Epidemiology (J Child Neurol 2002;17:S44)
- Most common szr disorder in children, affects ~2–5% between ages 6–60 mo
- Risk factors: 1st-/2nd-degree relative h/o febrile szr, peak temp, & rate of rise

Pathophysiology (J Child Neurol 2002;17:S44; Trends Neurosci 2007;30:490)
- Mechanism unclear, may be related to rate of rise of fever or actual peak temp (usually >102). Possible cytokine & temp effect on ion channels & neuronal tissue

Diagnostic Studies (Pediatrics 2011;127:389)
- In general, focus should be on fever workup and not workup of seizure itself
  - **1st simple febrile seizure:** No workup
  - **Complex febrile seizure:** CBC w/ diff, Chem 10, EEG; lumbar puncture (LP) (as below), neuroimaging if focal (MRI preferred)
- **LP:** Not routinely warranted for simple febrile szr but recommended for:
  - Signs suggestive of meningitis or intracranial infection. Be aware that meningeal sx may be absent in infants <12 mo and subtle in pts 12–18 mo
  - Infants 6–12 mo w/ unknown or deficient Hib or Strep pneumo vaccination status
  - Current or recent antibiotics use (risk of partially rx'd meningitis, can mask sx)
  - Febrile status epilepticus
- **EEG:** Not recommended in eval of neurologically healthy pts w/ 1st simple febrile szr
  - No assoc btw abnl EEG & future febrile szr or development of epilepsy
- **Neuroimaging:** Not recommended in routine eval of first simple febrile seizure
- **Laboratory studies:** No evidence that routine blood studies (Chem7, Ca, Mg, Phos, CBC, or blood glucose) are of benefit in eval of first simple febrile seizure

Treatment (Pediatrics 2008;121:1281; Pediatr Rev 2007;28:405)
- Most febrile seizures require no intervention and end within <10 min
- Anticonvulsant therapy is not recommended for simple febrile seizures
- For prolonged or recurrent febrile szr, rx for home rectal diazepam (0.3–0.5 mg/kg) may be provided for outpt treatment of szr lasting >5 min
- Children w/ complex febrile seizures are candidates for trial of antiepileptic drug (AED) prophylaxis, such as phenobarbital, benzodiazepines, or valproate. However, there is no evidence associating a reduced risk of epilepsy with prophylactic AED use
- Antipyretics have not been shown to ↓ risk of recurrence of simple febrile seizures

Complications (Pediatrics 2008;121:1281; J Child Neurol 2002;17:S44)
- Almost all w/ excellent prognosis. No evidence that simple febrile szr causes IQ decline
- May progress to febrile status epilepticus. Usually focal and often the pts' 1st febrile szr (Neurology 2008;7:170)
- Minimal ↑ risk of developing epilepsy. Simple febrile seizure carries 1% risk, same as compared to general pop. ↑ to 2.4% if multiple simple febrile seizures, <12 mo at the time of the 1st febrile seizure, or +family history of epilepsy
- Febrile szrs frequently recur. Risk ~30% if 1st szr occurs >12 mo or ~50% if 1st szr occurs <12 mo. Recurrence risk also ↑ if +FHx febrile szr, lower peak temp w/ 1st szr, and shorter duration of fever w/ 1st febrile szr

FIRST NONFEBRILE SEIZURE IN CHILDREN

Definition (Neurology 2000;55:616; Pediatr Rev 2007;28:363)
- 1 or more afebrile or otherwise unprovoked seizures (i.e., not 2/2 febrile illness, trauma, or other acute medical condition). Excludes children w/ previous dx of epilepsy
  - **Provoked seizure:** 2/2 acute condition, fever, stress, hypoglycemia, toxic ingestion, intracranial infxn, trauma, alcohol, recreational drug use or w/d, AED abrupt withdrawal related to compliance, & other precipitating factors
  - **Unprovoked:** W/o underlying condition. Idiopathic or 2/2 remote brain insult
- **Differentiating between seizures and seizure-like episodes**
  - **Pre-ictal sx** include aura, mood, or behavior Δs, vocal sx (cries, gasps, slurred words, garbled speech), motor sx (head or eye turning, eye deviation, posturing,

rhythmic jerking, stiffening, automatisms, generalized or focal mvmts), resp sx (Δs breathing pattern, apnea, cyanosis), autonomic sx (pupil dilation, drooling, Δ in RR or HR, incontinence, pallor, vomiting, LOC, inability to understand or speak)
- **Ictal sx:** Preserved or altered consciousness (simple vs. complex), unilat or bilat (generalized) involvement, ↑ tone (tonic), rhythmic or sporadic jerking (clonic, myoclonic), loss of tone (atonic), or other sx (sensory, autonomic, or psychic)
- **Post-ictal symptoms** include amnesia for events, confusion, lethargy, sleepiness, HAs and muscle aches, transient focal weakness (Todd paralysis), and N/V
- **Seizure-like episodes:** Breath-holding, syncope, GERD, pseudoseizure, panic attacks, parasomnias, TIAs, vestibular d/o, paroxysmal choreoathetosis, psychotic hallucinations/delusion, migraine, tics, benign myoclonus of infancy, and other nonepileptic events

Epidemiology (Neurology 2000;55:616)
- 25,000–40,000 children have 1st nonfebrile szr each yr. In US, 1% of children will have an unprovoked seizure by 14 yo. Most common etiology is idiopathic/cryptogenic

Diagnostic Studies (Neurology 2000;55:616)
- **EEG:** Std of care. Most sensitive within 24 hr of szr but may be scheduled as outpt. Repeat EEG should be obtained if initial EEG is non-diagnostic
- **LP:** Consider if concern for possible meningitis/encephalitis
- **Neuroimaging studies:** Emergent if prolonged focal postictal deficit or not back to baseline within few hrs. Strongly consider non-urgent imaging if cognitive or motor impairment of unknown etiology, abnl neuro exam, focal szr, abnl/non-benign EEG, or <1 yo. MRI is preferred over CT if possible
- Consider tox studies if any question of exposure or substance abuse
- Tests ordered on the basis of individual H&P. Routine labs in child >6 mo who returns to baseline and whose hx non-suggestive is generally not necessary

Treatment (Neurology 2003;60:166)
- AEDs generally not indicated after a 1st non-febrile seizure
- No difference in prognosis for long-term szr remission if started after 1st vs. 2nd szr

Complications (Pediatrics 1990;85:1076; Neurology 2005;64:880)
- Majority of children w/ 1st unprovoked afebrile szr have no or few recurrences (24% recurrence in 1 yr, 45% recurrence over 14 yr). Risk ↑ w/ abnl EEG findings & h/o remote brain injury (recurrence risk often >50%)

EPILEPSY

Definition (Pediatr Rev 2007;28:363; Epilepsia 2010;51:676)
- **Epilepsy:** ≥2 seizures w/o clear underlying cause
- **Focal seizures:** Unilateral hemispheric origin with *consistent* focal motor manifestations. Seizures often propagate and lead to global excitation
- **Associated syndromes:**
  - Benign partial epilepsy (benign rolandic): Presents 3–13 yo. Tonic or clonic mvmts, often unilateral paresthesias of lower face. Typical electrical correlate in sleep
  - Temporal lobe epilepsy: Presents childhood, may remit in adol, return in adulthood. Often w/ aura, psychic sx, and automatisms. May/may not arise from temporal lobe
  - Frontal lobe epilepsy: Frequently occurs in nighttime clusters. Often involves auras and bizarre automatisms (e.g., bicycle pedaling, pelvic thrusting)
  - Parietal lobe epilepsy: Often involves somatosensory sx, including paresthesia and detailed visual hallucinations
  - Occipital lobe: Often involves vague visual sx of flashes of light/colors
- **Generalized seizures:** Bilateral excitation with *inconsistent* localization and lateralization patterns. Motor manifestations bilateral and often synchronous
- **Subtypes:**
  - Absence: "Staring spells." Sudden brief LOC, +/− eye flickering. Ictal EEG shows 3 Hz spike/wave pattern. Activated by hyperventilation
  - Myoclonic: Sudden muscle contractions
  - Clonic: Asymmetric/irregular jerking
  - Tonic: Sustained contraction w/o clonic phase. Assoc w/ diffuse cerebral damage
  - Tonic–clonic: Has tonic, clonic, and postictal phases
  - Atonic: "Drop seizure." Brief lapse in muscle tone
- **Associated syndromes (Epilepsia 2010;51:2175; Lancet Neurol 2009;8:82):**
  - Infantile spasms: Usually presents 5–12 mo, remitting by ~3 yo. Symmetric, bilateral, brief, and sudden contractions of axial muscle groups. Assoc w/ poor neurocog outcomes

and Lennox–Gastaut syndrome. Freq ranges from few to 100s of szrs daily. Typical EEG correlate of hypsarrhythmia (Irregular, disorganized, high amplitude waves and spikes)
  • Lennox–Gastaut: Usually presents 2–8 yo. Characterized by mental retardation and multiple generalized seizure subtypes, particularly tonic and atonic. Typical EEG correlate is a slow spike–wave pattern with highest voltage in the frontal regions

Epidemiology (Pediatr Rev 2007;28:363)
• Prevalence of epilepsy ~1%. About 1/3 have developmental disabilities

Etiology (Pediatr Rev 2007;28:363)
• 65–70% idiopathic/cryptogenic, i.e., no identifiable structural abnormalities
• Remainders are "symptomatic," or with identifiable abnormality impacting brain function
  • **Inherited/genetic:** Channelopathies, chromosomal abnormalities, mitochondrial DNA disorder, metabolic disorder, hereditary neurocutaneous disorders
  • **Congenital:** Cortical malform & dysplasia, polymicrogyria, vascular malform, prenatal injury
  • **Acquired:** Trauma, infection, tumors, vascular disease, hippocampal sclerosis, neurodegenerative disorders, toxic disorders

Diagnosis (Pediatr Rev 2007;28:405; Epilepsia 2009;50:2147)
• **EEG:** Nml in 10–20%. Can induce szr w/ hypervent, photic stim, sleep depriv
• **Brain imaging:** Recommended in pts w/ focal szr. Not needed w/ generalized szr if nml neurodev, <2% w/ abnormality on scan. MRI is preferred modality
• **Neuropsych eval:** Better qualify learning diff assoc w/ epilepsy; target interventions

Treatment (Pediatr Rev 2007;28:405; Clin Pediatr (Phila) 2005;44:383; Pediatrics 2007;119:535)
AEDs:
• Choice of AED depends on age and szr type
  • Neonatal seizures: Phenobarbital and phenytoin
  • Focal seizures: 1st line – carbamazepine, phenobarbital, valproic acid, topiramate, phenytoin, lamotrigine, oxcarbazepine. 2nd line – gabapentin, levetiracetam
  • Generalized tonic–clonic: 1st line – carbamazepine, valproic acid, phenytoin, phenobarbital, topiramate. 2nd line – lamotrigine
  • Absence: 1st line – ethosuximide, valproic acid, lamotrigine. 2nd line – clonazepam
  • Infantile spasms: 1st line – vigabatrin, ACTH, prednisone
  • Lennox–Gastaut: 1st line – valproic acid, lamotrigine, clonazepam, carbamazepine, topiramate. 2nd line – ethosuximide (drop attacks)
• Several AEDs require regular monitoring of AED blood concentration to assess for dose-related toxicity, compliance, and potential drug–drug interactions
• Several AEDs affect liver metab. Carbamazepine, phenytoin, and phenobarbital are cytochrome p450 inducers & can ↑ metabolism of other AEDs and meds (e.g., OCPs, steroids, warfarin). Valproic acid is a cytochrome p450 inhibitor
Adverse Effects of AEDs (Pediatr Rev 1997;18:39; Pediatr Rev 2007;28:405)

Drug	Selected Adverse Effects
Carbamazepine	Dizziness, drowsiness, ataxia, diplopia, rash, liver dysfxn, blood dyscrasia
Clobazam	Somnolence, insomnia, agitation, ataxia, suicidal ideation, mood changes, UTI, Stevens–Johnson
Clonazepam	Drowsiness, hyperactivity
Ethosuximide	Drowsiness, blood dyscrasia
Gabapentin	Ataxia, fatigue, dizziness, HA, vomiting, nystagmus
Lamotrigine	Severe rash, ataxia, drowsiness, insomnia, headache
Phenobarbital	Cognitive impairment, drowsiness, rash
Lacosamide	Dizziness, HA, nausea, diplopia, AV block
Levetiracetam	Sedation, mood disturbance, agitation, wt loss, thrombocytopenia, neural tube defects
Oxcarbazepine	Sedation, HA, dizziness, rash, vertigo, ataxia, nausea, hyponatremia, diplopia, low serum T4, Stevens–Johnson, toxic epidermal necrolysis
Phenytoin	Hirsuitism, gum hypertrophy, ataxia, rash, Stevens–Johnson, nystagmus,
Rufinamide	Somnolence, vomiting, QT shortening
Sodium valproate	Wt gain, alopecia, tremor, liver dysfxn, osteopenia, ↑ NH₃, ↓ plts`
Topiramate	Wt loss, impaired cognition, paresthesias, HA, fatigue, drowsiness, depression, mood problems, decreased sweating, met acidosis
Vigabatrin	Agitation, drowsiness, wt gain, dizziness, HA, ataxia, retinal degen

- **Ketogenic diet:** High-fat, low-carb; assoc w/ improved szr control & awareness level. Long-term adverse effects: Renal stones, growth inhib, hyperlipid, vit def, constipation
- **Surgery:** Must have localizable seizure focus
- **Vagus nerve stimulator:** Adjunctive therapy for intractable partial seizures. Electric impulse to L vagus nerve.

Seizure precautions:
- Avoid common triggers (sleep depriv, hypervent, drugs/EtOH, photic light stim)
- Teach szr 1st aid. Put pt in swimmers ¾ prone position; keep mouth clear
- Basic safety precautions (e.g., water & helmet safety) & driving restrictions (vary by state)

STATUS EPILEPTICUS (SE)

Definition (Neurology 2006;67:1542)
- Min duration of 30 min or ≥2 sequential szrs w/o consciousness btw szrs
- Initiate treatment after 5 min for impending SE

Epidemiology (Lancet 2006;368:222; Epilepsia 2007;48:1652; Neurology 2010;74:636)
- Incidence ~20/100,000 children per yr. If hx of epilepsy, risk incr 9.1–27%
- 60% of affected children were previously neurologically healthy
- First presentation of epilepsy in ~10% of children
- Risk factors include hx of clustered focal seizures or prior SE, focal EEG abnl, neuroimaging abnl, and <1 yo

Etiology (Neurology 2006;67:1542)
- **Acute symptomatic:** More common in younger kids/infants, during acute illness. Etiology: Meningitis, encephalitis, electrolyte abnl, sepsis, hypoxia, trauma, intox
- **Remote symptomatic:** Occurs w/o acute trigger and in pt w/ prior CNS insult Etiology: CNS malform, prior TBI or insult, chromosomal disorder
- **Febrile:** No direct CNS infxn. Etiology: e.g., URI, gastroenteritis, sinusitis, sepsis
- **Progressive encephalopathy:** Underlying progressive CNS disorder. Includes mitochondrial disorders, CNS lipid storage diseases, amino/organic acidopathies
- **Idiopathic:** No definable cause

Diagnostic Workup (Neurology 2006;67:1542; Pediatr Rev 2007;28:405)
- **Labs:** Finger glucose, CBC, Chem10. Consider urine and blood cxs. LP if suspicion of CNS infection. Consider serum and urine tox and/or studies for inborn errors of metabolism and genetics if history suggestive or etiology unclear. Check AED levels for pts w/ epilepsy on AED prophy
- **EEG:** Consider if child p/w new onset or non-convulsive SE
- **Neuroimaging:** Consider if suspect ↑ ICP, focal deficits, or if unknown etiology

Treatment (Pediatr Rev 2007;28:405)
- ABCs: O₂ by mask, CV monitor. IV. Correct metabolic abnl. Monitor for resp depression
- **For children <1 wk old:** No universal protocols. The protocol at our institution:

Step 1	Phenobarbital 20 mg/kg IV bolus. May give up to 2 addl 10 mg/kg IV bolus
Step 2	Fosphenytoin 20 mg/kg IV bolus
Step 3	If unresponsive to AEDs, pyridoxine (100 mg IV) then folinic acid (2.5 mg IV)

- **For children > 4 wk old:**

Step 1 (0–5 min)	If IV access: Lorazepam 0.1 mg/kg (max 4 mg)
	If no IV access: Diazepam PR (0.5 mg/kg if 2–5 yo, 0.3 mg/kg 6–11 y/o, 0.2 mg/kg if >11 y/o)
Step 2 (5–10 min)	Repeat lorazepam IV or diazepam PR dose
Step 3 (10–15 min)	Phenytoin or fosphenytoin 20 mg/kg IV (max 1,250 mg)
	or
	Phenobarbital 10–20 mg/kg (max 300 mg)
Step 4 (15–30 min)	Consider "pentobarbital coma" and intubate with anesthesia present. Neuro should be involved with all cases of SE

Note: Levetiracetam 20 mg/kg IV often used in clinical practice, though there is little data.

Complications (Lancet Neurol 2006;5:769)
- Include hypoxemia, acidosis, hypo/hyperglycemia, ↑ ICP, vascular changes
- Mortality ~5%; excess metab demand → O₂ insuff and neuronal damage/necrosis
- Morbidity <15% for neurological sequelae, often 2/2 underlying cause of SE

DYSKINESIAS/MOVEMENT DISORDERS

Definitions (J Child Neurol 2003;18:S1)
- **Tics:** Sudden, "brief" involuntary (but suppressible), stereotyped mvmts/vocalizations
- **Tremor:** Involuntary, usually regular, oscillatory mvmts; may be limited to an extremity, may involve entire body including tongue
- **Chorea:** Hyperkinetic, invol, arrhythmic, nonrepetitive, random jerking mvmt. Typically expressed distally, but may involve entire body or extremities; may flow into a voluntary movement and possess a dancing quality
- **Ballism:** Violent, involuntary, usually high amplitude flailing mvmt of entire extremity
- **Athetosis:** Involuntary, alternating flexion/extension, writhing mvmts typically accentuate in distal extremities & perioral muscles; may involve entire body + tongue (not eyes)
- **Dystonia:** Tonic fixation of posture, not dependent upon contracture (not a mvmt)
- **Myoclonus:** Involuntary asym brief shock-like w/ recovery, muscle jerk may be limited to distal extr or involve entire body, sym in phase or multifocal and asym

Etiology
- **Tics:** Tourette syndrome (TS), transient tic of childhood, drug-induced
- **Tremor:** Hyperthyroid, hypoglycemia, essential tremor, drugs (AEDs, amphetamines, bronchodilators, antidepressants, caffeine, steroids), CP, Wilson dz, juvenile Huntington dz, and multiple other (esp of cerebellar and other central motor system relays and tracts)
- **Chorea:** Sydenham chorea, CP, drugs (AEDs, antidepressants, antihistamines, OCP, CCBs, digoxin), SLE, Wilson dz, post-pump cardiac surgery. PANDAS
- **Ballism:** Subthalamic nucleus damage/hemiballismus typically hypertensive small vessel infarct but other small causes of small focal disease rarely
- **Athetosis:** CP, host of degenerative infectious, metabolic disorders, ischemia, trauma
- **Dystonia:** Neuroleptic-induced, dopa-responsive dystonia (Segawa), Sandifer syndrome, dystonia musculorum deformans, CP, drugs (AEDs, antipsychotics, antihistamines, CCBs), Wilson dz, perinatal hypoxia, brain tumors, trauma
- **Myoclonus:** Benign neonatal sleep myoclonus/"sleep starts," epilepsy, drugs (AEDs, antidepressants), infxns (SSPE, HSV, HIV, Creutzfeldt–Jakob), autoimmune (MS), neoplastic/tumors, paraneoplastic (neuroblastoma), metabolic (most prevalent; renal failure, hyperglycemia), hypoxia

TICS & TOURETTE SYNDROME (TS)

Diagnostic Criteria (Neurol Clin 2002;20:1101; NEJM 2010;363:2332)
- **Transient tic of childhood** – single or multiple motor &/or vocal tics; duration of at least 4 wk but less than 12 mo
- **Chronic tics** – single or multiple tics but restricted to 1 class (either motor or vocal); duration at least 1 yr, no tic-free period greater than 3 consecutive mo
- **TS** – must include multiple motor & ≥1 vocal tic (not necessarily concurrently); onset before 18 yo, duration at least 1 yr, no tic-free period greater than 3 mo; must exclude other causes (e.g., drugs) & general medical conditions
  - Now viewed as neuropsych spectrum d/o often a/w OCD & ADHD (TS triad)

Epidemiology (Mov Disorder 2011;26:1149; Neurol Clin 2002;20:1101)
- Tics are the most common primary movement disorder in children
  - Transient tic disorders: 20–30% school-aged children
  - Chronic tic disorders: 2–5% of school-aged children
  - TS: Worldwide prevalence 1%, male predominance
  - %TS pts w/ comorbidities: None (TS only) 12%, ADHD 60%, OCD 27%, obsessive compulsive behaviors 32%, LD 23%, mood dis 20%, anxiety dis 18%, CD/ODD 15% (Dev Med Child Neurol 2000;42:436)

Pathophysiology (J Child Neurol 2006;21:630; Neurol Clin 2002;20:1101)
- Exact mechanisms still unknown but common factors include:
  - Basal ganglia dysfunction, dopaminergic overactivity, perturbation of corticostriatal–thalamocortical circuits
  - Likely involvement of other neurotransmitters affecting dopamine (serotonin, norepinephrine)
- Genetic component in TS: 50% concordance monozygotic twins, 8% dizygotic

Clinical Features & Natural History of TS (J Child Neurol 2006;21:630; NEJM 2010;363:2332)
- Pts often report premonitory urges (feeling of pressure that builds until tic occurs); differentiates tics from other hyperkinesias

- Tics may be suppressible for brief time & are exacerbated during periods stress/transition
- Simple motor tics (e.g., eye blinking, facial grimacing, shoulder shrugging) usually begin between 3–8 yo
- Simple vocal tics (e.g., throat clearing, sniffing) may follow motor tics by several yr
- Can include dystonic tics (slow twisting mvmt), tonic tics (isometric contractions such as abd tensing), complex tics (words, complicated purposeful looking mvmt). Coprolalia (obscene words) <50%
- Tics wax & wane over wks to mos; peak intensity at 7–14 yo; 1/3 resolve adolescence/adulthood, 1/3 improve, 1/3 no change
- Comorbid neuropsych disorders (ADHD & OCD) are often more impairing than the tics

Treatment (NEJM 2010;363:2332; Mov Disorder 2011;26:1149)
- Most patients do not require medication for tics. Do NOT medicate for an acute exacerbation; only if persistent
- Mild tic disorders (usually disappear by young adulthood): Education & reassurance
- Pharmacotherapy for tics:
  - Indicated if tics cause self-injury/pain, social impairment, functional impairment, classroom disruption
  - 1st tier: α_2 agonists (clonidine, guanfacine), consider topiramate
  - 2nd tier: Atypical antipsychotics (risperidone, ziprasidone, aripiprazole)
  - 3rd tier: Typical antipsychotics (haloperidol, pimozide, fluphenazine); highest efficacy but many short- & long-term side effects
  - Other: Tetrabenazine (depletes neuronal dopamine, as effective as typical neuroleptics w/o tardive dyskinesia risk, botulinum toxin (consider for single bothersome tic)
- Habit reversal training (HRT): Teaches pts to recognize premonitory urges & perform voluntary behavior that is incompatible w/ tics. Randomized controlled trial showed modest improvement in tic severity (JAMA 2010;303:1929)
- Deep brain stimulation (DBS): For severely disabling, medication refractory tics; optimal location of electrode placement (thalamus, GP, subthalamic nucl) still unclear
- Comorbid disorders: Important to tx as often more impairing than tics
  - OCD: CBT, SSRIs, atypical antipsychotics, DBS for severe cases
  - ADHD: Stimulants NOT contraindicated! Double-blind placebo controlled trial showed no difference in tic exacerbation w/ MPH (methylphenidate), clonidine or placebo; combo MPH + clonidine best for both ADHD & tics (Neurology 2002;58:527). Amphetamine derivatives, atomoxetine (NE reuptake inhib), guanfacine also proven effective. In practice, can see transient tic worsening after stimulant initiation but often abates w/ time
- Other: Education of family & schools, counseling & support services, educational accommodations, treatment of comorbid conditions (ADHD, OCD, anxiety disorders, learning disabilities)

ABNORMAL GAIT/ATAXIA

(J Child Neurol 2003;18:309; Pediatr Rev 2001;22:177)

Definitions
- Abnormal coordination of balance and movement
- May result from dysfunction in the cerebellum, sensory or motor pathways
- Classified as genetic vs. acquired; also acute, episodic, or chronic/progressive
- Dysmetria; disturbance of metric/rhythmic aspect of mvmt; incoord of volunt mvmt
- Dysdiadochokinesia; dysfunction of rapid alternating movements
- Can also see: Scanning speech: ↑ length btw syllables; titubation-ataxic, to-and-fro mvmt trunk and/or head

Clinical Manifestations
- **Cerebellar ataxia:** Wide-based swerving gait, sx unΔ w/ eyes open or closed, pendular DTRs, dysmetria, dysdiadochokinesia, over-/undershoot finger–nose test, scanning speech w/ fluctuation invol may be assoc w/ intention tremor (oscillatory, to-and-fro)
- **Sensory ataxia:** Broad-based (high-step) gait, +Romberg (sx worse w/ eyes shut)

Etiology
- **Acute ataxia:** Most common: Postinfectious cerebellitis (varicella up to 26%) and ADEM, drug ingestions/intox (AED, benzos, antihistamines, PCP, mercury, lead, thallium, alcohol, ethylene glycol)
  - Other: Trauma (vertebral artery dissect & postconcussion syndr), hydrocephalus, mass lesions, vascular event, labyrinthitis, Miller-Fisher/Guillain–Barré (sensory ataxia)

- **Episodic ataxia:** Basilar migraine, nonconvulsive szrs, metabolic d/o (pyruvate decarboxylase def, Hartnup dz, maple syrup urine dz), genetic episodic ataxias
- **Chronic/progressive ataxia:** Most common: Brain tumors and spinocerebellar deg (AD) other (Ataxia-telangiectasia, Friedreich ataxia, a-β-lipoproteinemia)

Pathophysiology
- Postinfectious cerebellitis: Sx occur during recovery from viral infxn; autoimmune demyelination by Ab; less commonly from direct cerebellar infxn
- ADEM (Acute postinfectious demyelinating encephalomyelitis): Similar to postinfectious cerebellitis, but demyelination multifocal → different clinical manifestations
- Paraneoplastic/neuroblastoma: Autoimmune

Differential Diagnosis
- Postinfectious cerebellitis: Sx max at onset; trunk > extrems; head titubation, truncal ataxia, dysmetria, nystagmus, intention tremor; opsoclonus & horizontal ocular flutter rare; no fevers or systemic signs; typically no MS Δ but small % reported w/ behavioral & cognitive affective syndrome (further studies needed) (Ann Neurol 1994;35:673)
- ADEM: Multifocal neuro abn, Δ MS, CN palsies, szrs, hemiparesis, systemic sx (HA, meningeal signs, fever); see Demyelinating section for further details
- Intoxications: Look for associated mental status changes; nystagmus, seizures
- Basilar migraines: Occipital HA, N/V, vertigo, hemiparesis, migrainous auras
- Metabolic d/o: Dev delay, vomiting, diarrhea, unusual odors, w/ lethargy/behavior Δ
- Brain tumor: Progressive ataxia (acute worsening due to 2/2 bleed or hydroceph), CN palsies and other focal deficits, papilledema, HA, personality Δ
- Paraneoplastic/neuroblastoma: Subacute, fluctuating ataxia; opsoclonus (multidirectional, chaotic, conjugate eye mvmts) may be transitory and drawn out by visual saccades or anxiety; myoclonus of head, trunk, and extremities

Diagnostic Evaluation
Detailed H&P, urine and serum tox screens (highest dx yield after H&P)
- **CT/MRI:** Eval mass lesion, r/o mass effect before LP; tumors (brain/chest/abd neuroblastoma), stroke, ADEM; usually nml in postinfectious cerebellitis;
- **Scintigraphy:** For neuroblastoma
- **CSF:** Usually nml in postinfectious; may have mild pleocytosis in some cases, postinfectious & opsoclonus-myoclonus; suspect meningitis/encephalitis if more marked pleocytosis; cytoalbuminologic dissoc in Miller-Fisher/Guillain–Barré, ADEM, CIDP
- **EMG:** If suspect sensory ataxia; **EEG;** often ↑ in postinfectious cases; nonconvulsive szrs
- **Urine catechol** (VMA/HVA); ↑ 47–60% opsoclonus-myoclonus neuroblastoma pts
- Metabolic and/or genetic w/u CBC, LFTs, serum NH_3, lactate, pyruvate, ketones, eval of acid/base balance, urine organic acids, urine and plasma amino acids

Treatment/Prognosis
- Acute postinfectious cerebellitis: Most recover w/o Rx but small % w/ persistent gait &/or neurobehavioral sx; limited case studies show IVIG &/or plasma exchange to be effective in these cases (Neurology 2004;62:1443)
- ADEM: Most spontaneously recover, more slowly than postinfectious cerebellitis; corticosteroids can accelerate recovery
- Intoxications: Varies according to substance; consider chelators, dialysis
- Opsoclonus-myoclonus/neuroblastoma: Surgical removal of tumor; however, neurologic paraneoplastic symptoms often do not improve w/ tumor removal
  - Efficacy of combo Rx w/ IVIG and/or high-dose steroids. Cyclophosphamide currently multicenter clinical trial under way. ACTH for opsoclonus-myoclonus-ataxia synd

WEAKNESS/PERIPHERAL NEUROPATHIES

Grade	Muscle Strength
0/5	No muscle mvmt
1/5	Visible muscle mvmt; no mvmt at joint
2/5	Mvmt at joint; not gravity
3/5	Mvmt against gravity; not resistance
4/5	Mvmt against resistance; < nml
5/5	Normal strength

- Distinguishing upper motor neuron and lower motor neuron patterns of weakness

Tendon Reflex Grading System	
Grade	Description
0	Absent
1+	Hypoactive
2+	"Normal"
3+	Hyperactive w/o clonus
4+	Hyperactive w/ clonus

Exam Findings	LMN	UMN
Tone	Decreased	Increased
Muscle bulk	Decreased/pseudohypertrophy	Decreased
"Pathologic reflex" (e.g., Babinski response)	Absent	Present
Fasciculations	Present in certain conditions (e.g., SMA)	Absent

- Examples of neuromuscular conditions with primary LMN pattern of weakness

Lesion Location in PNS	Acute Presentation	Chronic Presentation
Anterior horn cell	Poliomyelitis	SMA
Peripheral nerve	GBS/AIDP, Bell's palsy, metabolic (DM, hypothyroid, toxins), porphyria	Hereditary motor–sensory neuropathies, CIDP, Erb palsy, heavy metal poisons
Neuromuscular junction	Botulism, tick paralysis, organophosphate poisons	Myasthenia gravis (can p/w acute crisis), Lambert–Eaton
Muscle	Myositis, rhabdomyolysis, periodic paralysis	Muscular dystrophies, myotonic dystrophy, myopathies (metabolic, congenital, inflammatory, steroid-induced)

Duchenne/Becker Muscular Dystrophy (Pediatr Rev 2000;21:233; Pediatr Rev 2006;27:83)
- **Epidemiology:** Incidence 1 in 3,600–6,000 ♂ births; 1/3 cases 2/2 new mutations musc dystrophy; genetic d/o of skeletal muscle w/o 1° involve of CNS or PNS
- **Pathology/pathophysiology**
  - X-linked recessive (Duchenne & Becker)
  - Duchenne, Becker: Mutation in gene for dystrophin (deletion more common than duplication) → muscle damage & fibrosis
  - Muscle bx w/ inflammation, degeneration/necrosis, & regeneration
- **Clinical manifestations:** Progressive weakness of prox muscles; legs before arms
  - **Duchenne:** Asymptomatic at birth
    - Develop proximal muscle weakness at 3–5 yo: Waddling gait, toe walking, frequent falls, difficulty running/jumping/climbing stairs
    - As pelvic girdle weakness continues, develop Trendelenburg gait, lumbar lordosis, & "Gower sign" (stand from supine position "climbs up self")
    - Pseudohypertrophy of muscles, esp calves; feel rubbery & firm
    - Wheelchair by 8–12 yo, then fixed skeletal deformities; scoliosis, equinovarus
    - Declining resp fxn at 9–11 yo; progressive restrict defect, weak cough, ↑ risk PNA
    - Weakness of arms in mid-teens; difficulty feeding & caring for themselves
    - Cardiomyopathy in mid-teens; may be free of sx as wheelchair bound
    - Also demonstrate nonprogressive cognitive & emotional disturbances; deficits in verbal IQ, poor attention span, easily frustrated & distracted, OCD
    - Usually die in 2nd–3rd decade from pulmonary or cardiac failure
  - **Becker:** Similar clinically, but milder & slower progression; survive to adult
    - Presents later in childhood; able to walk w/o assistance beyond 16 yo
    - More severe cardiac dysfxn; 15% w/ cardiomyopathy <6 y & 75% pts >40 y
- **Diagnostic studies**
  - Muscle enzymes: CK ↑ 50–100 × s nml; highest levels early when asymp; ↓ over time
  - Mildly ↑ AST, ALT, & LDH; check GGT to verify that it is not of hepatic origin
  - Gene mutation analysis
  - 10–20% still need muscle bx for dx confirmation; needle or open bx; minimal histologic
  - Δ if pt very young; when older, test for ↓ /absent dystrophin
  - EMG changes nonspecific & not helpful in dx
- **Treatment:** Steroids preserve fxn & delay progression (QD prednisone or deflazacort)
  - PT/OT, bracing, night splints, nutrition guidance when non-ambulatory
  - Consider QD vit D & calcium for ↑ fracture risk from osteopenia of immobility

MUSC DYST 12-8

- Surgical tendon lengthening to prolong walking, scoliosis surgery
- Monitoring of pulmonary and cardiac functions

Guillain–Barré Syndrome (GBS) (Neurology 2011;76:294; Curr Treat Options Neurol 2011;13:590; Ped Rev 1997;18:10; Neurology 2003;61:736; Arch Dis Child Educ Pract Ed 2007;92:161)

- **Definition and epidemiology:** Annual incidence in pts >18 yo 0.5–2/100,000 pop
  - Acute inflammatory demyelinating polyradiculoneuropathy (AIDP)
  - Most common cause of acute generalized paralysis in all age groups
  - Male-to-female ratio = 1.5:1
- **Pathology/pathophysiology:** Immune-mediated segmental demyelination of peripheral nerves w/ inflammatory cell infiltration
  - **Variants:** (1) AIDP, (2) Miller-Fisher syndrome: Ophthalmoplegia, ataxia, & areflexia, (3) acute motor axonal neuropathy: Less common but often more severe, (4) acute motor and sensory axonal neuropathy
  - 50–70% w/ recent illness or vaccination w/i past 4 wk, URI or gastroenteritis; assoc w/ CMV, EBV, hepatitis, varicella, *Mycoplasma pneumoniae* and *Campylobacter jejuni* (most common preceding infxn; especially in Miller-Fisher variant)
- **Clinical manifestations:** Fever is atypical and suggests secondary infection
  - **3 phases:** Progression phase d to wks, plateau d to wks, recovery wks to mos
  - Progressive, ascending, symmetric muscle weakness starting in legs, ↓ DTRs
  - Sensory dysfxn: Pain or paresthesia (of back, extremities, or around mouth; may be in band distribution), ↓ position and vibratory sensation
  - Ataxia out of proportion to muscle weakness; bowel and bladder dysfxn are rare
  - CN involved (less common): Swallowing difficulty, facial weakness, ocular palsy
  - Dysautonomia (less common): Tachy/bradyarrhythmias, hyper/hypotension
  - Respiratory distress may progress to need for mechanical ventilation
- **Diagnostic criteria/studies**
  - Hx; recent illness, onset and progression of sx, exposure to ticks, toxins or meds
  - Exam w/ assessment of spinal tenderness and complete neuro exam w/ distribution and symmetry of strength, reflexes, and sensation
  - Suggested workup: CBC, ESR, ANA, U/A, CSF protein and cells, EMG
  - May also consider urine porphobilinogen, ALA, and heavy metal screen; quantitative immunoglobulins; *Campylobacter jejuni* Abs
  - **Required for dx:** Progressive motor weakness >1 limb, areflexia or hyporeflexia
  - **Supportive of dx:** Progression rapid but halts after 4 wk, relative symmetry, mild sensory deficits, CN involvement (facial weakness in 50%), autonomic dysfxn, initial absence of fever, recovery 2–4 wk after progression ceases
  - **Labs/studies supportive of dx:**
    - Albuminocytologic dissociation: ↑ CSF protein after 1 wk sx and CSF lymphs <10 per mm³; >50 cells/mm³ or PMN predom → alternative dx
    - Nerve conduction studies w/ prolonged F waves, slowing or block (unless variant)
  - **Features that cast doubt on dx:** Marked, persistent asymmetry, prolonged progressive phase >4 wk (likely CIDP) or recurrent = CIDP, persistent bowel/bladder dysfxn or dysfxn present at onset, discrete sensory level, (suggests transverse myelitis) CSF pleocytosis >50 wcc/mm³ (suggests infection)
  - **Features that exclude dx:** Recent Hx of hexacarbon abuse, porphyria, recent diphtheria, Hx/evidence of lead intox, pure sensory syndrome
- **Treatment:** Symptomatic Rx and supportive care
  - Measure FVC, negative inspiratory force and vital signs q6h until trend determined
  - Admit ICU if any of following: Severe rapid progression, flaccid tetraparesis, bulbar palsy, vital capacity ≤20 mL/kg, autonomic cardiovasc instability
  - Immunotherapy speeds recovery and lessens disability: Plasmapheresis (series of exchanges to total 250 mL/kg) or IVIg (2 g/kg divided over 2–4 d)
  - Pain management: Opioids, NSAIDs, carbamazepine, amitriptyline
  - **Corticosteroids may worsen or slow recovery!**
- **Outcome/prognosis:** 90–95% complete recovery in 3–12 mo; mortality <5%
  - 5%–10% retain severe permanent disability
  - Indicators of a poor prognosis: CN involvement, ventilatory dysfxn, rapid progressive tetraparesis, severe ↓ (<10% of nml) in compound muscle action potentials at 1st measurement, *C. jejuni* infection
  - Deaths 2/2 cardiac arrhythmias, resp failure, dysautonomia, pulmonary embolism

Bell's Palsy (J Child Neurol 2001;16:565; Clin Pediatr (Phila) 2010;49:411; Brain Dev 2011;33:644)

- **Definition and epidemiology:** Acute idiopathic lower motor neuron facial palsy
  - Incidence 2.7/100,000 in children <10 yo; 10.1/100,000 in those 10–20 yo

- **Pathology/pathophysiology**
  - Upper face innervated by fibers from both cerebral hemispheres while lower face innervated by corticobulbar fibers primarily from contralateral hemisphere
  - Lower motor neuron dysfxn (as in Bell's palsy) affects both upper and lower face, whereas upper motor neuron dysfxn affects lower face
  - Portion of CN VII w/i temporal bone is most commonly affected
- **Differential diagnosis**
  - Causes may be identified in up to 70% of children
  - Most common cause of acute facial palsy in kids: AOM, Lyme (50% in endemic area)
  - Infectious etiologies: HSV, Lyme, VZV (Ramsay Hunt), HIV, EBV, CMV, coxsackie, rubella, mumps, mycoplasma, TB
  - If gradual onset, consider neoplasm (cholesteatoma, schwannoma, meningioma, glioma, lymphoma/leukemia, parotid tumor)
  - Other: mastoiditis, trauma, GBS/MFS, toxins, vasculitis, sarcoidosis, HTN
- **Clinical manifestations**
  - Rapid onset is usually unilateral upper & lower facial weakness w/ facial sagging
  - Initial sx pain/tingling in ear canal. Typically aching is severe over mastoid
  - No facial sensory loss, although may report a "numb" feeling
  - May have disruption of taste on ant 2/3 tongue, hyperacusis, decreased tearing
  - Inability to close eyelid w/ risk of corneal injury if not lubricated and patched
- **Diagnostic studies:** If typical presentation, no need for diagnostic testing; full neuro exam, otoscopy, BP check and CBC recommended
  - Serologic testing for Lyme if endemic area
  - If <2 yo or atypical features (slow onset) consider w/u for ddx above with serum studies, tox screen, LP, urgent neuro-imaging
  - Consider neuroimaging if resolution does not begin within 1 mo
- **Prognosis and treatment:** ~80–90% pts recover completely or satisfactorily from cosmetic perspective, many w/l 2 mo and most w/l 6 mo
  - Evidence mixed if corticosteroids provide any benefit in children. Often prescribed in clinical practice (rx ideally begun w/i 72 hr onset symptoms)
  - Evidence mixed if antivirals (acyclovir/valcyclovir) w/ any benefit
  - Patch the eye and apply artificial tears several times a d

Myasthenia Gravis (MG) in Childhood (J Child Neurol 2009;24:584; Pediatr Rev 1990;12:73; J Child Neurol 1999;14:41)

- Includes **juvenile, congenital, and transient neonatal subtypes.** Hallmark feature is fatigable muscle weakness; sensation intact; DTR nml
- Childhood forms comprise 10–15% of all MG cases in N.America; incidence ~1.1/million
- **Juvenile MG**
  - Pathophysiology: Presents <19 yo. Classic **immune-mediated MG** w/ Ab against postsynaptic acetylcholine receptor at NMJ. AChR Ab accounts for ~80% cases; MuSK much less frequent and often assoc w/ more severe sx. Prepubertal children often seronegative. Thymoma/thymic hyperplasia identified in many cases
  - Clinical manifestations: Ptosis & diplopia typically initial sx of both forms; pupillary function wnl
- **Ocular MG:** 1°ly ocular sx w/ +/− mild weakness limbs & face; may progress to total ophthalmoplegia or relapses/remissions; no resp distress or deficits in swallowing or speaking; can progress to generalized sx (but less likely to progress if >1 yr w/ ocular sx only)
- **Generalized myasthenia:** Mod–severe limb & bulbar weakness; generalized weakness 1 yr after initial sx; dysphagia, facial diplegia, dysarthria, difficulty chewing, fatigable limb muscles; 1/3 w/ resp insufficiency → can lead to myasthenic crisis; permanent remission rare; ↑ incidence other autoimmune diseases
- **Diagnosis**
  - Tensilon test (edrophonium, an AChEI): + test w/ transient improvement in weakness
  - EMG – "decremental"; ↓ response w/ repetitive nerve stimulation (RNS)
  - Test anti-AChR Ab in serum; if negative, consider anti-MuSK Ab
  - Imaging for thymoma
- **Differential diagnosis:** Hypothyroidism, mitochondrial d/o, myopathy, GBS, ADEM, MS, botulism/other neurotoxins, Lambert–Eaton, tick paralysis, intracranial tumor
- **Treatment**
  - AChEIs first-line therapy (neostigmine, pyridostigmine) Other: Steroids, steroid-sparing agents. IVIG/plasma exchange and respiratory support for myasthenic crisis (acute severe weakness)
  - Consider thymectomy if thymoma present, or in anti-AChR + forms unresponsive to medications

- **Congenital myasthenic syndromes:** Associated w/ various genetic defects of NMJ jnctn. Not immune mediated, therefore not responsive to steroids, only some subtypes respond to AChEIs. Variable age of onset/dz severity. Usually presents in neonates/children, but can present in teens/adulthood
- **Transient neonatal myasthenia:** 2/2 to passive transfer of maternal Abs. Hypotonia & easy fatigability w/ feeding; weak cry, lack of facial expression; 15% w/ ocular findings; resp dysfxn uncommon; self-limited, worsens in first few d then usually resolves in few wks

DEMYELINATING DISEASES

Definition (Neurology 2007;68:S7; Neurology 2008;70:344; Ann Neurol 2011;69:292; Ann Neurol. 2012; 72: 211)

Disorder	Definition/Diagnostic Criteria (per 2007 Interntl Pediatric Consensus Criteria)	Additional Lab Info
CIS	<ul><li>1st inflam or demyelinating event affecting monofocal or multifocal areas CNS</li><li>No encephalopathy (except in bstem syndromes)</li><li>Mono vs. multifocal defined by clinical sx, not neuroimaging</li><li>Ex.: TM, ON, & dysfunction of bstem, cerebellum &/or hemispheres</li></ul>	
ADEM Mono-phasic	<ul><li>1st inflammatory or demyelinating event affecting multifocal areas of CNS; must be polysymptomatic & include encephalopathy (behavioral Δ or altered consciousness)</li><li>Must show improvement clinically or on MRI, though may have enduring deficits</li><li>New/fluctuating symptoms/MRI Δs w/in 3 mo still considered part of acute episode.</li><li>MRI w/ multifocal or focal lesions w/o prior Δs</li><li>Multiple (rarely single) large lesions >1–2 cm in WM (predom) or gray matter (esp basal ganglia / thalamus); may have confluent intramedullary lesion on spinal MRI</li></ul>	Variable ↑ CSF prot & WBC (can be >50) Occ CSF OCB Micro studies usually neg
ADEM Re-current	<ul><li>Recurrence of prior symptoms/signs ≥3 mo after 1st event & ≥1 mo after completion of steroid therapy</li><li>No new sx/ lesions by hx, exam, imaging; original MRI lesions may have ↑'d</li></ul>	Same as ADEM above
ADEM Multi-phasic	<ul><li>New ADEM event w/ new anatomic CNS lesion ≥3 mo after 1st event & ≥1 mo after completion of steroid therapy</li><li>Brain MRI *must* show new lesions *and* complete/partial resolution of prior lesions</li></ul>	Same as ADEM above
NMO	<ul><li>Dx requires both ON & TM, plus 1 of 2<ul><li>Serum +NMO IgG+ or</li><li>MRI spinal lesions encompassing ≥3 segments</li></ul></li><li>Can see brain lesions (usu hypothalamus, bstem, or diffuse cerebral WM)</li></ul>	+serum NMO IgG (sens 47%; ↑'s w/ relapses) +CSF NMO IgG Variable ↑ CSF prot & WBC (can be >50) Rare OCB
Pediatric MS (children/ adolesc <18 yo)	<ul><li>Multiple CNS demyelinating events disseminated in space and time (using either clinical or MRI criteria for each)</li><li>DIT (1 of 2 options):<ul><li>Clinical: Discrete clinical events ≥4 wk apart; or</li><li>MRI: New T2 or GAD+ lesions ≥3 mo after 1st clinical event (vs. adult 2005 McDonald Criteria w/ 3rd option of new T2 lesion any time after reference baseline MRI done ≥30 d after 1st event)</li></ul></li><li>DIS (1 of 3 options)<ul><li>Clinical/exam features of anatomically separated lesions; or</li><li>2 MRI lesions (at least 1 in brain) in combo w/ abn CSF (OCB or ↑ IgG index); or</li><li>Combo of 3 of 4 MRI features: ≥3 periventric lesions; ≥9 WM lesions or 1 GAD+ lesion; 1 juxtacortical lesion; 1 infratentorial lesion</li></ul></li><li>Clinical event cannot meet MS criteria</li><li>If 1st event c/w AEDM, then still need 2 more events meeting MS criteria, w/ all 3 events separated by 3 mo</li></ul>	<ul><li>CSF WBC <50!!</li><li>Frequent OCB, ↑IgG index</li></ul>

- **2010 Revised McDonald Criteria:**
  - New criteria for adult MS
  - Approved & being used by some for pedi MS but not yet validated
  - Allows dx of MS in some CIS pt's using only single MRI for DIT
  - DIT (1 of 3 options):
    - Clinical: Discrete clinical events ≥4 wk apart; or
    - MRI: New T2 or GAD+ lesion compared to baseline scan, regardless of timing of baseline MRI; or
    - MRI: Simult presence of GAD+ & GAD–lesions at any time on any 1 MRI
  - DIS (1 of 2 options)
    - Clinical/exam features of anatomically separated lesions; or
    - MRI: ≥1 T2 (do not need GAD+) lesion in 2 of 4 areas: Juxtacortical, periventricular, infratentorial, spinal cord (if pt has bstem or sp cord syndrome then symptomatic lesions excluded from count)
  - New study found PPV 76% in kids >11 yo, similar to PPV for adults; PPV only 55% in kids < 11yo (even excluding ADEM)

ADEM, Acute disseminated encephalomyelitis; DIS, dissemination in space; DIT, dissemination in time; GAD+, gadolinium enhancing; MS, multiple sclerosis; NMO, neuromyelitis optica; OCB, oligoclonal bands; ON, optic neuritis; TM, transverse myelitis; WM, white matter.

Epidemiology (Neurology 2007;68:S23; Neurology 2007;68:S37; Neurologist 2010;16:92)

- ADEM: More common in kids than adults; avg age: 5–8 ; no gender predom; seasonal (usually winter/spring); 70–77% report antecedent infection or vaccination
- MS: 2–5% of all MS pts w/ onset <16 yo;
  - Avg onset 8–14 yo; female predominance, lower F:M ratio in younger kids
  - Adult pattern: ↑ risk in Caucasians at ↑ distance from equator not proven in kids yet

Etiology/Pathophysiology (Lancet Neurol 2011;10:436; Neurology 2007;68:S23; Neurology 2007;68:S37)

- ADEM: Usually 2–21 d after infxn, may occur after vaccination
  - 2/2 immune-mediated inflammation, not direct infection of CNS
- MS: Evidence of autoimmune mechanism and reaction to prior infection, esp EBV
  - Risk likely inferred by interaction of genes and environment
  - Recent study showed ↑ risk w/ HLA-DRB1*15, remote EBV inf, low Vit D level

Clinical Manifestations (Neurology 2007;68:S7; Neurology 2007;68:S23; Neurologist 2010;16:92)

- ADEM: Rapid onset of encephalopathy and multiple neuro deficits; progresses w/i hrs to max deficits w/i days; +/– prodrome fever, HA, N/V, malaise
  - Kids more often w/ szrs and ongoing fever and HA; adults w/ sensory deficits & PNS
- MS: Present w/ sensory, motor & brainstem deficits; 0–50% w/ optic neuritis (uni- & bilateral); ataxia & szrs frequently in children <6 yo

Differential Diagnosis and Assessment (Neurology 2007;68:S13; Neurology 2007;68:S23)

- **Minimum dx testing** for 1st inflammatory demyelinating event:
  - Brain and C-spine MRI w/ and w/o gadolinium; consider imaging entire spinal cord
  - CBC/diff; ESR; ANA; CSF for cell count/diff, total protein oligoclonal bands, IgG index (simultaneous measurement of IgG and albumen in serum & CSF), cytology
- **Consider extended testing** according to presentation: MR angiography & spectroscopy, B12, Vit D level, TSH, ACE, NMO, IgG (serum +/– CSF), ophtho eval for visual dysfxn, evoked potentials (visual, brainstem auditory, & somatosensory evoked potentials) Exclude other etiologies; esp if atypical MS features (e.g., PNS involve, encephalopathy, fever, ↑ ESR, ↑ WBC, lack of CSF oligoclonal bands, notable CSF pleocytosis)
- **If acute encephalopathy**, rule out acute infxn of CNS and begin empiric Abx. Check:
  - CSF: GS/Cx, HSV, EBV, CMV, VZV, HHV-6, enterovirus, mycoplasma, Lyme, West Nile (seasonal)
  - Serum: GS/Cx, HSV, EBV, CMV, VZV, HHV-6, HIV, mycoplasma, Lyme, West Nile
  - Throat / nasal swab: Paraflu, RSV, influenza, mycoplasma, enterovirus
  - Stool: Enterovirus, viral Cx

Treatment (Neurology 2007;68:S23; Neurology 2007;68:S54)

- ADEM: High-dose steroids (IV methylprednisolone 10–30 mg/kg/d to max of 1 g/d) for 3–5 d, then oral steroid taper for 4–6 wk; achieves 50–80% recovery rate
  - Consider IVIG (1–2 g/kg single dose or divided over 3–5 d) alone or w/ steroids
  - Plasmapheresis has been used w/ some success when above treatments fail

- MS:
  - **Relapse therapy:** High-dose steroids (IV methylprednisolone 20–30 mg/kg/d) for 3–5 d, consider oral taper for ≤2–3 wk if incomplete res; IVIG(1 g/kg/d) for 2 d if steroids contraindicated; consider plasmapheresis or IVIG if freq attacks or steroid dependant
  - **Disease-modifying therapy** (none FDA approved in kids, off-label MGH approach)**:** 1st line are interferon β-1a and -1b and glatiramer acetate; 2nd-line natalizumab, fingolimod; 3rd-line cyclophosphamide, rituximab, mycophenolate, mito-xantrone, consider IVIG as alternative in ≤6 yo
  - **Symptomatic therapy** for spasticity (e.g., baclofen), fatigue (e.g., modafinil), tremor, bladder dysfxn (e.g., straight cath, antichol), cognitive impairment (donepezil)
- NMO (Eur J Neurol 2010;17:1019)
  - **Relapse/acute therapy** – high dose methylprednisolone as above; plasma exchange if fail steroids; IVIG not evaluated in NMO
  - **Disease-modifying therapy** – immunosuppressants (azathioprine, rituximab, cyclophosphamide, mitoxantrone, mycophenolate), interferon β ineffective for NMO

Outcome (Neurology 2007;68:S23; Neurology 2007;68:537)
- ADEM: ²/₃ recover completely w/o Rx, whereas Rx appears to speed recovery; 6–50% show behavioral or cognitive deficits
- NMO: Poor prognosis, mortality 20% in acute stage, 30–50% w/i first 5 yr
- MS:
  - >90% w/ relapsing remitting course (RRMS); 2.3–7% pediatric pts w/ 1° progres-sive course (PPMS)
  - Relapse rate ↑ in pediatric MS, sx more transitory & remit more quickly; most relapse w/i 1st yr of disease
  - Very young display more aggressive form w/ irreversible psychomotor deficits
  - Vs. adults, kids have lower disability scores, longer time to conversion to 2° progressive course (SPMS) & ↓ probability of converting to SPMS
  - Kids who do convert do so at a younger age & become disabled earlier
  - Even if no physical disabilities, children display significant cognitive deficits

CEREBRAL PALSY

Definition/Classification (Neurology 2004;62:851; Pediatr Rev 1995;16:411)
- Classified by syndrome of motor impairment, (including but not limited to): Spastic (hypertonic w/ inc DTRs), dystonic, athetoid, ataxic
- Nonprogressive d/o mvmt & posture 2/2 lesion/dysfxn in develop brain (often dxd <2 yo)
- Approx 70% have associated nonmotor impairments (commonly mental retardation)
- Not always permanent; many w/ mild motor dysfxn in infancy attain nml motor fxn later in childhood (but ¼ retain cognitive impairments)

Clinical Manifestations (Pediatr Rev 1995;16:411)

Spastic diplegia	All 4 ext can be affected, typically leg weakness > arm. Nml tone/hypotonic in 1st 4 mo, w/ progressive spasticity in 1st yr. "Army" crawl using arms, delayed sitting, toe-walking, tight heel cords, flexed knees, hyperflexia (+clonus, +up going toes, +crossed adductor reflex), scissoring (legs cross at thigh when vertically suspended)
Spastic hemiplegia	Unilateral limb weakness, asymmetry rarely evident in 1st few mos. Sustained fisting of 1 hand or abn focal posturing, delayed crawl/walk, non-alternating crawl using nml arm/leg & dragging contralateral arm/leg, hand dominance expressed early (NEVER NORMAL in <1 yo), asym tightness of elbow flexors & wrist pronator, diff w/ ankle dorsiflexion
Spastic quadriplegia	Usually affects all 4 ext, typically leg weakness > arm. Often assoc w/ severe dev delay, characteristic supine posturing (retracted head/neck, clenched hands w/ flexed elbows & extended legs) Persistent neonatal reflexes & hyperreflexia Dysphagia, seizures, cognitive impairment, speech-language d/os, hearing /vision defects commonly associated
Athetoid	If hyperbili, eval for sx kernicterus @ 3–5 d (high pitched cry, opisthotonos, ↑ DTRs); extensor hypertonicity gradually ↓ to nml then "floppy" at 3 mo w/ return of nml DTRs; oblig asym tonic neck reflex, delayed voluntary motor milestones, involve athetoid/dystonic posturing at 12–18 mo & change from hypotonia to rigid/cogwheel hypotonia
Dystonic	Dystonic posturing, tone nml to ↓ early in childhood, may evolve w/ time
Ataxic	Nml DTRs, hypotonicity of trunk & extremities, wide-based gait, infants rarely display overt ataxic signs (intention tremor, head titubation)

Epidemiology (Neurology 2004;62:851)
- Worldwide incidence 2/1,000 live births; 10,000/yr in US

Pathophysiology (Neurology 2004;62:851; Pediatr Rev 1995;16:411)
- Often multifactorial in etiology, which can occur in pre-, peri-, or post-natal periods
- Risk factors include (but are not limited to) prematurity, IUGR, cerebral infarction, hemorrhage, cystic encephalomalacia, brain malformations, genetic dzs, infxn, bilirubin encephalopathy, hypoxic ischemic injury, and trauma
- Preterm infant w/ periventricular leukomalacia is a common clinical scenario

Diagnostic Assessment (Neurology 2004;62:851)
- Confirm CP dx by H&P; assure no features of progressive/degenerative d/o, classify type of motor impairment
- Screen assoc conditions: Developmental delay, ophthalmologic/hearing impairments, speech/language disorders, feeding/swallowing difficulties
- EEG if H&P suggest seizures
- Neuroimaging if etiology is not established by perinatal imaging (MRI preferred to CT)
- Consider eval for coagulopathy if unexplained infarction in imaging
- Consider genetic/metabolic eval if malformation found on imaging

Treatment/Management (Pediatr Rev 1995;16:411)

Rehabilitation	PT/OT, speech therapy (for oromotor dysfxn), orthotic devices, serial casting, education, counseling, nutritional supplements
Botulinum toxin A injection	Used for temporary (4–6 mo) relief of localized or segmental spasticity. Level A evidence for effectiveness in rx of spasticity
Oral antispasticity meds	Used for rx of generalized spasticity: Diazepam, dantrolene, baclofen, tizanidine
Intrathecal baclofen pump	Used for rx of generalized spasticity. Complications include CSF leak, catheter related AEs, infection
Surgery	Tendon release for contractures, osteotomy for 2° skeletal deformities, selective post rhizotomy to ↓ spastic hypertonicity

HEADACHE (HA)

Definitions
- **Primary HA:** Includes migraine, tension, and cluster HAs
- **Secondary HA:** 2/2 underlying medical condition
  - Etiologies include infxn, substance use or w/d from substance (often analgesic overuse: >3–5 doses/wk), trauma, SAH/ICH, d/o of head and neck (e.g., tooth abscess, sinusitis, AOM, cranial pain), ↑ ICP or pseudotumor, vascular d/o, vasculitis, vasospasm, venous sinus thrombosis, PRES, psychiatric d/o, facial pain, refractive vision error, HTN

Diagnostic Studies (Pediatr Rev 2007;28:43; Neurology 2002;59:490; Pediatr Rev 1999;20:39; Neurology 2004;63:427)
- **HPI:** time patterns of HA, freq, duration, pre-HA sx, location, quality of pain, assoc sx, alleviating/exacerbating factors, degree debility 2/2 HA, sx btw Has, FamHx, SocHx
- **PE:** Assess vital signs, particularly BP
  - Examine fundi for papilledema (may indicate incr ICP)
  - Measure head circum (rapid growth may be sign of obstructive hydrocephalus)
  - Assess for focal neuro signs/sx & signs of infxn (fever, rash, pain w/ neck flexion)
  - Listen for cranial bruits 2/2 AVM (although absent in 50% of cases)
- **Neuroimaging:** Not recommended for recurrent HAs and normal neuro exam
  - Consider if abnl neuro exam (e.g., focal exam, signs of ↑ ICP, ∆MS, concurrent seizures), hx of acute onset of severe HA, ∆ in HA type
  - Urgent neuroimaging required if ↑ ICP suspected (papilledema, pain worse w/ lying flat, HA awakening pt from sleep, pain worse w/ maneuvers that ↑ venous pressure → Valsalva, cough)
- **Labs:** No specific recs for routine lab workup. Consider Chem7 & UA if ↑ BP or CBC & blood cx if suspect infectious etiology
- **EEG:** Not recommended
- **LP:** Not recommended unless suspicion of CNS infxn, SAH, or pseudotumor cerebri. Obtain neuroimaging 1st if suspect ↑ ICP

Migraine

Subtypes of Migraine (Pediatr Rev 2007;28:43; Neurology 2004;63:427)
- **Migraine w/o aura:** Often unilateral in frontal/temporal region, pulsating, mod or severe pain intensity, aggravated by physical activity. +/– N/V, photophobia, & phonophobia

- **Migraine w/ aura:** HA similar to migraine w/o aura. Auras most commonly involve visual disturbances (scotoma, distortion, hallucination, obscuration, visual field defects). Less common auras include sensory sx (e.g., numbness/tingling), dysphasic speech disturbances, hemiparesis, CN palsies (most common oculomotor → ptosis)
- **Basilar type migraine:** Usually preceded by dizziness, vertigo, visual disturbances, ataxia, diplopia, ↓ consciousness, ↓ hearing, bilateral paresthesias, tinnitus, dysarthria, or other bulbar symptoms

Epidemiology (Pediatr Review 2007;28:43)
- +FHx in ~80%; prev 1.2–3.2% in 3–7 yo; 4–11% in 7–11 yo, 8–23% in 15 yo
- Sex ratio: Prepuberty afflicts boys > girls, postpuberty afflicts girls > boys
- Migraine w/o aura is most common subtype (frequency 60–85%)
- May see in relation to cyclic vomiting syndrome or abdominal migraine

Pathophysiology (Pediatr Rev 2007;28:43; Pediatr Rev 1999;20:39)
- Exact mechanism unknown but evidence implicating calcium channels & 5HT changes
  - Altered neuronal calcium channels → "cortical spreading depression" whereby neurons undergo hyperpolarization followed by depolarization
  - Altered serotoninergic function → ? effect on vasculature or central pain pathways
- Triggers for migraine include sleep deprivation, stress/tension, lack of exercise, excessive caffeine, dehydration, dietary (e.g., cheese, chocolate, citrus fruits), analgesic overuse (>5×/wk), & hormonal factors (menarche, OCPs, premenstrual, pregnancy, premenopause)

Treatment (Pediatr Rev 2007;28:43; Neurology 2004;63:2215)
- **Acute treatment:** Tylenol and ibuprofen have proven efficacy and safety in children and adolescents. Nasal sumatriptan also proven efficacy in adolescents but is expensive, so oral sumatriptan more widely used in clinical practice. Limited data for other triptans, such as zolmitriptan and rizatriptan
- **Prophylaxis:** Consider if ≥3 HA per mo and/or functional disability from HA. However, no migraine-specific meds FDA approved for use in children
- Rx w/ antihistamine (cyproheptadine), AEDs (topiramate, valproic acid, gabapentin), TCAs (amitriptyline, nortriptyline), NSAIDs (naproxen sodium), CCBs (verapamil), BBs (propranolol)
- **Behavior modification:** Adequate sleep, stress mgmt, avoid known triggers, stop analgesic overuse, ↑ exercise and hydration

Tension Headache (Pediatr Rev 1999;20:39; Pediatr Neurol 2005;33:303)
- **Definition:** Diffuse, bilateral, tightening/pressing quality in "band-like" distribution, duration ranging from min to days, typically no N/V. Generally aches but is non-pulsatile & non-throbbing (Pediatr Neurol 2005;33:303)
- **Epidemiology:** More common in ♀; age of onset ~5 yo; prevalence ranges 11–72.8%
- **Etiology:** Often associated with psychological stress and/or analgesic overuse
- **Treatment:** Aimed at stress reduction through relaxation techniques, massage, etc. Avoid reliance on analgesic meds

Cluster Headaches (Pediatr Neurol 2005;33:303)
- **Definition:** Clustered intense periorbital or temporal pain, often unilateral, with autonomic sx (ipsilat rhinorrhea, tearing, congestion, eyelid edema, miosis, ptosis). Occurs in periods of wks to mos w/ long pain-free periods (up to 2 yr)
- **Epidemiology:** Affects <0.1% of children. Very rare in children <10 yo. Mostly in males
- **Treatment:** In adults, acute rx w/ O_2 lidocaine aqueous drops intranasally, olanzapine, dihydroergotamine, sumatriptan. Most common preventative rx is steroids

NEUROCUTANEOUS SYNDROMES

Tuberous Sclerosis
Diagnosis (Arch Neurol 2000;57:662; NEJM 2006;355:1345; J Child Neurol 2004;19:643)
- Need ≥2 major features or 1 major w/ 2 minor features. May emerge over time. Consider diagnosis if FamHx of TS and in infants w/ infantile spasms

Major Criteria	Minor Criteria
Facial angiofibromas or forehead plaques (75% pts)	Confetti skin lesions (multiple 1–2 mm hypomelanotic macules)
Shagreen patch (20–30% pts)	Gingival fibromas
≥3 hypopigmented macules (90% pts)	Multiple randomly-distributed pits in dental enamel
Nontraumatic ungula or periungual fibromas	
Lymphangioleiomyomatosis	Hamartomatous rectal polyps
Renal angiomyolipoma (75–80% pts)	Multiple renal cysts
Cardiac rhabdomyoma (66% pts)	Nonrenal hamartomas
Retinal nodular hamartomas (up to 87%)	Bone cysts
Cortical tuber (almost all pts)	Retinal achromic patch
Subependymal nodules	Cerebral white matter radial migration lines
Subependymal giant cell astrocytoma	

Epidemiology: Incidence is 1/5,000–10,000 live births (Neurol Clin 2003;21:983)

Pathophysiology (Arch Neurol 2000;57:662; N Engl J Med 2006;355:1345)

- Inheritance pattern: Autosomal dominant or sporadic (accounts for $^2/_3$ of cases)
- Genes involved: $TSC1$ on chromosome 9, $TSC2$ on chromosome 16. Encode cell cycle regulation proteins. Variable penetrance. TSC1 mutations often w/ milder phenotype
- Screening (Arch Neurol 2000;57:662; N Engl J Med 2006;355:1345)
  - Brain MRI yearly until 21 yo to evaluate for subependymal giant cell tumors
  - Renal imaging at least q1–3yr for emergence/growth of renal angiomyolipomas
  - Funduscopic exam to assess for retinal hamartomas
  - Dermatologic exam w/ Wood lamp to assess for assoc skin findings. Rpt if needed
  - Echo yearly to assess for growth of cardiac rhabdomyomas
  - Chest CT if pulm sx develop to assess for lymphangiomyomatosis. Annual PFTs in patients with known lymphangiomyomatosis
  - Neurodevelopmental testing

Complications (N Engl J Med 2006;355:1345)

- Neurologic: Epilepsy (in 70–80% of TS pts; infantile spasms strongly assoc w/ TS), mental retardation (affects ~50% TS pts), neurobehavioral d/o/autism 2/2 cortical tubers. ↑ ICP, hydrocephalus 2/2 subependymal giant-cell tumors
- Renal: Sudden hemorrhage 2/2 renal angiomyolipomas. HTN/CRI 2/2 renal cysts
- Pulmonary: Pneumothorax/dyspnea due to lymphangiomyomatosis
- Cardiac: Cardiac failure in infancy (very rare), dysrhythmias due to rhabdomyomas

Neurofibromatosis Type 1

Diagnosis (JAMA 1997;278:51; Pediatrics 2000;105:608; Pediatrics 2008;121:633)

- Requires at least 2 of following, can emerge over time:
  - ≥6 café-au-lait spots (1.5 cm ≥ postpuberty; 0.5 cm ≥ prepuberty). Most common feature in children, presents by 2 yo. Affects 99% of patients
  - ≥2 neurofibromas, or 1 or more plexiform neurofibromas. Occur in brain and/or periphery, including SC tissue. Plexiform neurofibromas usually congenital, and can have multiorgan involvement. Neurofibromas occur in 48% of pts by 10 yo; ↑ to 84% by 20 yo. 60% of NF1 pts have brain neurofibromas
  - Freckling in axilla or groin. 2nd most common feature in children. Commonly presents 3–5 yo. Present in up to 90% of patients by 7 yo.
  - Optic glioma (tumor of optic pathway). Presents in pts <6 yo. In up to 15% of pts
  - 2 or more Lisch nodules (benign iris hamartomas that are best appreciated on slit-lamp examination). Present in >70% of patients by 10 yo
  - Distinctive bony lesion (dysplasia of the sphenoid bone or dysplasia/thinning of long bone cortex.) Often apparent by 1 yo. Present in ~14% pts
  - A 1st-degree relative w/ NF1

Epidemiology: Prevalence is 1/2,000–1/4,500 (Pediatrics 2000;105:608)

Pathophysiology (JAMA 1997;278:51; Pediatrics 2008;121:633)

- 50% AD, 50% sporadic; high rate of penetrance
- NF1 is a tumor suppressor gene on long arm of chromosome 17 band q11.2

Complications (Pediatrics 2000;105:608; Pediatrics 2008;121:633)

- Most pts w/ NF1 are mildly affected. Serious complications occur in ~30% pts
- Growth abnormality, short stature, disfigurement 2/2 neurofibromas
- Vision loss, severe proptosis, hydrocephalus, precocious puberty 2/2 optic glioma, neurofibromas impinging on optic, hypothalamic, and pituitary tissues
- Malignancy: 5–10% of pts have malignant peripheral nerve sheath tumors, usually in adulthood. Less common malignancies include pheochromocytoma, rhabdomyosarcoma, leukemia, and CNS gliomas
- Gross organ damage due to plexiform neurofibromas
- HTN, ↑ stroke risk 2/2 vasc dysplasia; segmental vasculopathies, moyamoya
- Focal neurologic deficits, hydrocephalus, ↑ ICP 2/2 neurofibromas/gliomas
- Epilepsy (affects 5–7% pts)
- Learning disabilities in ~60%. MR in ~4% kids. Assoc w/ ADHD and autism

Screening (JAMA 1997;278:51; Pediatrics 2008;121:633; J Med Genet 2007;44:81)

- Routine imaging of the chest, abdomen, spine, and brain is not indicated
- Yearly ophtho exam until 7 yo to assess for optic glioma/associated vision defects
- Annual PE w/ BP check, neurodevelopmental assessment, skin exam to assess for progression of neurofibromas & underlying plexiform neurofibromas, skeletal exam to assess for scoliosis, vertebral angulation, limb abnormalities, tibial dysplasia, head circum to assess for hydrocephalus, and pubertal development to assess for precocious puberty

Neurofibromatosis Type 2
- Autosomal dominant. Less common than NF1
- Diagnostic criteria: Bilateral vestibular schwannomas (VS) or FHx NF2 (1st-degree relative) and unilateral VS or any 2 of following: Meningioma, glioma, schwannoma, juvenile posterior subcapsular lenticular opacities/juvenile cortical cataract

Sturge–Weber
- Congenital vascular capillary disorder, nonheritable. Characterized by port wine stain (facial capillary angioma) typically in distribution of trigeminal nerve 1st and 2nd divisions. Assoc w/ ipsilateral leptomeningeal angioma w/ risk of venous thrombosis and/or surrounding brain ischemia. Complications include szr, MR, & glaucoma

Von Hippel–Lindau
- Rare AD condition assoc w/ multiple neoplasms: RCC, pheochromocytomas, hemangioblastomas (often retinal, intracranial, or intraspinal), endolymphatic sac tumors, pancreatic tumors (neuroendocrine and serous cystadenomas), and papillary cystadenomas of the epididymis. Screening in VHL pts includes yearly ophtho exams, serum catecholamines, and MRI of brain/spine

Ataxia Telangiectasia
- Rare AR condition assoc w/ progressive cerebellar ataxia, immune def, abnl eye mvmt/impaired tracking, & oculocutaneous telangiectasias

ADHD

Definition & Dx Criteria (Postgrad Med 2010;122:97; Postgrad Med 2008;120:48)
- Neurobiologic condition w/ hyperactivity, impulsivity and/or inattention
- **3 subtypes:** Predominantly inattentive, predominantly hyperactive/impulsive, combined types
- **DSM IV criteria:** ≥6 of 9 inattentive and/or ≥6 of 9 hyperactive/impulsive sx
  - Sx must persist for ≥6 mo; be maladaptive & inconsistent w/ developmental level; present in ≥2 settings (school, home, etc); present before 7 yo; cause significant impairment in social, academic or occupational fxn; not be attributable to another physical, situational, or mental disorder
  - Might not be recognized until after 7 yo when school/work becomes more challenging (esp in inattentive subtype)
  - Anticipated DSM V will likely ↑ age limit for 1st symptoms from 7 yo to 12 yo

Inattentive	Hyperactive/Impulsive	
inattentive to detail/careless mistakes	fidgets w/ hands/feet, squirms in seat	Hyper-activity sx
difficulty sustaining attn	difficulty remaining seated	
not listen when spoken to directly	runs about/climbs excessively (adolesc w/ subjective restlessness)	
not follow through/finish tasks	difficulty playing/engaging in leisure activities quietly	
difficulty organizing	"on the go," "driven by motor"	
loses things	talks excessively	
avoids/dislikes tasks requiring sustained attn	blurts answers before questions completed	Impulsivity symptoms
easily distracted	difficulty awaiting turn	
forgetful	interrupts/intrudes on others	

Epidemiology & Comorbidity (Annu Rev Med 2002;53:113)
- Most commonly dx'd pedi neurobehavioral do; 4–12% school-aged children
- Kids w/ male predominance; in adults M:F ratio equal
- Combined subtype 50–75%, inattentive 20–30%, hyperactive/impulsive <15%
- Combined subtype most severe, greatest risk of comorbidities
- Common comorbidities: Anxiety disorders, depression, bipolar, ODD, conduct disorder, learning disabilities, substance abuse

Pathophysiology
- Heterogenous do w/ multiple contributing factors: Genetic, neuroanatomical, neurochemical, environmental

Clinical Features
- DSM symptom cluster req'd but somewhat simplified description
- Variable executive function deficits: Response inhibition, planning & organizing, working memory, self-regulation, frustration tolerance, complex problem solving, intrinsic motivation, goal-directed behavior ("procrastination")

- May develop demoralization & low self esteem 2/2 persistent impairments of untreated ADHD; often mistaken for depression

Evaluation & Workup (J Am Acad Child Adolesc Psychiatry 2007;46:894)
- Current AAP & AACAP guidelines require DSM IV criteria be met for ADHD dx
- AAP recently expanded guidelines from 6–12 yo to include children 4–18 yo
- **Complete Eval:** Interview of pt & parent(s), DSM criteria, developmental hx, FHx & psychosocial hx, physical/neuro exam, ancillary reports (daycare/teacher/coaches reports, academic records), various sx rating scales for ADHD & comorbid disorders (e.g., ADHD rating scale, Vanderbilt parent & teacher scales, Conners' rating scales–revised, Brown ADD rating scales, etc.)
- **Screen for comorbid do:** Psychiatric (anxiety/OCD, depression, ODD, CD, bipolar), developmental (learning, language, other neurodevelopmental disorders), neurologic (tics, szrs, ALD in boys), medical/physical (sleep apnea, lead exposure)

Treatment (Pediatrics 2011;128:1007)
- **Stimulants:** Methylphenidate-based (MPH) & amphetamine-based (AMP)
  - Side effects: ↓ appetite, insomnia, HA, abd discomfort, transient ↑ tics (*not* contraindicated in tic do), rebound phenomena (irritability, lowered mood)
  - CV effects: Rate sudden death in kids on stimulants not > base pop rate; obtain pt & FHx of CV dz (e.g., WPW, sudden death, HOCM, long Qt); if no significant hx, do *not* need screening EKG or echo
  - 65–75% pt's w/ clinical response; ↑ s to 85% if tried both MPH & AMP
  - Linear dose-response curve to stimulants; ↑ sx reduction w/ ↑ ing doses:
  - Start at lowest dose & titrate up every 3–7 d; long-acting preferred to short-acting for ease & ↑ adherence

Duration Action	MPH-based *(max 2 mg/kg/day except dex-MPH 1 mg/kg/day)*	AMP-based *(max 1.5 mg/kg/day)*
Short-acting	[3–5 hr] Ritalin, Methylin, Focalin (dex-MPH)	[4–6 hr] Dexedrine (dextro-AMP), Dextrostat
Intermediate-acting	[3–8 hr] Ritalin SR, Metadate ER, Methylin ER	[6–8 hr] Adderall (AMP mixed salts), Dexedrine spansules
Intermediate/long-acting	[8–10 hr] Metadate CD, Ritalin LA	
Long-acting	[10–12 hr] Focalin XR, Concerta, Daytrana patch	[8–12 hr] Adderall XR, Vyvanse (prodrug lisdexamphetamine)

- **Non-stimulants:** Often less effective than stimulants & delayed onset action; good if stimulant non-response/adverse effects or as adjunctive rx
  - Atomoxetine: Selective NE reuptake inhib (NRI); start 0.5 mg/kg/day × 2 wk, then ↑ 1.2 mg/kg/day; consider for ADHD w/ anxiety, tics, substance abuse
  - α-adrenergic agonists: Guanfacine ER (Intuniv) & clonidine ER (Kapvay); for ADHD w/ tics, anxiety, sleep disturbance, emotional dysreg, ODD
  - Non-FDA approved but demonstrated benefit: Buproprion, TCAs (imipramine, nortriptyline), modafinil (for arousal/motivation), melatonin (for sleep)
- **School- & home-based interventions:** Medication often ineffective for many executive fxn deficits; school accommodations (504 plan or IEP), extended time on tests, preferential seating, organizers, daily progress reports, tutors, home/classroom behavioral interventions, social skills remediation

Outcome & Prognosis
- **ADHD pts have ↑ risk/rates:** Smoking & substance abuse (SA), w/ SA more severe & longer lasting; psychosocial deficits; hospitalizations for accidental injuries; teen pregnancies; driving problems; academic difficulties; employment & family/marital problems

Hypoxia (see Respiratory Failure in PICU Chapter for additional information)
- Failure of oxygen delivery or an inability of tissues to use oxygen
- Severe hypoxia can lead to cyanosis which can be seen with 5 g/dL of deoxyhemoglobin
- **Hypoxemic hypoxia:** Low arterial partial pressure of oxygen. Five causes include low inspired FiO_2, hypoventilation, intrapulmonary and extrapulmonary shunt, V/Q mismatch and diffusion defect
- **Workup:** Pulse oximetry, ABG or arterialized capillary blood gas, hyperoxia test, CXR, CT, pulmonary function tests

Tachypnea (see next page for additional information)
- Pneumonia, asthma, pneumothorax, chest wall restriction, splinting, pulmonary embolism, anxiety, metabolic acidosis, upper airway obstruction, fever, FB (lower airway obstruction), chronic lung disease
- **Workup:** CXR, CT, CBC, glucose, nasopharyngoscopy, bronchoscopy, pulmonary function tests, lung biopsy

Stertor
- **Nasopharyngeal:** Choanal atresia, lingual thyroid or thyroglossal cyst, macroglossia or micrognathia, hypertrophic tonsils/adenoids
- **Workup:** Attempt to pass NG tube, lateral neck x-ray, nasopharyngoscopy

Stridor (see page 13-2 for additional information)
- **Inspiratory:** Extrathoracic. Laryngomalacia, tracheomalacia, bronchomalacia (chronic), croup, tracheitis, epiglottitis, retropharyngeal abscess (acute), laryngeal web/cyst, vocal cord paralysis, subglottic stenosis, foreign body, intraluminal tumor (subglottic hemangioma or laryngeal papilloma) or external compression (cystic hygroma or tumor), angioedema, traumatic intubation, laryngospasm (hypocalcemic tetany), psychogenic
- **Expiratory:** Intrathoracic; mimics asthma, but tracheal/bronchial origin. Tracheomalacia, bronchomalacia, vascular rings, extrinsic compression, foreign body, psychogenic
- **Workup:** AP/lateral neck film to assess upper airway anatomy, chest film if suspect foreign body aspiration, direct bronch for persistent sx or foreign body, CT to r/o extrinsic compression, barium swallow to r/o vascular compression, tumor, or GERD, EGD or pH probe to r/o GERD, PFTs

Cough (see page 13-3 for additional information)
- **Acute:** URI, pneumonia, aspiration
- **Chronic:** Postnasal drip, GERD, bronchitis, TB, bronchiectasis, cough-variant asthma, toxic exposure (cigarette smoke), CHF, drug (ACE-I), ILD, COP, bronchiolitis obliterans, bronchiectasis, habit (psychogenic) cough
- **Workup:** ENT exam for s/sx allergic rhinitis, CXR +/– sputum culture if suspect infection, CT scan if suspect bronchiectasis or chronic ILD, empiric antacid if hx c/w GERD

Wheezing (see page 13-5 for additional information)
- **Homophonous without signs of hyperinflation:** Upper airway. **Heterophonous with signs of hyperinflation:** Lower airway
- **Acute:** Asthma, bronchiolitis, anaphylaxis, toxic inhalation, medication induced (β-blocker, ASA, indomethacin), aspiration, foreign body
- **Chronic:** Asthma, GERD, protracted bronchitis, CHF, vascular rings, tracheomalacia, cystic fibrosis, bronchopulmonary dysplasia, vocal cord dysfunction
- **Workup:** Consider CXR, PFTs, pH probe, fluoroscopy, or bronchoscopy

Hemoptysis (see page 13-8 for additional information)
- Airway inflammation/infection, pneumonia, TB, tumor, trauma, idiopathic pulmonary hemosiderosis (IPH), Heiner syndrome (assoc w/ cow's milk), vasculitis (Wegener, Goodpasture, HSP, SLE), pulmonary HTN, pulmonary infarction, PE, AVMs, coagulopathies, complication in CF
- **Workup:** Rule out nasopharyngeal pathology and GI sources; CXR, CBC (including platelets), coags, ANA, ANCA, chest CT, bronchoscopy, nasopharyngoscopy, PPD, UA

Pleuritic Chest Pain (see page 13-9 for additional information)
- Pneumothorax, chest wall trauma, pneumonia, pleural effusion, pulmonary embolism, pericarditis, asthma
- **Workup:** EKG, chest x-ray, CT scan

Apnea (see page 13-11 for additional information)
- **Obstructive:** Obesity, tonsillar and adenoid hypertrophy, micrognathia, macroglossia, Pierre Robin sequence

- **Central:** Infection, intraventricular hemorrhage, shaken baby syndrome, apnea of prematurity, brainstem abnormalities, expiratory apnea, congenital or secondary central hypoventilation syndrome (Ondine's curse)
- **Workup:** Polysomnography (PSG), pneumogram, brain MRI, lateral neck films, nasopharyngoscopy

TACHYPNEA

Normal Respiratory Rates

	Infant (birth–1 yr)	Toddler (1–3 yr)	Pre-schooler (3–6 yr)	School aged (6–12 yr)	Adolescent (12–18 yr)
Breaths per min	30–60	24–40	22–34	18–30	12–16

Differential of Tachypnea
- Compensation for decreased tidal volume
  - Upper/lower airway obstruction, upper/lower respiratory infection, foreign body, restrictive lung disease or chest wall immobility, pain/splinting, fever
- Compensation for decreased oxygen supply
  - VQ mismatch: Pneumonia, pulmonary embolism, atelectasis
  - Decreased FiO_2: Altitude
  - Increased diffusion gradient: Pulmonary hypertension, interstitial lung disease
  - Shunt: Cardiopulmonary and intrapulmonary shunts
  - Anemia
- Compensation for metabolic acidosis
  - Sepsis, RTA, diabetic ketoacidosis, (MUDPILES)

Workup: CXR, CT, CBC with diff, glucose, nasopharyngoscopy, bronchoscopy, pulmonary function tests, lung biopsy

STRIDOR

Laryngomalacia (Pediatr Rev 2006;27:e33)
- Floppy tissue above vocal cords that falls into airway w/ inspiration
- Collapse of supraglottic structures (arytenoid cartilages and epiglottis) w/ inspiration
- **Epidemiology:** Most common cause of stridor in infants (~65–75% of all cases)
- **Clinical manifestations**
  - Symptoms appear during the first 2 mo of life; infant usually happy/thriving
  - Noises are inspiratory and may sound like nasal congestion
  - Exacerbated with crying, agitation, or during an upper respiratory infection
  - Prone position may diminish the stridor
- **Diagnostic studies:** History/physical, flexible laryngoscopy, and/or bronchoscopy
- **Prognosis**
  - Self-limited condition, usually resolves w/o Rx by 12–18 mo of age
  - In 10% of affected pts, upper airway obstruct severe enough to cause apnea or FTT; may have expiratory/biphasic stridor
  - May coexist with other airway malformations

When to refer: FTT, feeding difficulty, respiratory distress/apnea/hoarseness, cyanosis, atypical clinical course/persistent stridor, sleep disturbances
Interventions: Surgery: Supraglottoplasty, tracheostomy

Tracheomalacia (Pediatr Rev 2006;27:e33)
- Weakness of the airway cartilage that results in "floppiness" of airway
- Positive intrathoracic pressure can cause intrathoracic trachea to collapse and obstruct on expiration; extrathoracic trachea may collapse on inspiration
- May be secondary to compression to mediastinal mass or vascular rings/slings
- **History/exam**
  - Wheeze is often expiratory central, low pitched, and homophonous, possibly stridor
  - Unlike the wheezing heard in asthma (which tends to be diffuse, high pitched, and musical). Unlike asthma there are no signs of hyperinflation
  - Wheezing after β-agonist therapy remains unchanged or even worsens
  - Better in the prone position

- **Diagnosis:** H&P, CXR, chest CT with contrast, airway fluoroscopy, bronchoscopy
- **Prognosis:** Most improve spontaneously by 6–12 mo of age if primary tracheomalacia
- **Interventions**
  - Nasal CPAP can help maintain airway patency temporarily
  - Aortopexy or tracheostomy for long-term relief of obstruction
  - Treat coexisting conditions such as GERD; consider avoiding β-agonists; Atrovent

Croup (see ED section for evaluation and management of croup)
- **Laryngotracheobronchitis:** Inflammation & edema of subglottic larynx, trachea, bronchi
- Clinical diagnosis for acute onset of barky cough, stridor, and respiratory distress
- DDx for recurrent croup: Asthma, laryngomalacia, laryngospasm, subglottic stenosis

COUGH

Pneumonia
- Inflammatory condition of the lung affecting the alveoli typically associated with fever, respiratory symptoms, and consolidation on chest x-ray
- **Unilateral:** Bacterial – strep pneumo, aspiration (especially with RML), mycobacterial
- **Multifocal:** Atypical (mycoplasma), viral (RSV, paraflu, metapneumo, adeno)
- **Neonatal:** Afebrile more likely Chlamydia; febrile more likely GBS
- **Recurrent, same location:** Suggests anatomic abnormality: Foreign body or obstructive mass, CCAM, sequestration, focal bronchiectasis
- **Recurrent, different locations:** Aspiration, immunodeficiency, diffuse bronchiectasis (CF, primary ciliary dyskinesia), cardiac disease, pulmonary hypertension, underling interstitial lung disease
- **Workup:** CXR, CT with contrast (look for CCAM, sequestration, cardiac vessels) or without contrast (interstitial lung disease), fluoroscopy (diaphragmatic excursion), bronchoscopy (foreign body, airway mass, laryngeal cleft/aspiration), swallow study (aspiration), immunoglobulins and vaccine titer response (immune deficiency), PPD (if CXR or history is suggestive of TB)
- **Treatment:** See ID section for treatment of specific microbiology guidelines for pneumonia

Pertussis (http://www.cdc.gov/vaccines/pubs/pinkbook/pert.html)
- Highly contagious, toxin-mediated respiratory dz 2/2 the bacterium Bordetella pertussis
- **Symptoms:** Uncontrollable, violent coughing, after fits of many coughs sufferers often take deep breathes which result in a "whooping" sound, apnea in infants
- **Clinical course**
  - Incubation period: Commonly 7–10 d, with a range of 4–42 d
  - Catarrhal stage (1–2 wk): Characterized by coryza (runny nose), sneezing, low-grade fever, and mild cough
  - Paroxysmal stage (1–10 wk): Bursts of numerous, rapid coughs and difficulty expelling thick mucus; more common at night; post-tussive vomiting
  - Convalescent stage (wks to mos): Gradual recovery
  - 50% of infants <1 yr will be hospitalized; complications include pneumonia, convulsions, apnea, encephalopathy, and death
  - Adolescents and children partially protected by vaccine often have milder disease; inspiratory whoop is uncommon
- **Diagnosis**
  - Hx of cough for more than 2 wk with whoop, paroxysms, or post-tussive vomiting
  - Nasopharyngeal (NP) swab or aspirate for culture, PCR, &/or direct florescent assay
- **Treatment**
  - Primarily supportive
  - Antibiotics (azithromycin, erythromycin or trimethoprim–sulfamethoxazole) eradicate organism from secretion; decreasing communicability; may modify course of illness (if initiated early)
- **Epidemiology:** Incidence has been gradually increasing since the early 1980s
  - Children of parents who refuse pertussis immunizations are at higher risk for pertussis infection relative to vaccinated children (Pediatrics 2009;123:1446; JAMA 2000;284:3145)
  - State policies granting personal belief exemptions & states that easily grant exemptions are assoc w/ ↑ pertussis incidence (Amer J of Epi 2008;168:1389)
  - Geographic pockets of vaccine exemptors pose a risk to the whole community (JAMA 2006;296:1757)

Cystic Fibrosis

- Most common recessive genetic dz in Caucasians (1/25 carriers, 1/2,500 affected)
- **Pathophysiology**
  - CFTR gene mut (70% ΔF508) → ↓ [Cl] secretion, ↑ Na absorption across resp epithelium (reverse in sweat) → ↓ mucociliary clearance, viscous secretions, ↓ bacterial killing
  - Most important tissues affected: Airways, bile ducts, pancreatic ducts, & vas deferens
- **Physical exam:** Salty skin, weight loss, failure to thrive, wheezing, mid insp crackles, cough, clubbing, nasal polyps, steatorrhea
- **Diagnostic studies**
  - Sweat test (pilocarpine iontophoresis): Gold standard test > age 48 hr, need 2 separate tests to make dx, [Clsweat] >60 mEq/L is 95% specificity (J Pediatr 2008;153:S4)
  - Genetic testing
  - Stool collection for fecal elastase; nml >500 (indicator of pancreatic exocrine insuff)
  - PFTs: ↓ FEV1
  - CXR: Early – hyperinflated, patchy atelectasis. Late – bronchiectasis (upper lobes)
- **Management of lung disease** (BMJ 2007;335:1255)
  - Segregation to prevent spread of resistant organisms (especially *B. cepacia, P. aeruginosa,* MRSA)
- **Stage I:** Pre-infection
  - Airway clearance techniques: Chest PT, positive expiratory pressure (weak evidence)
  - Mucolytics: RhDNase (Cochrane Rev 2003;3:CD001127), hypertonic saline (New Eng J Med 2006;354:229)
  - Early eradication: Beneficial against P. aeruginosa (Cochrane Rev 2006;CD004197), uncertain benefit against S. aureus
  - Influenza vaccination
- **Stage II:** Chronic infection
  - Maintenance therapy (Am J Resp Crit Care Med 2007;176:957)
  - Airway clearance: Chest PT to keep airways open, facilitate mucus removal
  - Mucolytics, inhaled β_2-agonists (Cochrane Rev 2005;4:CD003428)
  - Eradication/reduction of bacterial load: Rx based on isolated organisms (i.e., *P. aeruginosa*: Inhaled tobramycin, colistin, cayston [aztreonam] (Cochrane Rev 2006:CD004197)
  - Reduce inflammation
    - Azithromycin (Cochrane Rev 2004;2:CD002203)
    - Ibuprofen, 20–30 mg/kg bid., goal serum peak 50 mcg/mL (J Pediatr 2007;151:249; Cochrane Rev 2007;4:CD001505)
    - Inhaled & oral corticosteroids w/o benefit unless treating asthma component
  - Acute exacerbations
    - Oral/inhaled antibiotics (tailor based on cultures/susceptibility, synergy studies useful for resistant organisms); common organisms include *P. aeruginosa,* non-typeable *H. influenza*
    - ABPA: Corticosteroids, antifungals
    - Atypical mycobacterial infxn: Ethambutol, rifampicin, azithromycin, amikacin
- **Stage III:** End stage, complicated CF
  - Severe hemoptysis: Bronchial artery embolization, lobectomy
  - Pneumothorax: Chest tube, pleurodesis (may complicate transplant)
  - Respiratory failure, heart failure 2/2 pulmonary HTN: Lung (+/– heart) transplantation
- **Extrapulmonary manifestations and management**
  - ENT: Nasal polyps (15%), recurrent sinusitis (~100%)
    - Nasal saline rinses, nasopolypectomy
  - GI: Meconium ileus (10%), distal ileal obstructive syndr (10–15%), rectal prolapse
    - Laxative, stool softeners. Pro-kinetic agents generally not helpful
  - GI: Pancreatic exocrine insuff (85%), chronic pancreatitis, Vit A, D, E, K def, malnut/FTT
    - Pancrelipase enzymes, A, D, E, K vitamins, high-fat/high-protein diet
    - Biliary cirrhosis (2%): Ursodiol
  - GI hyponatremia
    - Hydration, sodium chloride supplements
  - Endocrine: Pancreatic endocrine insufficiency (CF-related diabetes), osteopenia
    - Insulin, vitamin D
  - Reproductive: Male sperm transport defects (95% M infertility), amenorrhea/thick cervical mucus (20% F infertility)
    - In vitro fertilization
  - Renal: Renal failure (due to underlying abnormalities and accumulated renal toxicity of medications), kidney stones
    - Minimize renal toxicity, Urocit-K

WHEEZE

Asthma (EPR3: Guidelines for Diagnosis and Management of Asthma, NIH 2007)
- Chronic disorder of recurring symptoms resulting from airway inflammation, hyperresponsiveness, and obstruction
- **Important information to obtain in history**
  - Description of sx: Wheeze, nighttime cough, chest tightness, difficulty breathing
  - Pattern of symptoms: Continual/episodic, onset, duration, frequency
  - Precipitating/aggravating factors: Viral infection, environmental allergens (dust mites, cat/dog dander, cockroach, pollution), smoke exposure, exercise, emotion, meds (such as aspirin β-blockers), changes in environment, comorbid conditions (obesity, GERD, sinusitis, rhinitis)
  - Hx: # of hospitalizations, ICU admits, or intubations; age of dx; h/o prior airway injury (BPD, parental smoking, early PNA/RSV infection); meds used and compliance; need for oral corticosteroids and frequency of use; number of flares in last yr
  - Family history of atopy: Asthma, eczema, allergy, sinusitis, rhinitis, nasal polyps
  - Social history: Day care, social factors that may interfere w/ adherence, social supports, smoke exposure
  - Impact of asthma: Number of school days missed, limitations of activity
  - Assessment of patient's and family's perception of disease
  - Knowledge of asthma and Rx plan, ability to recognize severity of exacerbation
- **Examination**
  - Overall patient comfort, hyperinflated chest, accessory muscle use, wheeze or prolonged expiratory phase, nasal secretions or polyps, eczema
  - Respiratory rate & trend of respiratory rate is important; slowing can be sign of fatigue
- **Classification of asthma**

	Intermittent	Mild Persistent	Moderate Persistent	Severe Persistent
Sx or use of albuterol	<2/wk	>2 d/wk, but not daily	Daily	Throughout the day
Nighttime sx	0	1–2/mo	3–4/mo	>1/wk
Lung function	FEV_1 nml btw exacerbations FEV_1 >80% predicted	FEV_1 ≥80% predicted	FEV_1 = 60–80% predicted	FEV_1 <60% predicted
Management	Albuterol PRN	Low-dose ICS, cromolyn or montelukast	Medium-dose ICS, +/– LABA or montelukast	High-dose ICS and LABA or montelukast

ICS, inhaled corticosteroids; LABA, long-acting β-agonist.

- **Outpatient management of asthma**
  - Method of delivery, age of child, and ability to execute proper technique are important treatment considerations
  - Short-acting β-agonist: Albuterol (Proair, Proventil), levalbuterol (Xopenex). Mechanism: Bronchodilator. Side effects: Tachycardia, hypertension, tremor, nervousness, paradoxical bronchospasm, tachyphylaxis (with long-term use)
  - **Inhaled corticosteroids (ICS)** Budesonide (Pulmicort), fluticasone (Flovent), beclomethasone (Qvar), flunisolide, ciclesonide. Mechanism: Acts locally in the lungs to inhibit the inflammatory process. Side effects: Thrush (use spacer or valved holding chamber and rinse mouth with water to reduce the incidence), dysphonia/hoarseness (use spacer or valved holding chamber), reflex cough/bronchospasm (use spacer or valved holding chamber and slower rates of inspiration to reduce incidence), behavioral disturbances
    - Regular use of nebulized budesonide more effective than budesonide used only as needed (Arch Dis Child 2008;93:654–659)
    - Daily use of budesonide not superior to intermittent use in preschool children with wheezing (N Engl J Med 2011;365:1990)
    - Beclomethasone may be used as rescue plus albuterol as a step-down for children with mild asthma (Lancet 2011;377:650)
    - Doubling dose of ICS w/ URI not effective (J Allergy Clin Immunol 2011;128:278)
  - **Leukotriene inhibitors:** Montelukast (Singulair), zafirlukast (Accolate), & zileuton (Zyflo). Mechanism: Leukotriene receptor antagonists (LTRA) prevent leukotriene binding (montelukast/zafirlukast) or leukotriene receptor inhibitors (zileuton). Side effects: Elevated liver transaminases

- LTRAs provide modest improvement in lung fxn when used as monoRx in children as young as 5 & in asthma control outcomes (other than lung fxn) in pts as young as 2 (EPR3: *Guidelines for Diagnosis and Management of Asthma*, NIH 2007)
- Fluticasone vs. montelukast: Fluticasone more effective in improving pulmonary fxn, asthma symptoms, and rescue albuterol use (J Pediatr 2005;147:213–220)
- Montelukast can offer protection from exercise-induced bronchospasm (Treat Respir Med 2004;3:9; Ann Allergy Asthma Immunol 2001;86:655)
- **Long-acting β-agonist** (LABA) combined with ICS: Fluticasone/salmeterol (Advair), budesonide/formoterol (Symbicort). Mechanism: Long-acting bronchodilation. Side effects: Tachycardia, tremor
  - In adolescents & adults (not children), LABAs combined w/ low/med dose ICS may be beneficial for poorly controlled asthma (Cochrane Rev 2010;CD005533)
  - Black-box warning: Increased risk of death when LABA used alone, esp in African-American population (SMART, Chest 2006;129:15)
- **Tiotropium** (Spiriva): Mechanism: Anticholinergic, reduces smooth muscle contraction. Side effects: Hypersensitivity reaction, anticholinergic effects (dry mouth, urinary retention, blurred vision, mental status changes), constipation, thrush
  - Equivalent to fluticasone/salmeterol for step-up therapy in asthma (N Engl J Med 2010;363:1715)
- **Theophylline:** Mechanism: Methylxanthine, relaxes bronchial smooth muscle and anti-inflammatory. Side effects: Narrow therapeutic window, cardiac arrhythmias, seizures, tremors, agitation, nausea/vomiting, electrolyte abnormalities (hypokalemia and metabolic acidosis)
  - Oral xanthines as maintenance for pediatric asthma suitable in the absence of ICS or in conjunction w/ other therapies in severe asthma (Cochrane Rev 2006;CD002885)
- **Oral steroids** (Prednisolone, Prednisone): Mechanism: Anti-inflammatory. Side effects: Weight gain, hyperglycemia, mood changes, osteoporosis, adrenal insufficiency, immunosuppression, gastritis or ulcers, sodium/fluid retention & HTN
  - Used in acute setting in short bursts typically from 5 to 7 d–2 wk. More effective than inhaled steroids in severe acute asthma (N Engl J Med 2000;343:689)
  - Refractory asthma may require daily low-dose or alternate-day dose oral steroids
- **IgE mediators:** Omalizumab (Xolair) effective maintenance therapy for patients with severe, persistent asthma, which cannot be controlled even with high doses of corticosteroids. Mechanism: Recombinant DNA-derived humanized IgG1k monoclonal antibody that selectively binds to IgE. Side effect: Anaphylaxis, expensive (J Allergy Clin Immunol 2009;124:1210)
- **Cromolyn sodium** (Intal): Mechanism: Anti-inflammatory, mast cell stabilizer. Side effects: Non-specific
  - Inhaled corticosteroids more effective than cromolyn sodium for asthma control in adults and children (Cochrane Rev 2006;CD003558)
- **When to refer to pulmonologist**
- Patient has had a life-threatening asthma exacerbation
- Patient is not meeting the goals of asthma therapy after 3–6 mo of treatment
- Atypical signs and symptoms
- Complicating conditions (e.g., sinusitis, nasal polyps, aspergillosis, severe rhinitis, VCD, GERD, COPD)
- Need for additional diagnostic testing (e.g., allergy skin testing, rhinoscopy, complete pulmonary function studies, provocative challenge, bronchoscopy)
- Patient requires additional education and guidance on complications of therapy, problems with adherence, or allergen avoidance
- Patient is being considered for immunotherapy
- Patient has required more than two bursts of oral corticosteroids in 1 yr or has an exacerbation requiring hospitalization
- Patient has a history suggesting an occupational/environmental inhalant or ingested substance is provoking or contributing to asthma
- **Risk factors for status asthmaticus**
- Asthma history: Prior severe exacerbation: Intubation/PICU stay
- 2 or more hospitalizations for asthma or 3 or more ED visits for asthma in past yr, or hospitalization/ED visit for asthma in past mo
- Using >2 canisters/mo of inhaler
- Poor compliance/understanding
- Social history: Low SES, illicit drug use, psychosocial problems
- Comorbidities: Cardiovascular dz, other chronic lung dz, psychiatric dz

- **Management of status asthmaticus**
  - ABCs, medications (see below)
  - Consider NPPV or intubation (ketamine is the induction drug of choice) for persistent hypoxia/hypercarbia/WOB, altered mental status, FiO_2 >60%
  - Ventilation strategy: Treat obstruction/atelectasis, limit hyperinflation and barotrauma
    - Volume control preferred (ensures consistent min ventilation despite changing airway resistance)
    - Limit TV (8–10 cc/kg) & RR (8–12) w/ "permissive hypercapnia" (goal pH > 7.2)
    - Limit I-time (I:E 1.3–1.5) to allow complete exhalation and minimize auto-PEEP
    - Avoid paralysis
    - For refractory cases, consider inhalational anesthetics (e.g., isoflurane, halothane [bronchodilators of unknown mechanism] or ECMO)
- **Medications for status asthmaticus**

Name	Dose	Comments
Albuterol (β-agonist)	0.15 mg/kg neb q1h (2.5–5 mg) 10–15 mg/hr continuous minimum dose 2.5 mg	
Ipratropium	250–500 mcg neb × 3 then q2h prn	
Methylprednisolone anti-inflammatory	2–4 mg/kg/d PO div bid; 1 mg/kg IV q6h (max pedi 60 mg/d, adult 125 mg/d)	
$MgSO_4$: Inhibits Ca influx → bronchial smooth muscle relax	25–75 mg/kg IV (max 2 g)	Severe obstruction not responding to bronchodilators; unk effectiveness in less-severe cases (Chest 2002;122:489)
Terbutaline β2-agonist	10 mcg/kg IV load → 0.1–10 mcg/kg/min	Acute severe asthma not responding to bronchodilators
Aminophylline PDE inhibitor → smooth muscle relaxation	6 mg/kg IV load → 0.6–1.5 mg/kg/hr	Acute severe asthma not responding to bronchodilators. **Therapeutic level 10–20 mcg/mL (measure 6 hr post load). Risk tachycardia, arrhythmia, sz**
Heliox (80% He/20% O_2) Low density → reduced airway resistance	Nebulized (with or without bronchodilator)	Costly; no evidence for improved outcomes (PFTs, admits, need for intubation) may be beneficial in the most severe acute asthmatics. (Cochrane Rev 2003;(4):CD002884)

- **Complications**
  - Dynamic hyperinflation (auto-PEEP)
    - Progressive airtrapping → hyperinflation → alveolar rupture/hemodynamic compromise
    - To assess for auto-PEEP: Check plateau pressure (end-expiratory pressure = airway pressure; goal < 30), expiratory pause maneuver
  - Mechanical ventilation complications (PTX, HoTN, myopathy, VAP, GIB)
  - Prognosis: 2–3% mortality w/ mech ventilation (Crit Care Med 2002;30:581)

Bronchiolitis (Pediatrics 2006;118:1774)
- AAP Guidelines established for 1 mo–2 yo; excludes pt w/ immunodeficiencies or underlying lung or heart dz
- Swelling and mucus buildup in the smallest air passages in the lungs (bronchioles), usually due to viral infection
- **Pathophysiology**
  - Lower respiratory tract infection with acute inflammation, edema, and necrosis of epithelial cells lining small airways, inc mucus production, and bronchospasm
  - 2/2 viruses: RSV, human metapneumovirus, influenza, adenovirus, and parainfluenza, rhinovirus
- **History**
  - Assess for risk factors for severe disease: Age <12 wk, history of prematurity, underlying cardiopulmonary disease, or immunodeficiency
  - Viral URI prodromal symptoms, cough, wheeze, apnea
  - Ability to feed/remain hydrated, and ability of the family to care for the child
  - Response to any treatments
  - Prior episode of wheeze

- **Clinical manifestations**
  - Exam variable over time – need serial observations to assess
  - Rhinitis, tachypnea, use of accessory muscles, nasal flaring, grunting, apnea
  - Auscultation: Cough, crackles, wheezing
  - May have concomitant/secondary bacterial infxn: Pneumonia, acute otitis media, UTI
- **Diagnostic studies**
  - Pulse oximetry both awake and while sleeping
  - RSV viral test for cohorting patients
  - CXR, blood tests, urinalysis not typically recommended unless toxic or febrile
- **Treatment/course**
  - O_2 supplementation to keep O_2 >90%, IVF if dehydrated
  - Bulb suctioning of nares may provide some temporary relief
  - Hand washing/contact precautions, cohorting patients
- **Additional treatments**
  - Saline or hypertonic (3%) nebs: May cause bronchospasm; closely monitor response
  - Bronchodilators: 1 in 4 children treated with bronchodilators may have a transient improvement in clinical score, particularly if reactive component
  - Epi nebs: No effect on hospital stay/course of illness. (N Engl J Med 2003;349:27)
  - Corticosteroids: Not generally recommended, no difference in clinical scores or outcomes (Cochrane Rev 2008:CD004878)
  - Antibiotics: Not recommended unless secondary bacterial infection
  - Chest PT: Generally not recommended

HEMOPTYSIS

- Expectoration of blood that originated in the lungs or bronchial tubes
- **Differential**
  - Extrapulmonary: Oral, GI, epistaxis
  - Airways: Tracheobronchitis (most common cause), bronchiectasis (esp with CF), foreign body, tracheostomy related
  - Pulmonary parenchyma: PNA, cavitary lesions, tumor (often metastatic), trauma, TB
  - Pulmonary vasculature: IPH, Heiner syndrome (assoc w/ cow's milk), vasculitis (Wegener, Goodpasture, HSP, SLE), pulm HTN (arterial or venous), pulm infarction/ PE, AVMs, coagulopathies
- **Diagnostic studies**
  - Labs: CBC, ANA, anti-GBM, ANCA, U/A (eval for hematuria), BUN/Cr, PT/PTT, PPD
  - pH analysis of sample (hematemesis: ↓ pH vs. hemoptysis: ↑ pH)
  - Radiographic studies: CXR (patchy or diffuse alveolar opacities in DAH)
  - Consider helical chest CT
  - Consider echocardiography to r/o heart disease
  - Diagnostic procedures
  - Flex bronch/BAL: Hemosiderin-laden macrophages present from 3 d–wk after bleed
  - Open lung biopsy
- **Management**
  - Treat underlying cause once identified
  - Mild hemoptysis: No immediate treatment required
  - Massive hemoptysis: Provide O_2, decubitus position (w/ bleeding side down to promote oxygenation), selective intubation or main stem bronchus on nonbleeding side, bronchial artery embolization, rigid bronchoscopy, surgical resection

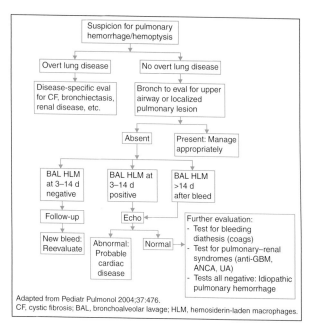

Adapted from Pediatr Pulmonol 2004;37:476.
CF, cystic fibrosis; BAL, bronchoalveolar lavage; HLM, hemosiderin-laden macrophages.

PLEURITIC CHEST PAIN

Pneumothorax (Pediatr Rev 2008;29:69)
- Air entering pleural space → pleural pressure → lung pressure → lung collapse
- **Pathophysiology**
  - Spontaneous: 1° (bleb rupture in young/tall/thin males; high-risk activities like diving/flying; smoking) or 2° (CF, abscess, TB, PCP, Marfan, Birt–Hogg–Dubé)
  - Traumatic: Lung puncture (trauma, thoracentesis, barotrauma from vent, CVC)
  - Tension: Tissues at point of air entry act as 1-way valve allowing air entry but no exit → eventually total lung/cardiac compression w/ hemodynamic collapse
- **Clinical manifestations**
  - Symptoms depend on baseline pulmonary status and PTX size: Sudden onset of SOB and pleuritic CP, hypoxia, absent or decreased BS on affected side
    - Small PTX (<15% of hemithorax) may have normal physical exam w/ only ↑ HR
    - Pain may radiate to ipsilateral shoulder
  - Tension PTX (life-threatening): Absent BS with tracheal/mediastinal shift away from affected side, JVD, hypotension, tachycardia, pulsus paradoxus
- **Diagnosis:** Exam and CXR (lat decubitus if not apparent on AP) or bedside ultrasound
  - Small PTX < 3 cm (space btw lung apex & ipsilateral dome of thoracic cavity)
- **Treatment**
  - Most reabsorb spontaneously in d to wks; follow w/ serial CXRs and vitals
  - Tension PTX (emergency): Immediate needle decompression followed by chest tube
  - Asymptomatic/small/1st occurrence: Obs, nitrogen washout (100% O_2) speeds absorb
  - Large/symptomatic/secondary occurrence: Chest tube insertion
  - VATS (w/ or w/o bullous resection/pleurodesis) considered for high-risk patients (divers, pilots), recurrent or bilateral PTX, or PTX not responding to other therapy
- **Prognosis:** 28–43% recurrence rate (2° > 1°, more common in smokers, tall/thin); VATS ↓ recurrence to 2–14%; 2° PTX tends to have worse course/outcome

Pleural Effusion (Pediatr Rev 2007;28:462; Pediatr Rev 2002;23:417)

- **Pathophysiology:** Fluid collection between visceral and parietal pleura
  - **Transudation:** Imbalance btw hydrostatic and oncotic forces with normal vasculature
    - CHF or pulmonary embolism → ↑ pulmonary venous pressure
    - Renal or liver dz → ↓ colloid osmotic pressure (can also see ascitic fluid; leakage across small defects in diaphragm)
  - **Exudation:** Secondary to leaky vasculature
    - Pneumonia, malignancy, connective tissue disorder → pleural inflammation, ↑ capillary permeability, at times w/ associated impaired lymphatic drainage
    - Parapneumonic effusions are the most common type of effusion
    - Exudative stage (uncomplicated): Protein-rich fluid 2/2 endothelial inflammation
      - Sterile fluid w/normal chemistries and PMN predominant
      - Fibropurulent stage: Bacterial growth; ↑ PMNs (↑ LDH), ↓ glucose &↑ lactic acid
      - Organization stage: Inc fibrin and collagen deposition w/ development of pleural "peel/rind" further impairing drainage
    - Most common organisms isolated = *Strep pneumoniae, Staph aureus* and GAS
    - Pleural-based metastasis in childhood: Nephroblastoma, Wilms tumor, hepatoblastoma, malignant germ cell tumors and rhabdomyosarcoma
  - **Thoracic duct:** Trauma or abnormality → ↓ lymphatic drainage (results in chylothorax; if above T5 results in L-sided chylothorax, if lower then R-sided)
    - Can be 2/2 congenital (Noonan, Turner, Down) or birth trauma (extension of spine)
- **Epidemiology** (Pediatr Rev 2002;23:417; Pediatr Emerg Care 2007;23:330)
  - PNA w/ parapneumonic effusion (50–70%) >> CHF (5–15%) > malignancy (5–10%)
  - Bacterial PNA most likely → effusion, viral & atypical infxn more common in kids
  - Empyema causes significant childhood morbidity but rarely causes death (3–6%)
  - Congenital chylothorax is the most common cause in newborns
- **Clinical manifestations** (Pediatr Rev 2002;23:417; Pediatr Emerg Care 2007;23:330)
  - If 2/2 PNA, cough, fever, chills SOB; w/o PNA often asymp until large then SOB
  - Can p/w sharp chest pain associated with inspiration or cough
  - Clinical exam w/ decreased breath sounds over area and dullness to percussion
  - Can note dec tactile fremitus and Hoover sign (lagging of chest wall movement)
  - Chest wall abscess and costal chondritis = empyema necessitatis
  - Early in development may hear a pleuritic friction rub (rare finding)
- **Diagnostic studies** (Pediatr Rev 2002;23:417)
  - CXR (PA, lat, and lat decub films with affected side down), ultrasound, chest CT (if loculation, empyema necessitatis, or malignancy is suspected)
  - Thoracentesis: For symptomatic relief or diagnostic evaluation
    - Precautions: Demonstrate layering on lateral decubitus film to ensure that fluid is not loculated (>10 mm fluid is safe for tap); best if done w/ U/S guidance
    - Standard studies: Cell count/diff, pH (send heparinized, on ice), glucose, total protein/albumin, LDH, Gram stain and culture, cytology; also send serum protein/albumin, LDH, and glucose for reference at the same time
    - Color can give info as well: Pale yellow → transudate; milky white → chyle; bloody → malignant, infectious, PE, or traumatic; chocolate brown → amebiasis
    - Other studies: Cholesterol & trigs (if suspect chylothorax), amylase (2/2 esophageal rupture), adenosine deaminase (>40 U/L is 90% sens for TB), IFN-γ (↑ in TB), serum NT proBNP (↑ in CHF) galactomannan (aspergillus), hemothorax if hematocrit of fluid >50% of serum hematocrit
- **Interpreting pleural fluid studies** (N Engl J Med 2002;346:843)

	Transudate	Exudate
Appearance	Serous, pale yellow	Cloudy, pus if empyema
Cell count	Few cells	WBC >10,000
pH	>7.45	<7.3
Glucose	>60 mg/dL	<60 mg/dL
Protein (pleural fluid)	<3 g/dL	≥3 g/dL
Protein: Fluid/serum[a]	<0.5	>0.5
Albumin: Serum–fluid	>1.2 g/dL	<1.2 g/dL
LDH[a]	Fluid/serum LDH <0.6	Fluid/serum LDH >0.6
	Absolute LDH <200 IU/mL	Absolute LDH >200 IU/mL
Cholesterol (fluid)	<45 mg/dL	>45 mg/dL

[a]Light's criteria.
Adapted from Ann Intern Med 1972;77:507.

- **Management** (Pediatr Emerg Care 2007;23:330)
  - Transudate: Diuresis (may increase concentration of pleural fluid, creating pseudoexudate), afterload reduction/inotropy, pleurodesis if refractory/recurrent
  - Exudate/parapneumonic effusion: Empiric antibiotics until susceptibilities known (3rd-gen cephalosporin, anti-staph covering MRSA), chest tube if complicated effusion (pH <7.2, LDH >1,000 U/mL, glucose <40 mg/dL, frank pus, + GS)
  - Surgical decortication for organized empyemas

APNEA

Apnea of Prematurity (NeoReviews 2007;8:e214, NeoReviews 2002;3:e59)
- Cessation of breathing >15 sec usually associated with desats and bradycardia. Characterized as obstructive, central, or mixed
- Occurs in 85% neonates less than 34 wk gestation; can persist up to 42 wk
- **Pathophysiology**
  - Immaturity of the central respiratory drive in response to hypercapnia, hypoxia and exaggerated inhibitory response to stimulation of airway receptors
  - Premature infants are predisposed to upper airway obstruction and desats during sleep due to poor airway stability
  - Periodic breathing: Benign condition consisting of regular, recurring cycles of breathing of 10–15 sec duration interrupted by pauses of at least 3 sec. More common in premature infants. Respiratory pauses are self-limited and ventilation continues. No treatment necessary
  - Apnea of infancy: Apnea that persists beyond 37 wk gestation
- **Diagnosis**
  - Often evident on continuous cardiorespiratory monitoring. Definitive diagnosis with pneumogram. Rule out infection
- **Treatment**
  - Supplemental O_2, nasal CPAP to prevent airway collapse and alveolar atelectasis
  - Caffeine (loading dose 20 mg/kg followed by maintenance of 5–10 mg/kg q24h) to stimulate CNS and respiratory muscle function
  - Consider treatment of GER

Central Apnea
- Pauses in respiration due to lack of signal from brain to initiate breath. Usually related to abnormality within brainstem or congenital
- **Causes**
  - Congenital central hypoventilation syndrome (CCHS, Ondine's curse). Associated with Hirschprung disease, neural crest tumors. Often due to PHOX2B mutation
  - Acquired central hypoventilation, such as a stroke or tumor of the brainstem
  - May be associated with cerebral palsy, tumors or other structural brainstem abnormality
- **Diagnosis**
  - Polysomnogram: Distinguishes obstruct vs. central apnea
  - Treatment: Bipap, tracheostomy and vent. Supplemental oxygen will treat desats with apnea but will not address ventilation

Obstructive Sleep Apnea (Arch Pediatr Adolesc Med 2005;159:775; Pediatrics 2002;109:704)
- Breathing disorder during sleep w/ prolonged partial upper airway obstruct and/or intermittent complete obstruct (obstructive apnea); disrupts ventilation and sleep
- Needs to be distinguished from 1° snoring, defined as snoring w/o obstructive apnea, frequent arousals from sleep, or gas exchange abnormalities
- **Clinical manifestations**
  - Chronic snoring, daytime fatigue/sleepiness, sleepwalking/-talking, enuresis, periodic limb movement, headaches
  - Mouth breathing, nasal obstruct w/ wakefulness, adenoidal facies, hyponasal speech
  - Neurocognitive deficits: Poor learning, behavioral problems, ADHD
- **Risk factors:** Adenotonsillar hypertrophy, obesity, craniofacial anom, neuromuscular d/o
- **Diagnosis**
  - PSG: Can distinguish 1° snoring from OSAS, assess severity and stratify patients likely to have post-tonsillectomy complication, allows titration to optimal level of CPAP

- **Treatment**
  - Weight loss
  - Adenotonsillectomy: The most common treatment for children with OSAS. Resolution occurs in 75–100% after adenotonsillectomy
  - CPAP: Used indefinitely
  - Surgery: Mandibular extraction, hypoglossal nerve stimulation
- **Complications**
  - Neurocognitive impairment, behavioral problems, FTT, cor pulmonale
  - Metabolic sequelae (HTN, insulin resistance, dyslipidemia) in obese children
  - Caution with sedation, surgery–increased risk of airway compromise. Risk of post-obstructive pulmonary edema following T&A

DIAGNOSTIC STUDIES

Pulmonary Function Tests
- **Basic spirometry with lung volumes**
  - **Indications:** Evaluate dysfunction – obstructive, restrictive, or mixed; location; degree of progression of known disease; response to bronchodilators
  - **Relative contraindications:** Hemoptysis of unknown origin, pneumothorax, recent eye surgery (as there is increased intraocular pressure during forced expiratory maneuvers)

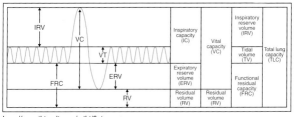

http://en.wikipedia.org/wiki/Spirometry

Parameter	Normal	Obstructive	Restrictive
FVC	≥80% predicted	↔↓	↓↓
FEV1	≥80% predicted	↓↓ bronchodilator responsive: ↑12% or 0.2 L)	↔↓
FEV1/FVC	85% for 8–19 yo	↓↓	↔↓
RV		↑↑	↓↓ (early)
TLC		↑↑ or normal	↓↓
RV/TLC		↑↑	↓↓

FVC, max volume expired during forced expiratory maneuver; **FEV1**, volume expired in 1st second after a deep inspiration; **FEV1/FVC**, measure of airflow obstruction; **FEF25–75**, mid flow rate of FVC (reflects small airways obstruction, less effort dependent, but highly variable); **DLCO**, diffusion capacity of CO; **PEFR**, peak expiratory flow rate.

Normal pattern

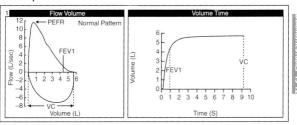

Obstructive pattern: Asthma, bronchiectasis, cystic fibrosis

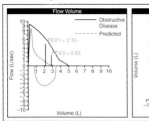 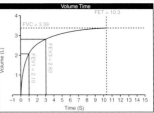

Restrictive pattern: Thoracic (ILD, pneumothorax, edema, consolidation, fibrosis) and extrathoracic (obesity, resp muscle weakness, neuromuscular weakness, thoracic deformities, pleural disease)

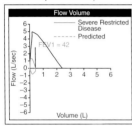 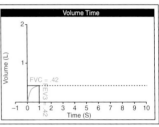

- **Diffusion capacity**
  - **Indications:** Eval for parenchymal dz (DLCO measures "efficiency" of gas exchange)
  - DLCO dependent on TLC and Hgb; any process that ↓ them will ↓ DLCO as well
  - ↓ DLCO can be 2/2: Parenchymal or pulm vascular dz, extrapulm restriction (lung resection, scoliosis), anemia (adjust for Hgb mathematically), tachycardia
  - ↑ DLCO can be 2/2 pulmonary hemorrhage
- **Bronchial provocation testing**
  - **Indication:** Suspect asthma, but spirometry normal, exercise-related symptoms
  - **Procedure:** Spirometry before/after progressive doses of methacholine, histamine, exercise, mannitol, or hyperventilation/cold air
  - **Positive test:** FEV1 reduced 20% after challenge
- **Respiratory muscle strength**
  - **Indication:** Rule out muscle weakness as a cause for respiratory insufficiency
  - **Procedure:** Pt breathes against shutter valve, measure max inspiratory pressure (MIP) and max expiratory pressure (MEP); perform at least 10× for consistency
  - **Implications:** Compare to age norms, MEP <50 cm H_2O suggests insuff cough to clear secretions; MIP <−80 and MEP >+80 cm H_2O r/o signif weakness (adults) (Thorax 1984;39:535)

- Cough into peak flow meter; may need face mask if facial muscle weakness
- **Indications:** Neuromuscular disease; assess for effective cough
- **Findings**
  - >270 L/min effective cough
  - 160–270 L/min. Introduce cough assist device w/ goal of raising cough peak flow to >270 L/min
  - <160 L/min cough ineffective to clear secretions and will need assistance, such as cough assist device, to aid clearance of secretions daily, or more frequently during times of respiratory illness

Bronchoscopy
- **Flexible bronchoscopy:** Dynamic view of airways with ability to reach lower airways, often done in conjunction with bronchoalveolar lavage, endo- or transbronchial biopsy, bronchial brushings

- **Indications:** Unexplained/persistent cough, persistent wheeze, persistent or recurrent pneumonia, dyspnea, aspiration, hemoptysis, foreign body, persistent infiltrate, atelectasis, or other radiologic changes
- **Findings:** Malacia or floppiness of airways, compression by vascular ring or extraluminal mass, narrowing by intraluminal mass, mucous, nodularity, tracheal bronchus (aka pig bronchus, bronchus suis), airway hemangioma, tracheoesophageal fistula, laryngeal clefts, subglottic stenosis, foreign body
- **BAL analysis:** Cell count and differential, cultures (bacterial, mycobacterial, fungal, viral), cytology (lipid-laden macrophages or hemosiderin-laden macrophages)
- **Rigid bronchoscopy:** Visualize the oropharynx, larynx, vocal cords, and tracheal bronchial tree; large lumen facilitates suctioning and the removal of debris, or for interventional procedures such as insertion of airway stents
  - **Indications:** Bleeding or hemorrhage, foreign body extraction, dilation of tracheal or bronchial strictures, relief of airway obstruction in trachea or proximal bronchus, insertion of stents, mechanical tumor ablation

Sweat Test
- Collection of sweat with pilocarpine iontophoresis and by chemical determination of the chloride concentration
- DNA testing is used for confirmation of patients with intermediate sweat chloride results and for prognostic and epidemiologic purposes
- **Indications**
  - Infants with positive CF newborn screening results
  - Infants with symptoms suggestive of CF (e.g., meconium ileus)
  - Older children and adults with symptoms suggestive of CF
  - Siblings of a patient with confirmed CF
- **Findings**
  - For infants under 6 mo
    - ≤29 mmol/L: Normal (CF very unlikely)
    - 30–59 mmol/L: Intermediate (possible CF)
    - ≥60 mmol/L: Abnormal (diagnosis of CF)
  - For infants >6 mo, children, and adults
    - ≤39 mmol/L: Normal (CF very unlikely)
    - 40–59 mmol/L: Intermediate (possible CF)
    - ≥ 60 mmol/L: Abnormal (diagnosis of CF)

Polysomnography (Sleep Med Clin 2009;4:393)
- **Indications:** Obstructive or central sleep apnea, neuromuscular disease, chronic lung disease, cpap titration, trach decannulation, parasomnias
- **Parameters measured:** EEG, EMG (mandible, tibial), electrooculogram, ECG, nasal pressure, oronasal airflow, end tidal CO_2, pulse oximetry, chest and abdominal wall motion, body position, audio and video
- **Central apnea:** Apnea >20 sec or assoc with 3% desat
- **Obstructive apnea:** Airflow obstruction despite resp effort lasting 2 breaths, associated with arousal or 3% desat
- **Hypopnea:** 50% reduction in airflow × 2 breaths with associated arousal or 3% desat
- **Apnea–hypopnea index (AHI):** 5–15/hr = Mild; 15–30/hr = Moderate; & >30/hr = Severe

Pneumogram
- **Indications:** Infants with significant apnea or bradycardia or at risk for ALTE. Can distinguish between central, obstructive, and mixed apnea. May be used in conjunction with pH probe to diagnose reflux
- **Parameters measured:** Typically 12–24 hr of continuous monitoring of HR, breathing effort, respiratory airflow, pulse oximetry, esophageal pH probe

URINALYSIS

Evaluation (Pediatr Clin North Am 2006;53:325)

Urine Dipstick Test Finding	Nonpathologic Causes	Pathologic Causes
Specific gravity (low)	Polydipsia	DI, renal tubular dysfunction
Specific gravity (high)	Dehydration	Volume depletion
pH (low)	High-protein diet	Acidosis
pH (high)	Low-protein diet; recent meal	RTA (inappropriate renal response); UTI (i.e., *Proteus*)
Blood present (can represent RBCs, Hgb, myoglobin)	Menses, traumatic catheterization, exercise	Glomerular d/o, tubular d/o, UTI, stones, hyperCa, urinary tract trauma, tumor, rhabdo, hemolysis
Protein present	Orthostatic proteinuria, fever, exercise	Glomerular disorders, tubular disorders, UTI
Glucose present	Renal glycosuria (SGLT2 transporter defect)	Diabetes mellitus, Fanconi anemia
Ketones	Restricted carbohydrate intake	Diabetes mellitus starvation, EtOH
Bilirubin present	None	Hepatitis, biliary obstruction
Urobilinogen present	Low amounts: Systemic abx rx	Hepatitis, intravascular hemolysis
Nitrite present	None	UTI (Enterobacteriaceae only)
LE present (from PMNs)	Fever	UTI, glomerulonephritis, pelvic inflamm, sterile pyuria

- Urine protein/Cr ratio correlates w/ total daily protein excretion based on g/1.73 m^2 BSA. Low Cr in cachectic child or ↓ muscle mass (e.g., myopathy, myelomeningocele) may overestimate ratio. Nml ratio <0.2 mg protein/mg Cr
- Urine albumin/Cr ratio correlates w/ excretion of albumin in timed sample. Ratio >30 mg/g Cr abn. Nml albumin excretion <20 mg/d, and microalbuminuria defined as 30–300 mg/d, and not typically detected on U/A
- Urine calcium/Cr ratio correlated w/ excretion of Ca^{++} in a timed sample. Nml ratio depends on age; in school-aged children and adolescents, it should be <0.21

ACUTE KIDNEY INJURY (AKI)

Definition (Adolesc Med Clin 2005;16:1)
- Sudden onset, inadeq renal fxn to clear metab waste, maintain nml fluid and electrolyte balance. May be oliguric (30%; <1 cc/kg/hr for infants) or nml to ↑'d urine output (70%)

Epidemiology (Pediatr Rev 2009;24:253; Am J Kidney Dis 2005;45:96)
- Epidemiology of renal failure changed in face of advances in pediatric ICU care, ↑ assoc w/ congenital heart surgery and pediatric oncology/bone marrow transplantation
- Retrospective review at 3° care pedi hospital w/ most common causes AKI to be renal ischemia (21%), nephrotoxic medications (16%), and sepsis (11%)
- In developing countries, 3 most common causes of AKI are: Hemolytic–uremic syndrome (31%), glomerulonephritis (23%), prerenal ischemia (18%)

Etiology (Pediatr Rev 2009;24:253; Adolesc Med Clin 2005;16:1)
- **Prerenal:** Renal hypoperfusion (intravasc volume loss 2/2 dehydration, trauma, capillary leak from sepsis/burns/nephrotic syndrome, poor cardiac function)
- **Postrenal:** Structural/obstructive causes (rare, 2/2 pelvic mass or ureteral obstruct)
- **Intrinsic renal:** Underlying kidney injury or dz
  - Endogenous toxins: Hgb, myoglobin, or uric acid in tumor lysis
  - Exogenous toxins: NSAIDs, abx, antifungals, chemo, contrast, ACE-I in some
  - Allergic rxn/interstitial nephritis
  - Infxn: Pyelo, postinfectious syndromes, such as poststreptococcal GN or HUS
  - Immune-mediated vasculitides: SLE, polyarteritis, Wegener, Goodpasture
  - Vascular; renal artery or vein thrombosis of a single or transplanted kidney

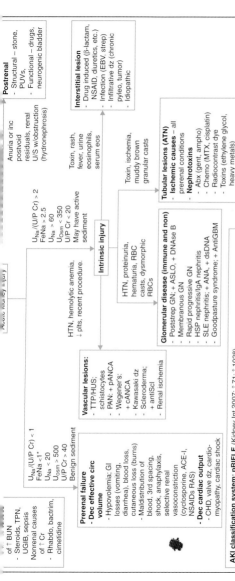

of ↑ BUN
- Steroids, TPN,
UGIB, sepsis
Nonrenal causes
of ↑ Cr
- Rhabdo, bactrim,
cimetidine

Acute kidney injury

Prerenal failure
- **Dec effective circ volume**
  - Hypovolemia: GI losses (vomiting, diarrhea), blood loss, cutaneous loss (burns)
  - Maldistribution of blood, 3rd spacing, shock, anaphylaxis, selective renal vasoconstriction (cyclosporine, ACE-I, NSAIDs RAS)
- **Dec cardiac output**
  - CHD, valve dz, cardiomyopathy, cardiac shock

U_{Na} (U/P Cr) < 1
FeNa <1*
U_{Na} < 20
U_{Osm} > 500
U/P Cr > 40
Benign sediment

HTN, hemolytic anemia,
↓ plts, recent procedure.

Intrinsic injury

U_{Na} (U/P Cr) > 2
FeNa > 2.5
U_{Na} > 60
U_{Osm} < 350
U/P Cr < 20
May have active sediment

Vascular lesions:
- TTP/HUS; schistocytes
- PAN; + pANCA
- Wegener's: + cANCA
- Kawasaki dz
- Scleroderma; + antiScl
- Renal ischemia

HTN, proteinuria,
hematuria, RBC
casts, dysmorphic
RBCs

Glomerular disease (immune and non)
- Poststrep GN; + ASLO; ↑ DNAse B
- Membranous GN
- Rapid progressive GN
- HSP nephritis/IgA nephritis
- SLE nephritis; + ANA, + dsDNA
- Goodpasture syndrome; + AntiGBM

Toxin, rash,
fever, urine
eosinophils,
serum eos

Interstitial lesion
- Drug induced (β-lactam, NSAID, diuretics, etc.)
- Infection (EBV, strep)
- Infiltrative dz (chronic pyelo, tumor)
- Idiopathic

Toxin, ischemia,
muddy brown
granular casts

Tubular lesions (ATN)
- **Ischemic causes** – all prerenal conditions
- **Nephrotoxins**
  - Abx (gent, ampho)
  - Chemo (MTX, cisplatin)
  - Radiocontrast dye
  - Toxins (ethylene glycol, heavy metals)
  - Pigment – Hgb, myoglobin

Anuria or inc
postvoid
residuals, renal
U/S w/obstruction
(hydronephrosis)

Postrenal
- Structural – stone, PUVs
- Functional – drugs, neurogenic bladder

* Other causes of FeNa <1%; Vascular occlusion, glomerulonephritis, vasculitis, early postrenal failure, pigment nephropathy, radiocontrast nephropathy, hepatorenal syndrome

AKI classification system: pRIFLE (Kidney Int 2007; ↑ 71; ↑ 1028)
- **R:** Risk for renal dysfunction; eCrCl ↓ by 25%; UOP < 0.5 mL/kg/hr for 8 hr
- **I:** Injury to kidney; eCrCl ↓ by 50%; UOP < 0.5 mL/kg/hr for 16 hr
- **F:** Failure of kidney; eCrCl ↓ by 50% or < 35 mL/min/1.73 m², UOP < 0.3 mL/kg/hr for 24 hr or anuric × 12 hr
- **L:** Loss of kidney function; Persistent failure > 4 wk
- **E:** End stage renal disease: Persistent failure > 3 mo

AKI 14-2

Diagnostic Evaluation (Pediatr Rev 1995;16:101; Pediatr Rev 2002;23:47)
- Complete H&P focused on narrowing the above differential
- Initial labs: U/A w/ microscopy & culture, CMP, CBC, sediment
- Fractional excretion (FE) Na = (PCr × UNa)/(BUN × UCr) (inaccurate w/ diuretics)
  - PCr is plasma conc of Cr; PNa is plasma conc of Na
  - UCr is urinary conc of Cr and UNa is urinary conc of Na
  - FENa <1%; ↓ renal perfusion, w/ hypovolemia, low cardiac output states
  - FeNa >2%; spilling Na, makes intrinsic renal dz more likely (i.e., ATN)
- FE urea − (PCr × UUN)/(BUN × UCr); <35–40% prerenal (use if on diuretics)
- Glomerular filtration rate (mL/min/1.73 m²) calculated as length (cm) × (K/plasma Cr conc), (K is coefficient 0.413 via the Schwartz formula); more often used for CKD
  - Creatinine clearance (CrCl) is a surrogate marker of GFR
- Consider: Albumin, cholesterol, serum complement, antinuclear Ab, streptococcal serologies, blood and stool cultures, toxicology screen
- Imaging may include ultrasound, CT, MRI/MRA; biopsy may be indicated

Therapy (Adolesc Med Clin 2005;16:1; Pediatr Rev 2009;24:253)
- Etiology dependent; please see sections on specific dx under proteinuria/hematuria
- Diuretics do not alter course of AKI, need for renal replacement or mortality; no data for benefit of dopamine (though fenoldopam, a dopamine-1 R agonist, may have a role)
- Monitor BP, volume status, serum chemistries (specifically hyperkalemia) and acid–base status (specifically, AKI produces metabolic acidosis)
- Avoid nephrotoxic agents and dose all meds according to estimated CrCl
- Renal replacement Rx (dialysis, CVVH) indicated for life-threatening and treatment unresponsive **A**cid–base disturbance, **E**lectrolyte abn, toxin **I**ngestion, volume **O**verload, & complications of **U**remia (pericarditis, encephalopathy), aka **AEIOU**

Prognosis (Arch Pediatr Adolesc Med 2002;156:893)
- Dependent on etiology, worse if multiorgan involvement; >50% mortality if ≥3 organs are involved; ~10% ped pts w/ AKI develop CKD in 1–3 yr (Am J Kidney Dis 2012;59:523)

CHRONIC KIDNEY DISEASE

Definition (Pediatr Rev 2008;29:335)
- CKD now classified as any kidney damage or GFR <60 mL/min/1.73 m² for >3 mo
- KDOQI Group classified CKD into 5 stages. Stage 1: Kidney damage w/ nml/↑ GFR (>90). Stage 2: ↓ GFR to 60–89. Stage 3: ↓ GFR to 30–59. Stage 4: ↓ GFR to 15–29. Stage 5: Kidney failure w/ GFR <15. All GFR in mL/min/1.73 m² and for pts >2 yo

Etiology (Pediatr Rev 2008;29:335)
- ~30–33% w/ urologic anomalies, 25–27% w/ glomerulopathies, 16% w/ hereditary nephropathies and ~11% w/ renal hypoplasia and dysplasia

Complications (Pediatr Rev 2008;29:335; Pediatr Nephrol 2003;18:796)
- Infections prompt 45% of hospital admissions in one series
- Other complications include: Anemia (keep Hgb 11–12 mg/dL w/ Fe & Epo), HTN, bone disease (rx'd w/ Vit D), electrolyte abn (met acidosis rx'd w/ NaBicarb, hyperK)
- Growth retardation is a major complication; degree matches age of onset of CKD, likely 2/2 effect on GH & IGF-1 axis; treatment w/ nutritional support +/– GH therapy

Prognosis (Pediatr Nephrol 2008;23:705; J Am Soc Nephrol 2016;27:96)
- CKiD is large prospective cohort study of pts aged 1–16 yr to identify risk factors for progression and the effect of ↓ GFR on cognition, growth, behavior, cardiovasc risk factors (Clin J Am Soc Nephrol 2006;1:1006)
- Intensive (50th percentile) BP control w/ ACE-I slows GFR ↓ (N Engl J Med 2009;361:1639)
- Proteinuria, low Hct, hypoalbuminemia, hypoCa, hyperphos, hyperPTH all assoc w/ rate of progress to ESRD, as is age at dx and the dx itself
- Rx of anemia, hypoCa, and hyperphos leads to improved outcomes in the short term
- Glomerular disorders, including FSGS, increase risk of progression to ESRD
- Cardiac and vascular abn (LVH, diastolic dysfxn, ↑ carotid intima-media thickness, Mönckeberg sclerosis) are progressive and may be related to ↑ calcium–phosphorus product (Nat Rev Nephrol 2011;7:624)

Management (N Engl J Med 2009;361:1639; Curr Opin Pediatr 2010;22:170)
- ESCAPE trial, fixed-dose ACE-inhibitor + additional anti-hypertensives to ↓ BP 3–4 mm Hg
- R-A blockade may also benefit by ↓ proteinuria, correction of acidosis, hyperuricemia
- W/ Stage V CKD ultimate management is renal transplantation

SECONDARY HYPERTENSION

Definitions (Pediatr Rev 2007;28:283; Pediatrics 2004;114(2 Suppl, 4th Report):555; JAMA 2003;289:2560)
- 2° HTN (BP >95th percentile for age and ht) – ↑ BP 2/2 underlying, identifiable cause
- Stage 1 = BP at 95th %ile – 5 mm Hg above 99th %ile; Stage 2 = BP >5 mm Hg above 99th %ile
- Hypertensive urgency = HTN w/o severe sx or evidence of end organ damage
- Hypertensive emergency = HTN w/ severe sx + evidence of end organ damage (in children, retinopathy, encephalopathy—lethargy, coma, sz—more common than CHF, pulmonary edema) (Arch Dis Child 1992;67:1089)

Etiology & Dx (Nat Rev Cardiol 2010;7:155; Pediatr Rev 2007;28:283)
- Evaluation begins with thorough H&P & exam. 75% cases 2/2 renal parenchymal dz
- Hypertensive emergency in children is most likely renal in origin
- **Meds** (amphetamines, corticosteroids, OCP, cyclosporine, others) can cause HTN
- **Renovascular disease** (may be assoc w/ high renin levels but not a consistent finding)
  - Ultrasonography can show decreased flow; renal arteriography is "gold standard"
  - MRA, CTA, and captopril-MAG 3 scanning each have strengths and limitations
- **Renal parenchymal disease** (evidence of glomerular or tubular dysfxn, dec GFR)
  - US shows size, location, echogenicity. Scarring can cause HTN and is a more common cause of 2° hypertension than glomerulonephritis
  - **Renal scarring** occurs 2/2 multiple, often overlapping etiologies; congenital dysplasia, vesicoureteral reflux, and infxn. Regardless etiology, scarring is prerequisite to develop HTN as sequelae (J Urol 2005;173:697)
- 5–44% of children with **ADPKD** have secondary HTN (Lancet 2007;369:1287)
- **Steroidogenic enzyme defects** (11-β-hydroxylase def, 11-α-hydroxylase def), hyperaldo, apparent mineralocorticoid excess, and nonsteroidal defects (Liddle syndrome, Gordon syndrome) can be assoc w/ low renin levels
- Cardiovascular disorders (**coarctation, midaortic syndrome**); 4 extremity blood pressures, differential cyanosis, echocardiography can be diagnostic
- Other: Umbilical artery catheterization, collagen vascular dz, SLE, hyper-/hypothyroid, Williams syndrome (and assoc renal vasc dz), Turner syndrome (and assoc coarctation), Cushing syndrome (and assoc steroid excess), neurofibromatosis (renovasc HTN, pheochromocytoma), lower extremity traction
- Possible assoc exists btw hyperuricemia and HTN (uric acid >5.5 mg/dL found in 89% of children w/ essential HTN but 30% 2° HTN); mechanism unknown

Therapy (Pediatr Nephrol 2009;24:1101; Pediatr Rev 2007;28:283)
- Based on underlying etiology
- Hypertensive urgency – tx w/i hours
- Hypertensive emergency – must continually monitor BP & avoid excessively rapid reduction (↓ 1/3 of tot reduction in 6 h, 2/3 tot by ~24 h, to maintenance by ~48–72 h) using short-acting agents (labetalol, nicardipine most studied, no agents proven in children)
- See Cardiology Chapter and (J Pediatr 2006;149:746) on treatment of hypertension

HEMATURIA, NEPHRITIC SYNDROMES

Definition (Pediatr Clin North Am 2001;48:1519)
- Macroscopic hematuria is visible to the naked eye (Pediatr Clin North Am 1997;44:1191)
- Microscopic hematuria definitions vary by study, >5–10 RBCs/high-power, midstream collection (Adolesc Med Clin 2005;16:229)

Epidemiology (Pediatrics 1977;59:557; J Pediatr 1979;95:676)
- Macroscopic hematuria has an estimated incidence of 1.3 per 1,000
- Prevalence of microscopic hematuria 0.5–2% depending on population—incidence of microscopic hematuria 0.32% in girls and 0.14% of boys

Etiology (Urol Clin North Am 2004;31:559)
- In 342 children w/ **asymptomatic microscopic hematuria:** 81% idiopathic, 16% hyperCa, 1% PSGN; of 228 children w/ **gross hematuria:** 38% idiopathic, 22% hyperCa, 15% IgA nephropathy, 4% structural abnormalities (Arch Pediatr Adolesc Med 2005;159:353)
- Mimics include meds (chloroquine, iron, isoniazid, rifampin), foods (beets, blackberry), pigments/toxins (**bile, hemoglobinuria, myoglobinuria,** lead, phenol, porphyria, urates)

- **Glomerular dz:** Recurrent gross hematuria (IgA nephropathy, benign familial hematuria, Alport syndrome), acute postinfectious GN (PIGN), membranoproliferative GN (MPGN), SLE, membranous nephropathy (MN), rapidly progressive GN (RPGN), Henoch–Schönlein purpura, Goodpasture dz
- **Interstitial and tubular Dz:** Acute pyelonephritis, acute interstitial nephritis, TB, hematologic (sickle-cell dz, coagulopathies including von Willebrand dz, renal vein thrombosis, thrombocytopenia), meds (AGs, NSAID, amitriptyline, anticonvulsants, chlorpromazine, coumadin, cyclophosphamide, diuretics, PCN, thorazine)
- **Urinary tract:** Bacterial or viral (adenovirus) infxn related, urolithiasis and hypercalciuria, structural anomalies (including polycystic kidney disease), trauma, tumor, exercise

Evaluation (Urol Clin North Am 2004;31:559)
- Careful history and physical examination, including family history
- **Macroscopic hematuria w/o significant proteinuria or RBC casts: Likely non-glomerular bleeding;** requires urine cx (exclude infxn), renal & bladder U/S (exclude malig or cystic renal dz), CT (urolithiasis), &/or cystoscopy (exclude malig, other process)
- **Hematuria plus any of the following is suggestive of glomerulonephritis:** Edema, HTN, significant proteinuria. Initial eval: CBC (HUS), CMP, sediment, throat cx, streptozyme panel, & complement levels (PIGN)
- See Proteinuria section for eval and Rx of disorders, for which this is a primary feature

Dx & Management of Specific Disorders (Urol Clin North Am 2004;31:559)
- **Postinfectious GN:** Up to 7–21 d after inciting infxn, often skin or soft tissue
  - Infxn w/ Group A *Strep* or other infections; w/ supportive care, excellent prognosis
  - Dark, tea-colored urine is common
  - Pts can be asymptomatic, or have malaise, fatigue, HTN, edema, or oliguria
  - C3 levels low during illness, improve over 6–8 wk
  - Antistreptolysin O titers may be neg at first, streptozyme pos w/i 10 d
- **Henoch–Schönlein purpura:** (See Rheumatology chapter) w/ renal involvement ~50% cases, extent variable (proteinuria, hematuria, nephrotic syndr, glomerulonephritis, AKI)
  - Relapses can occur, long-term prognosis depends on degree of renal compromise
- **IgA nephropathy** common cause hematuria, path w/ mesangial deposition of IgA
  - Poor prognostic indicators: HTN, nephrotic range proteinuria, renal insufficiency
  - Controversy exists regarding utility of biopsy
- **Rapidly progressive glomerulonephritis:** AKI, glomerular crescents on biopsy
  - **EMERGENCY:** Need prompt Rx w/ pulse steroids, can still progress to ESRD w/i wks. Aggressively pursue/address underlying condition

URINARY TRACT CALCULI

Epidemiology (Kidney Int 2011;80:1278)
- Nephrolithiasis accounts for 1 in 1,000 to 1 in 7,500 pediatric hospital admissions
  - Prevalence ↑ ing in US, Caucasians more affected than AAs (J Pediatr 2010;157:132)
  - Stone recurrence 6.5–54%, time to recurrence 3–6 yr (Urol Clin North Am 2004;31:575)
  - Metabolic disorders increase the rate of stone formation

Clinical Manifestations (Urol Clin North Am 2004;31:575)
- P/w abd/flank/pelvic pain (50%), hematuria (33%), incidental radiology findings (15%), infection (11%); younger children (<5 yo) more likely p/w radiographic findings and infection than older children
  - Family history of stones is present in 37% of pediatric patients
  - In US, 75% of pediatric stones are renal, 10% ureteral, 10% bladder

Etiology (Kidney Int 2011;80:1278; J Urol 2002;167:670)
- >75% urinary tract calculi in US. Ca-oxalate or Ca-phos; infectious stones 15–25%
  - Metabolic or urinary tract abn account for 30–50% of pts w/ urinary tract calculi
  - Hypercalciuria w/ or w/o hypercalcemia most common cause (34%) of pedi urolithiasis
    - Genetic hypercalciuria causes: Familial idiopathic hypercalciuria, distal RTA, Bartter syndrome, hypercalciuria/hypomagnesemia, Dent disease
  - Other causes: Uric acid urolithiasis (as in ketogenic diet, lymphoproliferative disorders, some inborn errors of metabolism), struvite stones (infectious), cystinuria (2–7%), hyperoxaluria (i.e., Crohn's), hypocitraturia
  - Acidic urine promotes formation of calcium oxalate, uric acid, and cystine stones
  - Alkaline urine promotes formation of struvite and calcium phosphate stones

- Serum: CBC, Chem10, alk phos, uric acid, PTH, Vit D (25-OH and 1,25-OH₂)
- Urine studies: U/A w/ pH, urine cx; 24 hr urine for Ca++, Phos, Mg, oxalate, Na, uric acid, citrate, cystine, Cr, volume (spot measure 2–4 hr after milk if child is not toilet trained)
- Stone analysis
- Radiography: Noncontrast helical CT most sens for urolithiasis; ↓ radiation dose by routine surveillance in asymp children w/ flat plate plain films & renal U/S
  - Radiation from stone protocol CT at MGH equivalent to 4.5 KUBs

Therapy and Prognosis (Urol Clin North Am 2004;31:575)
- At all ages, ureteral stones ≥5 mm rarely pass w/o help; may need intervention
- Pain control and hydration for sx; pharmacologic Rx depends on etiology of stone

NEPHROTIC SYNDROME

Definition (Kidney Int 2004;66:1294)
- Constellation of edema, proteinuria, hypoalbuminemia, and ↑ plasma cholesterol levels

Etiology (Kidney Int 2004;66:1294)
- Heterogenous disorder with mutations in multiple slit diaphragm and podocyte proteins now identified (N Engl J Med 2006;354:1387)
- Minimal change dz used to account for ~60–85% of nephrotic syndrome; followed by idiopathic focal segmental glomerulosclerosis (FSGS), mesangial prolif (MP), membranoprolif glomerulonephritis (MPGN), and membranous nephropathy (MN)
- ↑ing fraction attributable to FSGS in recent past, particularly w/ African-Americans

Evaluation (Kidney Int 2004;66:1294)
- Bx may be indicated for those p/w typical features of FSGS (HTN, hematuria, renal insuff) or for those failing to respond to steroids
- Adolesc may be biopsied before steroids as FSGS and MN are more common

Therapy (Pediatr Nephrol 2011;26:881)
- Initial rx prednisone 60 mg/m²/d divided doses. 12 wk course may ↓ rate of relapse
- Steroid responsiveness confers favorable prognosis; check PPD before Rx
- W/ failure to respond to steroids, may use cytotoxic agents, calcineurin inhibitors (cyclosporine, tacrolimus; all require long-term tx), or mycophenolate mofetil and assoc w/ worsening renal fxn over time; choice of subsequent therapy may depend on bx results

RENAL TUBULAR ACIDOSIS

Definition (Int J Biochem Cell Biol 2005;37:1151)
- Metabolic acidosis 2/2 impaired renal acid excretion

Clinical Manifestations (Int J Biochem Cell Biol 2005;37:1151)
- Often p/w hyperchloremic metab acidosis w/ nml/near-nml AG & w/o diarrhea
- Can also present with hypokalemia, medullary nephrocalcinosis, recurrent calcium phosphate stone disease, growth retardation/rickets

Classification/Etiology (Int J Biochem Cell Biol 2005;37:1151)
- Isolated tubular defects can be due to drugs, autoimmune disease, obstructive nephropathy, or any cause of medullary nephrocalcinosis
- Can be genetic, associated with deafness, osteopetrosis, or ocular abnormalities
- **Distal (Type 1 RTA)** 2/2 impaired distal acid excretion. Acidosis may not be present. HypoK can occur. Bone dz and nephrocalcinosis can occur w/ hypercalciuria
  - Type 1 RTA can be acquired; 2/2 autoimmune dz (Sjögren syndrome or SLE)
- **Proximal (Type 2 RTA)** leads to bicarb wasting and high urine pH; eventually more acidic as plasma HCO_3^- levels ↓ and less filtered. ↑ frac excretion of HCO_3^- (>15%) characteristic. Osmotic effect of HCO_3^- can lead to loss of K as well
  - Type 2 RTA can be part of generalized tubular defect, (i.e., Fanconi syndrome [proximal cell dysfxn]: Prox renal tubular acidosis (bicarb wasting), hypophos (phos wasting), polyuria (Na wasting), glucosuria, and aminoaciduria)
  - Type 2 RTA can occur in cystinosis, hereditary fructose intolerance, and Wilson disease, or can be caused by ifosamide, acetazolamide

- **Type 4 RTA** also a distal RTA assoc w/ hyperK instead of hypoK (effective hypoaldo), and can be 2/2 sickle-cell dz, urinary tract obstruct, amyloidosis, xplnt
  - Can be 2/2 drugs: Aldosterone inhibitor diuretics such as spironolactone, ACE-I/ARBs, trimethoprim, heparin, pentamidine, NSAIDs

Diagnosis & Rx (Rose & Post. *Clinical Physiology of Acid-Base and Electrolyte Disorders*; 5th ed., McGraw-Hill; 2001)

	Type I – Distal	Type II – Proximal	Type IV
Pathology	Dec distal acidification	Dec prox HCO_3 reabsorp	Aldosterone def/resistance
FeHCO₃ at nml [HCO₃][a]	5–10% in children <3% in adolescents	>**15–20%**	<3%
[K⁺]	Low or normal	Low or normal	**High**
Urine pH[b]	>**5.3**	Variable	Usually <5.3
Serum [HCO₃]	Can be <10 mEq/L	14–20 mEq/L	Usually >15 mEq/L
HCO₃ dose to replace	4–14 mEq/kg qd in children; 1–2 in adol	10–15 mEq/kg qd	1–3 mEq/kg qd only if ↑ K corrected
Complications	Nephrocalcinosis and stones	Rickets/osteomalacia	None
Rx[b]	Oral alkali supplements often corrects hypoK and hypoCa	Oral alkali supps w/ K and Vit D supplements	Alkali supplements +/− diuretics

[a]Measured at normalized serum [HCO₃].
[b]Measured while patient is acidemic.
Adapted from *Int J Biochem Cell Biol* 2005;37:1151.

VESICOURETERAL REFLUX

Definition (Pediatr Clin North Am 2006;53:413)
- "Abnormal retrograde flow of urine from bladder into ureter and possibly kidney"

Grade I	VUR does not reach renal pelvis
Grade II	VUR extends up to the renal pelvis without dilation
Grade III	Mild/mod dilation of ureter and renal pelvis. No/slight blunting of fornices
Grade IV	Mod dilation of ureter, renal pelvis, and calyces. Complete obliteration of sharp angle of fornices but maintenance of papillary impression in most calyces
Grade V	Gross dilation/tortuosity of ureter, renal pelvis, and calyces. Papillary impressions not visible in calyces

Epidemiology (Pediatr Clin North Am 2006;53:413)
- Prevalence ~1% of nml kids, changes w/ age as VUR may resolve w/ time
- VUR in 20–40% of kids w/ UTIs & in 10–20% of infants w/ antenatal hydronephrosis

Diagnosis (Pediatrics 2011;128:595)
- Febrile infants w/ UTI should undergo renal U/S to assess for anatomic abnormalities
- Voiding cystourethrogram (VCUG) should not be performed for infant w/ 1st febrile UTI, it is indicated if renal U/S shows hydronephrosis, scarring, or other signs of high-grade VURVCUG allows grading, anatomic eval; direct radionuclide cystography can be used for f/u eval (↓ rad exposure but poorer anatomic detail)
- Antenatal hydronephrosis; f/u U/S at 1 mo (relative ↓ in urinary flow in 1st mo may result in false neg if sooner) unless severe hydronephrosis noted prenatally

Clinical Manifestations (Pediatrics 2011;128:595; Pediatr Clin North Am 2001;48:1505)
- Clinical consequences: UTI, reflux nephropathy or scarring, though can occur w/o VUR
- Congenital ureteropelvic junction obstruction (UPJO) can p/w hydronephrosis & nml renal function in asymptomatic infant

Natural History and Complications (Pediatr Clin North Am 2001;48:1505; J Urol 2002;168:2594)
- Grades I & II reflux resolves in >80% of pts (10–25% resolution/yr); Grade III reflux resolves in 50% (Grade IV resolved in ~30%, & Grade V rarely spontaneously resolves)
- Reflux nephropathy can produce renal failure, proteinuria, and hypertension

Management (Pediatrics 2011;128:595)
- AAP guidelines abx ppx no longer indicated for recurrent UTIs as evidence that ppx not effective in pts w/ or w/o VUR (Pediatrics 2008;122:1064; N Engl J Med 2009;361:1748)
- Grade V reflux almost always requires surgical correction; Grade III or IV reflux can be managed medically unless recurrent UTIs and progressive scarring

CONGENITAL RENAL MALFORMATIONS

(Avner, Harmon & Niaudet, *Pediatric Nephrology* 5th edition, 2004 p83–86)
- Bilateral agenesis – oligohydramnios w/ fetal or perinatal death
- Unilateral agenesis – 1/2,900 live births, ↑ w/ maternal DM, usually asso'd w/ ipsilateral ureter agenesis, often asymptomatic
- Primary hypoplasia – multiple hereditary forms, renal coloboma syndrome (PAX2), branchiootorenal syndrome (OMIM 113650), VATER, VACTERL, vitamin A deficiency
- Multicystic/dysplastic kidney – unilateral, 1/4,000 live births, bilateral rare, may be isolated to a single pole
- Ectopic kidney – mostly pelvic, uni- or bilateral (often w/ fusion leading to *pancake* or *discoid* kidney), generally hypoplastic, often asymptomatic, but may p/w infection or calculi
- Horseshoe kidney – fusion of kidneys at lower poles (usually w/ fibrous isthmus), often kidneys in pelvis or lower vertebral level (below IMA), may p/w obstructive uropathy, calculi, UTI; associated w/ Wilms, RCC, & other tumors

JUVENILE IDIOPATHIC ARTHRITIS (JIA)

Definition (Lancet 2011;377:2138; Lancet 2007;369:767)
- Dx of exclusion; previously JRA, now JIA per Internat League of Assoc for Rheum(ILAR)
- Includes all forms of arthritis (swelling or limitation of motion of joint w/ heat or pain) <16 yo, >6-wk duration and of unknown cause (Pediatr Clin North Am 2005:413)
- Must exclude infectious and postinfectious etiology, hematologic and neoplastic dz, connective tissue disease, vasculitis, and other inflammatory conditions

Epidemiology (Lancet 2007;369:767)
- Most common chronic rheumatic dz in children, prevalence 16–150 per 100,000
- Oligoarthritis most common in the US, W. European countries, polyarthritis in Costa Rica, India, New Zealand, and South Africa
- Occurs as frequently as juvenile DM, 4× more freq than CF & sickle cell anemia, & 10× more than ALL, hemophilia or musc dystrophy (Pediatr Rev 2006;27:e24)

Clinical Manifestations (BMJ 2010;341:c6434; Lancet 2007;369:767)
- **Systemic arthritis:** 10% of all cases of JIA; polygenic autoinflam syndrome w/ ↑ IL1 & 6
  - Arthritis + quotidian fever of at least 2 wk duration + ≥1 of the following: Classic transient blanching macular or maculopapular rash, HSM, generalized LAD, or serositis. Fever and/or rash may precede arthritis by wks to mos
  - Fever peak (usually >102.2°F in evening or morning) may coincide w/ appearance of rash, occ assoc w/ abd pain, myalgias (Pediatr Rev 2006;27:e24)
  - Systemic sx often abate, polyarticular arthritis can develop late in disease course
  - 2 types based on resp to anti-IL-1 Rx; one w/ complete resp, other resistant/interm
  - 5–8% develop macrophage activation syndrome(MAS) which is life-threatening; sudden onset sustained fever, pancytopenia, HSM, liver insuff, coagulopathy w/ hemorrhagic signs & neuro sx (labs: Paradoxically ↓ ESR, ↑ Trigs, ↓ Na, ↑ ferritin, ↑ PT/PTT)
- **Oligoarthritis:** 40% of all cases JIA; ≤4 joints during 1st 6 mo of disease
  - Asym arthritis, onset <6 yo, ♀ predilection, often +ANA, w/ ↑ risk iridocyclitis (chronic, nongranulomatous, anter uveitis affects iris and ciliary body can cause visual impairment; affects 30%, flare/onset do not follow arthritis course
  - Exclude if w/ psoriasis, FHx psoriasis, HLA B27 dz in 1st-degree relative, +RF, or occurs in a male >6 yo (consider psoriatic or enthesitis-related arthritis)
  - Usually knee > ankles, 30–50% 1 joint at presentation
  - Often w/ swollen warm joint, limp worse at AM, after nap (Pediatr Rev 2006;27:e24)
  - 50% w/ upper limb joint involved and ↑ ESR at onset predicts more severe outcome
  - Can have leg-length discrepancy, initially sustained ↑ blood flow to growth plate w/ ↑ growth, then chronic inflamm w/ early epiphyseal closure
- **Polyarticular onset:** 25% of all cases of JIA, divided into RF+ and RF–
  - **RF+** (5%) affects ≥5 joints in 1st 6 mo of dz and +IgM RF, also assoc w/ +anti-CCP, at least 2× >3 mo apart; same as adult RF + RA and seen mainly in adolescent ♀
  - Symmetric polyarthritis, affects small joints of hands & feet, unlike adult RA in that often w/ growth retardation or accelerated growth at affected joint
  - Large joints, usually knees and ankles, can be affected, but usually w/ small joints
  - Rheumatoid may occur, often extensor surfaces of joint
  - **RF neg:** Heterogenous subtype affects ≥5 joints in 1st 6 mo of dz and IgM RF neg
  - Can be asymmetric, early age at onset, female predomination, frequently +ANA, ↑ risk of iridocyclitis and assoc w/ HLA DRB1*0801
  - Can be overt symmetric synovitis of large and small joints, onset in school age, ↑ ESR, neg ANA, variable outcome
  - Can have dry synovitis (min joint swelling), stiffness, flexion contractures nml–↑ ESR
  - **Spondyloarthropathies** (HLA B27 assoc; psoriatic, IBD, reactive arthritis): Usually asymm, 6–14 yo, ♂ predom, affects large joints, assoc w/ enthesitis, sacroiliitis
    - Psoriatic arthritis can occasionally lead to aortic stenosis as adults

Etiology and Pathogenesis (Lancet 2011;377:2138)
- Unknown; autoimmune, possible infectious trigger. Heterog group of disorders
- Genome-wide scan of kids suggests several genes, also HLA A2, B27, DRB1, & DP

Diagnostic Studies (Lancet 2011;377:2138; Lancet 2007;369:767)
- Eval is dependent on history (associated symptoms and signs) and physical exam (PE)
  - PE sens 64% & spec 86%; screen w/ U/S for subclin dz (J Rheumatol 2011;38:2671)
- Systemic arthritis labs: ↑ WBC w/ ↑ PMNs, ↑ ESR, ↑ CRP, thrombocytosis, ↑ ferritin, ↑ vWFag
- Oligoarthritis labs: Acute phase labs nml–↑, + ANA (70–80%; risk for iridocyclitis)
- Polyarthritis lab features: RF+/– variable as above
- Radiographic eval w/ U/S & MRI often beneficial (↑ sens)

- Joint asp to r/o infxn only if it appears septic. Crystal dz very rare. If WBC >100 × 10^3 mL (100 × 10^9/L) and 90% polys, infxn likely. Send fluid for cx, consider Lyme PCR

Management (BMJ 2010;341:c6434)
- Combo of drugs, physical and occupational Rx, and psychosocial support
- Periodic x-rays of affected joints to document progression of erosive disease
- Oligoarticular–intraarticular steroids can be very beneficial
- Classic use of NSAIDs w/ delayed DMARDs/steroids; new data favor DMARDs early
- NSAIDs mainstay of Rx: Avg time to sx improv 1 mo, up to 25% w/ no improv until 8–12 wk; approx 50% w/ improv to 1st NSAID, 50% w/ relief w/ next NSAID
- $^2/_3$ children w/ persistently active joint dz require DMARDs or steroids. MTX most commonly prescribed w/ ~70% responding. Biologic agents used: Etanercept, adalimumab, infliximab, golimumab, rituximab, abatacept, anti-IL-1 & anti-IL-6 used for systemics (anakinra, tocilizumab)
  - ~1/3 w/ excellent resp (inactive dz or remission) w/ etanercept (JAMA 2011;306:2340)
- Other agents, sulfasalazine, leflunomide, cyclosporine, cyclophosphamide, hydroxychloroquine, thalidomide, intraarticular steroids often helpful

Prognosis and Outcome: Studies have inconsistent results
- Systemic arthritis: Variable course
  - 50% monocyclic or intermittent; w/ fever, remits when systemic sx controlled
  - 50% unremitting, often systemic sx resolve and pt has chronic arthritis; severe w/ joint destruct. Rx w/ steroids can cause growth retard and osteoporosis
- Oligoarthritis: Best outcomes, joint erosion more freq in pts w/ polyartic course
- If w/ iridocyclitis at risk for post-synechiae, band keratopathy, cataract, and glaucoma
- Polyarthritis: RF+: Progressive and diffuse involv; x-ray Δs early esp in hands and feet
  - RF–: Variable outcome
- JIA pts w/ 2–4× inc risk malig; ? 2/2 MTX/anti-TNF rx (Nat Rev Rheumatol 2011;7:6)

Poststrep Reactive Arthritis
- Distinct from arthritis assoc w/ rheumatic fever
- At least 1–2 wk btw acute strep infxn and onset + anti-DNAse B/ASLO titer/cx
- Response to aspirin and NSAIDs is poor
- Modified Jones criteria usually not met and there is no evidence of carditis
- Duration prolonged or recurrent and of ↑ severity and w/ tenosynovitis and renal abn
- No clear definition or Rx guidelines: No consensus on prophy PCN

Arthritis in Rheumatic Fever
- Most freq and least specific sx of rheumatic fever
- Migratory arthritis: Usually affects large joints, lower, then the upper extremities
- Joint involvement early in illness, more common and severe in adol and young adults
- Polyarthritis painful, but transient, inflammation lasts 2–3 d in each joint and 2 wk total
- X-ray may show slight effusion but otherwise normal
- Self-limited, resolves without sequelae and responds well to NSAIDs

REACTIVE (ENTHESITIS-RELATED) ARTHRITIS

Definition (J Adolesc Health 2009;44:309; Clin Microbiol Rev 2004;17:348)
- Arthritis associated with a recent, prior, or coexisting extraarticular infection
- Can refer to post-infxn arthritis, urethritis, and conjunctivitis; w/ 3:1 ♂:♀ predominance
- Per ILAR; reactive arthritis in pt <16 yo now known as enthesitis-related arthritis

Pathophysiology (Curr Opin Rheumatol 1999;11:238)
- Classic pathogens: *Campylobacter, Chlamydia trach, Salmonella, Shigella, Yersinia*
- Bacterial antigens in synovium, trigger T-cell resp → immune-mediated synovitis
  - Chlamydial DNA and mRNA have been found in synovial membrane biopsies
  - *Campylobacter, Salmonella, Shigella, Yersinia* antigens present in synovial fluid
- 30–70% w/ HLA B27, perhaps because HLA B27 cells allow bacteria to persist

Epidemiology (Clin Microbiol Rev 2004;17:348)
- Uncommon disorder, estimated at 0.1% prevalence; 2nd–4th decade of life
- May be underdiagnosed because of asymptomatic prior infection
- Following GU infxn (male to female 9:1) or enteric infection (male to female 1:1)

Clinical Manifestations (Clin Microbiol Rev 2004;17:348)
- Latent period from infection to onset of symptoms from a few days to 6 wk
- Extraarticular findings include

- Conjunctivitis (30%), often coincides with flares of arthritis, is mild, lasts 1–4 wk
- Urethritis, usually painless, clear discharge; can involve other GU structures
- Dermatologic findings: Balanitis circinata & keratoderma blennorrhagica
- Articular findings: Asym, mono- or oligoarthritis, predominantly lower extremities

Symptoms	Sens	Spec	Comments
Asym oligoarthritis	44%	95%	Avg of 4 joints (knee, ankle, toes, wrist, fingers); nondestructive
Sausage digit	27%	99%	Occurs in 16% of pts
Heel pain	52%	92%	A result of enthesitis
Low back pain	71%	77%	Predictor of more severe disease

Diagnostic Studies (Clin Microbiol Rev 2004;17:348)
- No established diagnostic criteria
- 1996 Third International Workshop on Reactive Arthritis
  - Typical peripheral arthritis (predominantly lower limb, asym oligoarthritis)
  - Evidence of preceding infection
    - If diarrhea or urethritis laboratory confirmation desired, not essential
    - If no clinical infection, laboratory confirmation is necessary
    - Positive confirmatory testing includes: +stool cx; +chlamydia trachomatis
    - Pts w/ other causes (Lyme dz, septic arthritis, spondyloarthritis) are excluded
- Routine HLA B27 screening is not helpful
- Eval: X-rays (usually nml) of affected joints to r/o trauma, joint aspiration to r/o septic arthritis & gout, U/A, Chlamydia PCR, stool cx, Lyme serology, RF, HIV test

Management (Clin Microbiol Rev 2004;17:348)
- NSAIDs (1st line Rx w/ 70–75% response rate), intraarticular corticosteroids, DMARDs (2nd line for refractory arthritis)
- Orthotics for enthesitis if present, gentle ROM exercises and avoidance of overuse
- No controlled data, but sulfasalazine, MTX, azathioprine have shown some efficacy
- Antibiotics: Rx of urethritis can ↓ risk of reactive arthritis and ↓ relapse
  - Rx of enteric infections does not affect development of reactive arthritis

Complications (Rheumatology 2000;39:117)
- Most recover in 2–6 mo w/o destructive Δs; 4–19% w/ chronic (>6 mo) arthritis
- Worse prognosis assoc w/: ♂ gender, FHx ankylosing spondylitis, presence of HLA B27, ESR > 30, poor response to NSAIDs, onset < 16 yo. (Clin Microbiol Rev 2004;17:348)

SYSTEMIC LUPUS ERYTHEMATOSUS

Definition (Pediatr Rev 2012;33:62)
- **SLE:** Chronic, episodic, multisystem, AI dz w/ presence of antinuclear auto-Abs to ds-DNA & w/ widespread vascular & connective tissue inflammation; more severe in children
- **Neonatal lupus syndrome:** Passively transferred AI dz in 1% of neonates born to moms w/ AI dz (SLE, Sjögren), by transplacental passage of maternal anti-Ro or anti-La Abs; clinically w/ congenital heart block (30%), rash, and rarely hepatobiliary or hematologic manifestations (anemia, thrombocytopenia)
- **"Drug-induced lupus" syndrome:** Variant form of lupus that resolves w/i d to mos after w/d of drug in pt w/ no underlying immune dysfxn. Most commonly w/ hydralazine, procainamide, quinidine, isoniazid, diltiazem, phenytoin, α-methyldopa, ethosuximide, trimethadione, carbamazepine, and minocycline

Epidemiology
- 20% of cases dx'd <20 yo; avg onset is at 12 yo; pre-puberty 3:1 ♀:♂, post-puberty 9:1
- Incidence and severity greater in AA, Hispanics, and Asians compared to Caucasians
- With aggressive therapy 5 yr survival in pediatric SLE 100%; 10 yr survival 86%

Pathophysiology
- Combination of hormonal and environmental factors in predisposed individuals
- 10% patients w/ +1st-degree family member w/ SLE
- Autoreactive B- and T-cells → antigen–Ab complexes in circulation and deposit in tissues, such as renal glomerulus, dermal–epidermoid junction, and choroid plexus
- Immune complexes activate complement system, resulting in hypocomplementemia during the active phase and presence of complement activation products

- Dx based on ACR criteria used for adults w/ 4+ criteria simultaneously or serially
- W/ +ANA titers, 4 classifications exist: Classical SLE (many criteria), definite SLE (≥4 criteria), probable SLE (3 criteria), possible SLE (2 criteria present)
- ACR criteria for dx of SLE from (Arthritis Rheum 1982;52: revised in 1997)

Criterion	Definition (% prevalence)
Malar (butterfly) rash	Fixed erythema, flat or raised, over the malar eminences, tending to spare nasolabial folds (70%)
Discoid-lupus rash	Erythematosus raised patches with adherent keratotic scaling and follicular plugging; atrophic scarring in older lesions (70%)
Photosensitivity	Skin rash as a result of unusual reaction to sunlight, by history or physical exam (70%)
Oral ulcers	Oral or nasopharyngeal ulceration, usually painless, on physical exam (70%)
Arthritis	Nonerosive arthritis involving 2 or more peripheral joints, characterized by tenderness, swelling, or effusion (64%)
Serositis	Pleuritis: Hx of pleuritic pain, rub or evid of effusion (77%); or pericarditis
Renal	Persistent proteinuria >0.5 g/d, or 3+ qualitatively; or cellular casts (red cell, Hgb, granular, tubular, or mixed) (50%) 6 classifications of lupus nephritis: Class I – minimal mesangial lupus nephritis (nml glomeruli, nml immune deposits), Class II (25%)– mesangial proliferative (mesangial hypercellularity or expansion), Class III (41%) – focal proliferative (<50% glomeruli w/ GN), Class IV (~65%) – diffuse proliferative (>50% glomeruli with GN), Class V (29%) – membranous, (subepithelial immune deposits), Class VI – advanced sclerosing (>90% glomeruli are sclerosed)
Neurologic	Encephalopathy (szrs or psychosis) in the absence of any other organic cause (offending drugs or metabolic derangements such as uremia, ketoacidosis, electrolyte imbalances)
Immunologic	Positive antiphospholipid antibody, or anti-DNA antibody, or anti-Sm antibody, or false-positive serologic test for syphilis known to be positive for at least 6 mo and confirmed by Treponema pallidum immobilization or fluorescent treponemal antibody absorption test
Hematologic	Hemolytic anemia with reticulocytosis, or leukopenia (WBC < 4,000/mm^3) on 2 or more occasions; lymphopenia (<1,500/mm^3), or thrombocytopenia (<100,000/mm^3) in the absence of offending drugs (28–35%)
Antinuclear antibody	Abnormal ANA titer at any point in time and in the absence of drugs known to be associated with "drug-induced lupus" syndrome

Adapted from prevalence data from French multicenter study published in J Pediatr 2005;146:648.

Diagnostic Studies
- **Autoantibodies in SLE** (N Engl J Med 2008;358:929); ANA+ in 99% pts w/ SLE

Autoantibody	Prevalence (%)	Main Clinical Effects
Antidouble-stranded DNA	70–80	Kidney disease, skin disease
Antinucleosomes	60–90	Kidney disease, skin disease
Anti-Ro	30–40	Kidney disease, skin disease, fetal cardiac problems
Anti-La	15–20	Fetal cardiac problems
Anti-Sm	10–30	Kidney disease
Anti-NMDA receptor	33–50	CNS disease
Antiphospholipid	20–30	Thrombosis, pregnancy loss
α-actinin	20	Kidney disease
C1q	40–50	Kidney disease

- Dx based on ACR criteria. Other abn labs: ↓ C3 and C4, ↑ ESR and CRP, ↑ serum Cr, ↓ serum albumin, ↓ Hgb, WBC or Plts, abn values found on 24-hr urine collection for calc of CrCl and quantification of proteinuria, GN, or mesangial dz on renal bx

Management
- Mild SLE: NSAIDs, hydroxychloroquine 200–400 mg qd, low-dose corticosteroids, dapsone may be used for dermatologic manifestations
- Mod SLE: Longer-term corticosteroids, mycophenolate mofetil, azathioprine, MTX
- Severe SLE: IV cyclophosphamide, mycophenolate mofetil, Rituximab (anti-CD-20 monoclonal Ab), stem cell transplantation, renal transplantation

Complications
- Risk for Libman–Sacks endocarditis and superimposed bacterial endocarditis
- Early atherosclerosis and coronary artery disease
- Antiphospholipid Abs ↑ risks of VTE (2–6× ↑), risk further ↑'d w/ OCP/pregnancies
- Morbidity & mortality in children primarily affected by degree of renal involv, in adults morbidity & mortality is most affected by long-term cardiovascular dz

VASCULITIDES

Practical Classification of Pediatric Vasculitis (Curr Rheumatol Rep 2009;11:402)
- 1° vasculitides: Classification based on International Consensus Conference, Vienna
- Large vessel vasculitis: Takayasu arteritis
- Medium vessel vasculitis: Kawasaki dz, cutaneous & systemic polyarteritis nodosa
- Small vessel vasculitis:
  - Granulomatous: Wegener granulomatosis & Churg–Strauss syndrome (CSS)
  - Nongranulomatous: Henoch–Schonlein purpura, microscopic polyangiitis, isolated cutaneous leukocytoclastic vasculitis, hypocomplementemic urticarial vasculitis
- Other vasculitides: Behcet' dz, Cogan's syndrome, unclassified, and 2° vasculitides 2/2 infection, malignancy, drugs or those associated with CTD

Clinical Manifestations
- Focal hypoperfusion: Claudication, HTN, CVA, abdominal pain
- Organ dysfunction: MI, myocarditis, neuropathy, myositis, sensory changes, cutaneous/ microvascular effects (palp purpura, GN, pulmonary–renal syndrome)
- Can result in vascular tissue injury w/ vascular leak, aneurysm formation, stenosis, occlusion, rupture & necrosis, Kawasaki disease (mucocutaneous lymph node synd)
- **Definition** (Pediatr Rev 2008;29:308; Pediatrics 2004;114:1708)
  - Acute self-limited vasculitis w/ fever, bilateral nonexudative conjunctivitis, erythema of lips and oral mucosa, extremities swelling, rash, and cervical LAD
  - Coronary artery aneurysms or ectasia develop in 15–25% of untreated children
- **Epidemiology:** Susceptibility assoc w/ ITPKC gene. (Nat Genet 2008;40:35)
  - 15 cases per 100,000 <5 yo/ median age 2 yr in the US; incidence highest in Asians
  - 85% pts <5 yo; pts <6 mo or >8 yo less common but ↑ risk coronary art aneurysm
- **Diagnostic criteria** (AHA/AAP Guidance Reports; updated 2007)
  - Confirmed by fever ≥5 d and 4 of the 5 criteria below, and no other explanation
    - Extremities Δs: Acute (erythema of palms, soles; edema of hands, feet); subacute (periungual peeling of fingers, toes in wk 2 and 3)
    - Polymorphous exanthem
    - Bilateral bulbar conjunctival injection (limbic sparing) without exudates
    - Mucosal changes: Erythema, lips cracking, strawberry tongue
    - Cervical lymphadenopathy (>1.5 cm diameter), usually unilateral
- **Exceptions:** Pts w/ fever ≥5 d and <4 criteria dx'd w/ Kawasaki if cardiac involvement
- **Other clinical manifestations:** Pericarditis, noncoronary aneurysms, hydrops of gallbladder, aseptic meningitis, urethritis/meatitis, anterior uveitis
- **Modified AHA/AAP algorithm for "incomplete" (atypical) Kawasaki**
  - Fever at least 5 d and at least 2 clinical criteria for Kawasaki, no other explanation and lab findings consistent with severe systemic inflammation

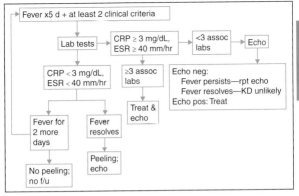

Flowchart:
- Fever x5 d + at least 2 clinical criteria
  - Lab tests
    - CRP ≥ 3 mg/dL, ESR ≥ 40 mm/hr
      - <3 assoc labs → Echo
      - ≥3 assoc labs → Treat & echo
      - Echo neg:
        - Fever persists—rpt echo
        - Fever resolves—KD unlikely
      - Echo pos: Treat
    - CRP < 3 mg/dL, ESR < 40 mm/hr
      - Fever for 2 more days
        - No peeling; no f/u
      - Fever resolves
        - Peeling; echo

- **Laboratory findings suggestive of KD include the following**
  - CRP ≥ 3 mg/dL or ESR ≥ 40 mm/hr; WBC ≥ 15,000, anemia (normocytic, normochromic), sterile pyuria (≥10 WBC/HPF), ALT > 50, albumin ≤ 3.0 g/dL, after 7 d of illness Plts > 450,000
- **Diagnostic studies: Echo** – aneurysms, findings c/w coronary arteritis (perivascular brightness, ectasia, and lack of tapering of coronary arteries), ↓ LV contractility, mild valvular regurg (1° mitral valve) and pericardial effusion
- **Treatment** (Pediatr Rev 2008;29:308)
  - **IVIG and Aspirin (ASA):** Single dose of 2 g/kg of IGIV over 10–12 hr; best w/l 1st 10 d
    - ASA 80–100 mg/kg/d in 4 divided doses during acute phase
    - Re-Rx w/ IVIG (2 g/kg) and cont ASA Rx may be indicated for persistent fever (>36 hr) or recurrent fever after initially afebrile ≤48 hr; infliximab has been used
    - After fever controlled 4–5 d, ASA dose ↓ to 3–5 mg/kg/d
    - ASA d/c'd if no coronary artery abn by 6–8 wk after onset of illness
    - Low-dose ASA Rx continued indefinitely in those w/ coronary artery abn
    - Even w/ appt Rx, 5% cor artery dilation 1% w/ giant aneurysm; vs. 20–25% w/o Rx
  - **Cardiac care:** Check echo early in acute phase of illness 2 & 6 wk after onset
    - F/u by cardiologist in 1st 2 mo assess for arrhythmias, CHF, and valvular regurg
    - Development of giant coronary artery aneurysms (≥8 mm in diameter) may need anticoagulant Rx, such as warfarin, to prevent thrombosis

Henoch–Schönlein Purpura
- **Definition** (Curr Opin Rheumatol 2010;22:598)
  - Leukocytoclastic vasculitis of small vessels w/ deposition of IgA1 in vessel walls and renal mesangium; most common vasculitis of childhood
- **Epidemiology:** 10–20 cases per 100,000 children/yr
  - Typically presents btw 3–10 yo; 50% cases at or before 5 yo; M:F 2:1
- **Pathophysiology** (BioDrugs 2001;15:99)
  - Assoc w/ a wide variety of microbial pathogens, drugs, environmental agents; significant minority of pts w/ evidence of recent group A strep infection
  - Skin findings w/ subepidermal hemorrhages and dermal necrotizing vasculitis
  - The vasculitis can also occur in organs, such as the gastrointestinal tract
- **ACR criteria for classification of Henoch–Schönlein purpura**
  - Need ≥2 of the 4 criteria. Presence ≥2 of criteria yields sens 87.1% and spec 87.7%

Criterion	Definition
Palpable purpura	Slightly raised "palpable" hemorrhagic skin lesions; not related to thrombocytopenia
≤20 yo at disease onset	Patient age ≤20 yr at onset of symptoms
Bowel angina	Diffuse abd pain, worse after meals, or dx of bowel ischemia, +/– bloody diarrhea
Wall granulocytes on bx	Histologic changes showing granulocytes in the walls of arterioles and venules

- **Clinical manifestations:** Usually p/w tetrad of rash, arthralgias, abd pain, & renal dz
  - Rash; typically nonblanching, in groups (can persist 3–10 d), most on legs and arms
  - Polyarthralgia; >80% pts. Most commonly affects knees and ankles, often w/ edema
  - Resolves after a few d and leaves no permanent damage
  - Abd pain; >1/2 pts, often colicky. Dev w/i 8 d of rash. Usually w/ N/V, diarrhea; blood and mucus often w/ stool. Rarely c/b intussusception
  - Renal dz: ~40–50% pts, p/w mild GN w/ proteinuria, microhematuria, and +/– RBC casts. Usually resolves spont but progressive renal dz may develop; those w/ persistent proteinuria likely w/ worsening renal damage
    - Renal failure is the most common cause of death in pts who die w/ HSP
- **Treatment** (Curr Rheumatol Rep 2004;6:195; J Pediatr 2006;149:241)
  - **Suggested management of HSP (See the table below)** (Curr Rheumatol Rep 2009;11:402)
  - RCT of 1 mg/kg/d pred ×2 wk then 2 wk taper for severe abd pain ↓ ineffective for purpura, development of nephritis, ↓ing duration of dz or ↓ing recurrence. Usu steroids are not used for joint pain/rash alone
  - Rx options for severe renal dz in HSP: High-dose corticosteroids +/– IS (AZA, cyclophosphamide, or cyclosporine); high-dose IVIG; plasma exchange or plasmapheresis; corticosteroids w/ urokinase and warfarin; renal xplant

Table 1 Vasculitides – Henoch–Schönlein Purpura							
Sx	Support	NSAIDs	PO Steroid	IV Steroid	IV Pulse Steroids	Steroids + IS Drugs	Plasma-pheresis
Mild sx	X						
Rash and arthritis	X	X					
Rash and mild edema	X						
Rash and severe edema	X		X				
Severe colicky abd pain	X		X				
Abd pain w/ N/V	X			X			
Scrotal/testicular involve	X		X				
Nephrotic proteinuria	X				X		
RPGN	X					X	X
Pulmonary hemorrhage	X					X	X

Steroids, corticosteroids; IS, immunosuppressive; RPGN, rapid progressive glomerulonephritis.

Polyarteritis Nodosa (PAN) (Curr Rheumatol Rep 2009;11:402)

- **Definition:** Systemic vasculitis involving small and medium muscular arteries
  - 1/3 w/ cutaneous PAN w/ limited dz restricted to skin, muscle, joints & periph nerves
- **Epidemiology** (J Pediatr 2004;145:517): Peak onset ~9–11 yo (1–16 yo), ♂ > ♀ slightly
- **Etiology:** Unknown; infxns (i.e., viral hepatitis, strep and parvo) implicated. Assoc w/ FMF
- **Criteria for classification** (1990 American College of Rheumatology Criteria)
- Commonly w/ fever, weight loss, malaise, and non-specific abdominal pain
- Classification criteria of ACR not validated for children; 3 of the following
  - Unexplained weight loss >4 kg; livedo reticularis; testicular pain or tenderness; myalgias (except shoulder and hip girdle), muscle weakness, leg muscle pain; mononeuropathy or polyneuropathy; new onset DBP >90 mm Hg; ↑ BUN (>40 mg/dL) or Cr (>1.5 mg/dL); hepatitis B virus infection; characteristic arteriographic abn; bx of small or medium-sized artery w/ PMNs
- **Diagnostic studies:** Labs— ↑ ESR/CRP, ↑ WBC, ↑ immunoglob, can also see proteinuria, hematuria, inc BUN/Cr, complement usually nml. +HBsAg (30%), p-ANCA (<20%)
  - **Angiogram:** Aneurysms and focal vessel narrowing
  - **Bx** (sural nerve or skin): Vasculitis with fibrinoid necrosis without granulomas
- **Rx:** Mainstay Rx is steroids and IS agents (cyclophos, MTX, MMF, anti-TNF, rituximab)
  - HBV-related PAN is treated with antiviral therapy

ANCA-related Vasculitis

- **Definition** (Pediatr Nephrol 2010;25:205): Aberrant interaction btw neutrophils & vascular endothelial cells; includes Wegener granulomatosis, microscopic polyangiitis, renal-limited microscopic polyangiitis, CSS and drug-induced vasculitides (antithyroid Rx, hydralazine, minocycline)
- **Epidemiology:** Can occur at any age but typically in young and middle-aged adults
- **Clinical indications for testing for ANCA** (Am J Kidney Dis 1991;18:184)
  - Glomerulonephritis, especially rapidly progressive glomerulonephritis
  - Pulmonary hemorrhage, especially pulmonary–renal syndrome
  - Cutaneous vasculitis, especially with systemic features
  - Multiple lung nodules; chronic destructive disease of the upper airways
  - Long-standing sinusitis or otitis; subglottic tracheal stenosis
  - Mononeuritis multiplex or peripheral neuropathy; retro-orbital mass
- **Wegener granulomatosis Classification** (2005 EULAR/PRES Criteria, updating 1990 ACR Criteria) (Arthritis Rheum 2009;60:3413)
  - Needs 3 of the 6 criteria. Yields sens of 73.6% and a spec of 73.2% in pediatric pts
  - Nasal or sinus inflamm (painful/painless ulcers, purulent or bloody nasal discharge)
  - Abn CXR or chest CT scan (w/ presence of nodules, fixed infiltrates, or cavities)
  - Abn U/A: Microhematuria (>5 RBCs/HPF) or significant proteinuria
  - Granulomatous inflamm on bx/necrotizing pauci-immune GN
  - Subglottic, tracheal, or endobronchial stenosis
  - Anti-PR3 ANCA or cANCA staining
- **Churg–Strauss vasculitis Classification** (1990 ACR Criteria; no EULAR/PRES Criteria)
  - 4 or more of the 6 criteria w/ sens 85% and spec 99.7%
  - Asthma: History of wheezing or diffuse high-pitched expiratory rhonchi
  - Eosinophilia: >10% on differential WBC count
  - Mono- or polyneuropathy: Glove/stocking distribution
  - Pulmonary infiltrates that are nonfixed: Migratory or transitory
  - Paranasal sinus abn: Hx acute/chronic sinus pain x-ray opacification of sinuses
  - Extravascular eosinophils: Demonstrated via bx of artery, arteriole, or venule

Diagnostic Testing

- Antineutrophil cytoplasmic antibody (Kidney Int 2000;57:846)

IF Pattern	Antigens	Disease Associations
C-ANCA – pattern w/ diffuse staining throughout the cytoplasm	PR3 (majority; occasionally MPO)	Wegener granulomatosis (80–90%), microscopic polyangiitis (20–40%), primary pauci-immune crescentic glomerulonephritis (20–40%), Churg–Strauss syndrome (35%)
P-ANCA – staining pattern around nucleus	MPO (majority; occasionally PR3)	Microscopic polyangiitis (50%), primary pauci-immune crescentic glomerulonephritis (50%), Churg–Strauss syndrome (35%)
Atypical-ANCA	HMG1/2. Catalase, Enolase, Actin, Lactoferrin, Lysozyme, Elastase, Cathepsin G, Defensin	Drug-induced systemic vasculitis, IBD, rheumatoid arthritis, cystic fibrosis, primary sclerosing cholangitis

IF, immunofluorescence; C-ANCA, cytoplasmic staining ANCA; P-ANCA, perinuclear staining ANCA; PR3, proteinase3, MPO, myeloperoxidase.

- **Wegener:** CXR or CT chest (for nodules, infiltrates, cavities), sinus CT for sinusitis, BUN/Cr, U/A (proteinuria, hematuria, sediment w/ RBC casts, dysmorphic RBCs for renal dz), bx (nec granulomatous inflamm of vessels)
- **Microscopic polyangiitis:** CXR, U/A (similar to Wegener), bx (necrotizing, pauci-immune inflammation of arterioles, capillaries, and venules)
- **Churg-Strauss syndrome:** CXR (pulm infiltrates), bx (microgranulomas, fibrinoid necrosis, and thrombosis of small vessels w/ eosinophilic infiltrates)

- **Clinical features** (Am J Med 2004;117:39)

Features	Wegener	Microscopic Polyangiitis	Churg–Strauss
ANCA positivity	80–90%	70%	≤50%
ANCA specificity	PR3 >> MPO	MPO > PR3	MPO > PR3
Histology	Leukocytoclastic vasculitis w/ granulomas	Leukocytoclastic vasculitis w/o granulomas	Eosinophilic vasculitis, w/ granulomas
Ear/nose/throat	Nasal septum perforation, saddle nose deformity, hearing loss, subglottic stenosis	Absent or mild	Nasal polyps, allergic rhinitis, conductive hearing loss
Eyes	Orbital pseudotumor, epi/scleritis, uveitis	Occ eye disease, epi/scleritis, uveitis	Occ eye disease, epi/scleritis, uveitis
Lungs	Nodules, infiltrates or cavitary lesions, alveolar hemorrhage	Alveolar hemorrhage	Asthma, transient infiltrates, alveolar hemorrhage
Kidney	Segmental necrotizing GN	Segmental necrotizing GN	Segmental necrotizing GN
Heart	Occ valvular lesions	Rare	Heart failure
Peripheral nerve	Vasc neuropathy (10%)	Vasc neuropathy (58%)	Vasc neuropathy (78%)
Eosinophilia	Rarely and mild	None	Very often & severe

MPO, myeloperoxidase; PR3, proteinase 3.

- **Treatment** (Pediatr Nephrol 2010;25:205)
  - **Wegener granulomatosis or microscopic polyangiitis**
    - Generalized non-organ–threatening dz = remission w/ MTX 0.3 mg/kg BW qwk orally + prednisone 1 mg/kg qd; MTX & pred for maintenance as well
    - Generalized organ-threatening dz – cyclophosphamide (15 mg/kg IV pulse q2wk × 6 mo) w/ oral prednisone 1 mg/kg tapered to 0.2 mg/kg by 6 mo effective, continued till 15 mo then tapered to 0.15 mg/kg × 3 mo more for remission
      - Addition of infliximab allows remission 6 wk earlier w/ dec steroid exposure
      - Azathioprine and w/ prednisone commonly used for maintenance
    - Severe renal disease and immediate life-threatening disease (DAH) = pulses of methylprednisolone and IV cyclophosphamide (3–4 mg/kg daily), consider plasma exchange
- **Churg-Strauss syndrome:** Initially w/ prednisone 1 mg/kg daily monotherapy
  - In severe dz addition of cyclophosphamide used (heart, CNS, GI, kidney involved)

DERMATOMYOSITIS/POLYMYOSITIS

Definition (Curr Rheumatol Rep 2011;13:216)
- Dermatomyositis: Weakness in proximal muscles and pathognomonic skin rashes
- Polymyositis: The skin is spared polymyositis; very rare in childhood

Pathophysiology (Pediatr Rev 1990;12:117; Pediatr Rev 1984;6:163)
- **Dermatomyositis:** 2/2 formation of thrombi from lesions of endothelial cells of intramuscular capillaries, arterioles, and veins resulting in infarct of muscle
  - Perivascular infiltrates generally present on biopsy. Vasculitic involvement
- **Polymyositis:** Inflammatory infiltrates, including lymphocytes and plasma cells, in perivascular regions and w/ muscle fascicles; bx may show muscle necrosis and phagocytosis, but endothelial cells of the blood vessels are normal

Epidemiology
- Dermatomyositis is the most common idiopathic inflam myopathy of childhood (80% cases)
- Bimodal distribution: 5–14 yo (avg age 7 yr) and 45–64 yo; 2:1 F:M predominance
- Combined freq 1–3.2 cases per 1,000,000 children <17 yo; Caucasian > Hispanic > AA
- Dermatomyositis is 10–20× more common than polymyositis

Criteria for Diagnosis (Curr Rheumatol Rep 2011;13:216)
- Exclusion of other rheumatic diseases
- Dermatomyositis: Characteristic rash (heliotrope dermatitis and Gottron's papules) and 3 of the following, sym prox muscle weakness, ↑ muscle enzymes, muscle

histopathology on bx; EMG w/ denervation & myopathy. MRI w/ contrast often used in place of EMG/biopsy in typical cases. Pyomyositis essentially as above but w/o dermatologic findings

Clinical Manifestations (Curr Rheumatol Rep 2011;13:216)
* Gottron's rash (91%), Heliotrope rash (83%), nail fold capillary Δs (80%), malar/facial rash (42%), myalgia/arthralgia (25%), dysphonia or dysphagia (24%); only 16% p/w fever
* Weakness usually prox and symmetrical (hip and shoulder girdles), LE > UE (difficulty climbing up stairs, getting up from chair, or combing one's hair)
* Motor weakness seen in ~100% of pts; DTRs may be absent, nml, or hyperactive
* Extraocular and facial muscles almost never involved but do see dysphagia/dysphonia
* Skin manifestations: Erythematous areas over MCP and IP joints (Gottron's papules), violaceous scaly rash often w/ lichenification, and violaceous discoloration of upper eyelids w/ periorbital edema (heliotrope rash), nail fold capillary Involvement, can also see ulcerative disease (<10% and predicts a severe course of illness & persistent weakness)
* Lipodystrophy develops in 14–25%, hypertriglyceridemia & insulin resistance (50%)
* Vasculopathy can affect any part of GI tract and 1/3 pts w/ pulmonary involvement 2/2 respiratory muscle weakness

Diagnostic Studies (Pediatr Rev 1990;12:117; Pediatr Rev 1984;6:163)
* Look for genetic disorders in family, which excludes dermatomyositis/polymyositis
* ↑ in muscle enzymes (CPK, aldolase, LDH, SGOT, SGPT); ↑ CPK is the most frequently seen. Inc vWF ag sugg active vasculitis
* MRI w/ contrast of quadriceps useful to eval for muscle inflammation
* Abn EMGs; nml nerve-conduct studies; fibrillation potentials, sharp waves at rest
  * Short duration and abundant single motor unit potentials on min volitional mvmt
  * High-frequency bizarre discharges
  * Muscle bx generally of biceps, quadriceps, or deltoid muscle; abn in ~90%
  * Findings include perivascular infiltrates, basophilia, moth-eaten appearance of many muscle fibers, and +alkaline–phosphatase reaction—not always done
* Skin bx can be done if normal mm enzymes
* Ancillary studies including ESR, neopterin, PFTs, UA, or HLA B8 may be helpful
* DMS in children not assoc with inc malignant risk as in adults

Management (Curr Rheumatol Rep 2011;13:216; Lancet 2008;371:2201)
* Prednisone 1st line, usually w/ initial induction phase w/ high dose of steroids followed by a lower dose for mtnce; Rx for 2–6 mo. Hydroxychloroquine for skin
  * One suggested regimen; 2 mg/kg IV divided q8 × 6 wk, when improved strength/rash and normalized muscle enzymes taper to bid then daily and tapered 10% q2wk
  * W/ dysphagia/dysphonia, pulmonary or GI dz then IV methylpred pulses
* Often methotrexate added as steroid-sparing agent. IVIG in severe cases
* Rituximab failed to show benefit in RCT, however has helped some patients. Cyclophosphamide & cyclosporine effective

Complications (Pediatr Rev 1990;12:117; Pediatr Rev 1984;6:163)
* Untreated pts can develop respiratory involvement, GIB, joint contractures, severe muscle wasting, calcinosis, and death
* Calcinosis can occur if unRx'd or Rx'd → pain, ↓ motion, skin ulcer, and abscesses
* Generally 4 diff patterns: Small nodules on skin, subcutaneous masses usually near joints, sheet-like deposits in fascial planes, and a pattern resembling an exoskeleton
* Relapses reported in pts w/ dermatomyositis several yrs after treatment
* Steroid-induced complications
* Dz can be monophasic or chronic; monophasic often can do well
* Outcome does not appear to correlate with age or sex; since introduction of steroids mortality rate <10% w/ improved functional outcomes

Intrapartum Fetal Heart Rate Monitoring

- Baseline fetal HR: Normal HR is 110–160 bpm
  - **Fetal tachycardia:** HR > 160 bpm. Causes: Maternal or fetal fever/infxn, fetal hypoxia, thyrotoxicosis, maternal meds (β-agonists and parasympathetic blockers)
  - **Fetal bradycardia:** HR < 110 bpm, w/ severe bradycardia <90 bpm. Causes: Hypoxia, complete heart block, maternal meds (β-blockers)
  - **Variability:** Absence of beat-to-beat variability may indicate: Severe hypoxia, anencephaly, complete heart block, maternal med effect (narcotics, MgSO₄)
  - **Accelerations:** Are associated with fetal movement and indicate fetal well-being
  - **Decelerations**
    - **Early:** Assoc w/ uterine compression of fetal head. Benign; not assoc w/ compromise
    - **Variable:** Assoc w/ umbilical cord compression. Can cause perinatal depression, but if beat-to-beat variability is maintained, then fetus is not compromised
    - **Late:** Assoc w/ uteroplacental insuff. If beat-to-beat variability maintained, fetus usually well compensated. If not, then may represent significant fetal hypoxia
- Fetal heart rate interpretation
  - Category I: Normal (ALL of: HR 110–160, moderate variability, +/– accels, no late or variable decels, may have early decels → routine care)
  - Category II: Indeterminate (any abnormality, requires surveillance and re-eval)
  - Category III: Abn (sinusoidal pattern OR absent variability w/ recurrent late decels, recurrent variable decels, or brady. Resolve cause expeditiously)

APGAR Scoring

	0	1	2
Heart rate	Absent	<100 min	>100 min
Respiratory effort	Absent	Weak cry; hypoventilation	Good, crying
Muscle tone	Flaccid	Some flexion	Active motion
Reflex irritability	No response	Grimace	Cry or active withdrawal
Color	Blue or pale	Acrocyanotic	Completely pink

Gestational Age and Birth Weight Classifications

Maturity by Gestational Age		
Preterm: <37 wk	Term: 37–42 wk	Post-term: >42 wk
Birth weight		
Low birth weight (LBW) : <2,500 g		
Very low birth weight (VLBW): <1,500 g		
Extremely low birth weight (ELBW): <1,000 g		
Birth Weight/Length for Gestational Age		
Small for gestational age (SGA): Weight or length <2 SD		
Appropriate for gestational age: Weight or length within 2 SD		
Large for gestational age: Weight or length >2 SD		
Asymmetric IUGR (delayed fetal weight gain with sparing of length and head growth) acute malnutrition or placental insufficiency; has potential for catch-up growth		
Symmetric IUGR (delayed fetal weight gain w/ comparable delays of length and head growth) prolonged malnutrition, genetic processes, or congenital anomalies; has less potential for catch-up growth		

Adapted from Pediatr Rev 2006;27:224.

- Be sure to plot length, weight, and head circumference on every infant
- New Ballard score to assess neuromuscular and physical maturity of infants, especially in those that are premature or if dates are unknown (J Pediatr 1991;119:417)
  - Can be obtained online at www.ballardscore.com
  - For preterm growth charts, go to www.medcalc.com/growth

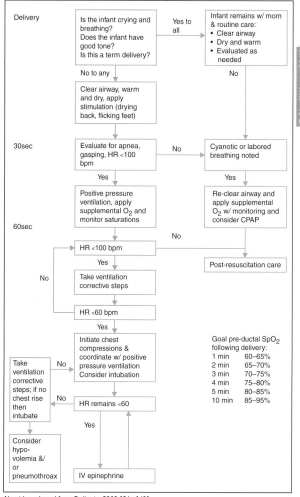

Algorithm adapted from Pediatrics 2010;126:e1400.

Neonatal Resuscitation (Pediatrics 2000;106:E29)
- When preparing for a high-risk delivery, have an estimated weight and GA so that appropriate ETT, umbilical catheter size, and drug doses can be calculated
  - Suggested ETT size and depth of insertion according to weight and GA
  - Depth of insertion can be estimated by weight in kg + 6 cm
  - <1,000 g or <28 wk: ETT 2.5; w/ depth of insertion 6.5–7 cm from upper lip
  - 1–2 kg or 28–34 wk; ETT 3; inserted 7–8 cm from upper lip
  - 2–3 kg or 34–38 wk; ETT 3.5; inserted 8–9 cm from upper lip
  - >3 kg or >38 wk; ETT 3.5–4; inserted ≥9 cm from lip

Sepsis Rule-out Algorithms
- Management of asymptomatic infants born at ≥35 wk gestation with risk factors for early-onset sepsis; protocols vary per institution
- Indications for intrapartum antibiotic prophylaxis (IAP)
  - +GBS cx unless elective C-section w/o labor or ROM
  - GBS bacteriuria in current pregnancy unless C-section w/o labor or ROM
  - Prior baby w/ invasive GBS disease
  - Maternal temp >100.4°F, even w/ negative GBS culture
  - GBS status unknown and ROM >18 hr, labor <37 wk or maternal temp >100.4°F

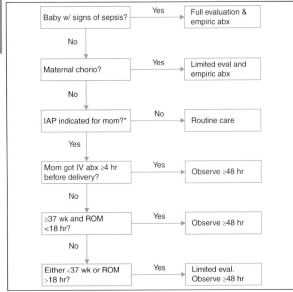

Adapted from CDC 2010 GBS Prevention Guidelines.
*See above for IAP guidelines.
Full eval = CBC w/ diff, blood cx, CXR (if resp sx) and LP (if baby stable enough).
Limited eval = CBC w/ diff, blood cx.

- MGH guidelines: Management of asymptomatic newborn at risk for sepsis
  - Abnormal WBC: Total WBC <5,000 or >30,000 or I:T ratio >0.2
  - I:T = number of immature PMNs/total number of PMNs
  - IV Abx
    - Ampicillin >2 kg give 50 mg/kg/dose q8; ≤2 kg give 50 mg/kg/dose q12
    - Gentamicin ≥35 wk GA → 4 mg/kg/dose q24h, <35 wk GA → 3 mg/kg/dose q24h
  - Of note, maternal fever w/i 1 hr of delivery should be Rx'd as intrapartum fever
  - Mother w/ prior child w/ GBS dz; baby should have CBC/diff, bld cx, and Abx if IAP <4 hr or if intrapartum fever >100.4°F
- The above are for management of asymptomatic infants born ≥35 wks' gestation
- Remember that these are only guidelines and do not replace clinical judgment

BASIC NICU MANAGEMENT

NICU Calculations and Formulas
- For a number of excellent online NICU calculators go to **www.nicutools.org**

Ventilatory Support and ECMO
(See PICU chapter)

Vascular Access
(Formulas may not be appropriate for SGA or LGA infants)
- Always check placement with babygram
- **Umbilical artery catheter** (UAC): For arterial BP monitoring or freq ABGs
  - Low line (cm) $\cong$ BW (kg) + 7 (want L3 − L5, just above aortic bifurcation)
    - Assoc w/ more vasospasms of the lower extremities
  - High line (cm) $\cong$ (3 × BW [kg]) + 9 (want T6 − T10, above diaphragm)
    - Assoc w/ risk HTN and ↑ risk IVH, ↓ incidence of cyanosis of lower extremities
- **Umbilical vein catheter** (UVC):
  - Normal: (0.5 × UA [cm]) + 1 (want above ductus venosus, at or below RA)
  - Low line: Insert to point of initial blood return (for emergent use)

NICU Testing Guidelines (Pediatrics 2006;117:572; Am Fam Physician 2007;75:1349; Arch Dis Child Fetal Neonatal Ed 2005;90:452)

Routine Neonatal Testing Guidelines	
Test	Gestational Age
Cranial Ultrasound	<32 wk; d of life: 3, 10, 30, then monthly until discharge
Ophthalmologic exams	≤31 wk or <1,500 g or 1,500–2,000 g and high risk; screen at 31 wk corrected GA, but not sooner than 4 wk chronologic age
Hearing tests	BAERS; for all infants before discharge
Car seat tests	<37 wk or <2,500 g or with respiratory instability

Fluids, Electrolytes, and Nutrition
- Growth parameters and expected weight gain
  - Weight <2 kg: Expect gain of 15–30 g/d or 10–20 g/kg/d
  - Weight >2 kg: Expect gain of >20 g/d
  - W/ preterm, may have initial weight loss of ≤15% (up to 20% in ELBW)
  - In term infants, may have initial weight loss of ≤10%
- Fluid requirements: Premature infants have greater ECF volumes
  - Initial fluid requirements: 60–120 mL/kg/d
    - Term infants ~60 mL/kg/d
    - ELBW ~120 mL/kg/d (assuming that they are in Giraffe incubators)
  - Goal after fluid stabilization: 100–150 mL/kg/d
  - Fluid restriction may be needed w/ PDA, BPD, CHF, renal failure, cerebral edema
  - Insensible loss inc w/: Inc skin permeability, inc BSA: weight ratio, phototherapy, radiant warmer beds, respiratory distress syndrome, cold stress, inc activity
  - Insensible water loss decreases with double-walled incubators
  - Monitor fluid status by daily weights, UOP, and serum Na, Hct, and BUN levels
  - Fluid loss also results from vomiting, diarrhea, ostomy output, chest tube drainage
  - Inadequate hydration can lead to hyperosmolarity and may be a risk for IVH
- Parenteral nutrition in preterm infant (NeoReviews 2011;12:e130)

NICU − BASICS 16-4

Carbohydrate

- GIR (mg/kg/min) = (% glucose in solution × rate of infusion per hr)/(6 × weight [kg]); OR = (% glucose concentration × cc/kg/d)/144
- Initial glucose rate: 4–6 mg/kg/min
- Adjust by 2 mg/kg/min as tolerated, advancing to meet nutritional need
- Limit to <14 mg/kg/min to prevent overfeeding, fatty liver, increased CO_2 production

Protein

- Infants <1,500 g BW: Begin at 2–3 g/kg/d, advance by 0.5–1 g/kg/d to goal of 3.5–4 g/kg
- Infants >1,500 g BW: Begin at 2–3 g/kg/d, advance by 1 g/kg/d to goal of 3 g/kg

Fat

- Begin at 1 g/kg/d and advance by 1 g/kg/d to goal of 3 g/kg
- May run lipid via central or peripheral access over 20–24 hr
- Monitor with serum triglyceride, normal range <200 mg/dL
- Essential fatty acid deficiency may occur in <1 wk without lipid source; provide minimum 0.5 g/kg/d 2–3 × per wk to prevent
- May need to limit to 2 g/kg/d with extreme hyperbilirubinemia

Total Energy Needs

- 90–100 kcal/kg/d for VLBW and SGA infants
- 80–90 kcal/kg/d for >28 wk and AGA

Additives*	
Na: 2–4 mEq/kg/d	Phos: 47–70 mg/kg/d
K: 2–4 mEq/kg/d	Cl: 2–3 mEq/kg/d
Ca: 60–90 mg/kg/d	Mg: 4.3–7.2 mg/kg/d

*Ca/phos ratio should be 1.7/1.

Modified from *Manual of Pediatric Nutrition*. 4th ed.

- Common total parenteral nutrition orders at MGH
  - Fluid orders on DOL #1: NPO and for
    - Term infants: $D_{10}W$ at a rate of 60–80 cc/kg/d
    - Preterm: $D_{10}W$ at a rate of 80–100 cc/kg/d
  - Add electrolytes after adequate UOP & after checking serum lytes at 12–24 hr
  - TPN labs
    - Daily: Na, K, Cl, CO_2, glucose
    - Weekly: Above tests plus Ca, Mg, P, alkaline phosphatase, BUN, creatinine, triglyceride, total protein, albumin, bilirubin, AST, ALT, hematocrit
  - "Feeder – Grower" labs
    - Hct and retic: 24–28 wk GA: Weekly; >28 wk GA: Every other wk
    - Chem 10, alk phos
      - Breast-fed <32 wk: Weekly Na, K, phos, Ca, alk phos
      - Formula-fed <32 wk: Weekly Ca, phos, alk phos
      - All breast-fed with supplement: Weekly lytes, Ca, phos
      - All infants on ProMod: Weekly BUN

Enteral Feeds *(Manual of Pediatric Nutrition, 4th ed)*

- Preterm neonates do not establish coordination of suck, swallow, and breathing until 32–34 wk GA; until then, enteral feeding via NGT (bolus vs. continuous) needed
- Enteral nutrition should generally begin as soon as the infant is clinically stable
- Initiation and advancement based on BW w/ attention to feeding tolerance
- Most premature infants start w/ trophic feeds (low vol; 10 mL/kg/d) to stim GI hormones, motility, and maturation and to prevent gut atrophy
- Option of pasteurized donor human breast milk: <31 wk, <1,500 g, after NEC or bowel surgery when mother's milk not available
- Once stable, volumes increased slowly as tolerated w/ increments ~10–20 mL/kg/d, allows for gut adaptation and minimizes risk of complications
- Signs of feeding intolerance include inc gastric residuals > 2 × previous hr's rate (continuous feed) or >$^1/_2$ previous bolus, inc in abd distention, vomiting, or bilious residuals, heme+ or frank blood in stools, ↑ in apnea or bradycardia with feeds

Criteria	Pre-made PN Initiation	Initiation	Advancement	Goal	Maximum	Comments
Amino Acids (gm/kg/d)	≤1,800 g and/or 34 wk					*Estimated Protein Requirements:*
	3 g/kg	3 g/kg	↑ 0.5–1 g/kg	3–4 g/kg	3.5–4 g/kg	• ≤1,500 g: 3.2–4 g/kg/d • >1,500 g: 3–3.5 g/kg/d • 4 g/kg if condition warrants (GI disease, surgery, or other protein-losing states)
Dextrose **GIR** (mg/kg/min)	7.5% (3.1 mg/kg/min)	4–6 mg/kg/min	↑ 1–2 mg/kg/min	10–12 mg/kg/min	14–18 mg/kg/min	• 45–60% of total calories • May exceed max GIR if clinical condition warrants
Intralipid (g/kg/d)	0	1 g/kg	↑ 0.5–1 g/kg	3 g/kg	0.12–0.15 g/kg/hr	• 25–40% of total calories (do **not** exceed 60%) • Minimum of 0.5 g/kg to prevent EFA deficiency (can develop within 2–3 d) • Decrease by 0.5–1 g/kg if TG >200–250
Fluids	60–80 cc/kg Pre-made PN volume is standard at 60 cc/kg	Begin with 60–80 cc/kg and advance total fluids per clinical status				
Miscellaneous	GIR 4.5 mg/kg/min: Pre-made PN with D$_{10}$W at 20 cc/kg					*Estimated Calorie Requirements:* • ≤1,500 g: 90–115 kcal/kg • >1,500 g: 90–100 kcal/kg *Lab Monitoring:* • Chem 10 — 2–3×/wk initially then weekly once stable • Baseline TG once receiving 2 g/kg IL × 24 hr • LFTs/TG weekly while on PN

- Trophic feedings should be initiated as soon as possible. Transitional feeding occurs generally between 2–14 d where the enteral feeding advances as TPN decreases to maintain fluid homeostasis. Enteral Feeding Guidelines should be followed. Monitor glucose during transition. TPN can usually be discontinued when enteral feedings reach 100 cc/kg

Respiratory Syncytial Virus (RSV) Prophylaxis (Pediatrics 2009;124:1694)

- Synagis 15 mg/kg IM monthly during RSV season. 1st dose 1 mo before RSV season
- Recommended at discharge (not while in NICU) for
  - Infants with chronic lung disease (CLD) (5 doses)
  - Infants born before 32 0/7 wk gestation (5 doses)
  - Infants born between 32 0/7 and 34 6/7 wk gestation w/ anticipated child care attendance or sibling less than 5 yr old (3 doses or until they reach 90 d old)
  - Infants with hemodynamically significant congenital heart disease (5 doses)
- Risk factors: School-aged siblings, day care, exposure to air pollutants, severe neuro-muscular dz, congenital abnormalities of the airways, LBW (<2,500 g), crowded living conditions, multiple birth, family history of asthma

Morbidity and Mortality with BW and GA (N Engl J Med 2008;358:1700)

Outcome	Birth Weight			
	501–760 g	751–1,000 g	1,001–1,250 g	1,251–1,500 g
Overall Survival	55%	88%	94%	96%
Survival w/ Complications*	65%	43%	22%	11%

*Complications include bronchopulmonary dysplasia, severe intraventricular hemorrhage, necrotizing enterocolitis, or bronchopulmonary dysplasia and severe intraventricular hemorrhage combined.

PULMONARY/RESPIRATORY

Etiologies of Respiratory Distress (NeoReviews 2005;6:e290)

Parenchymal Conditions
- Transient tachypnea of the newborn
- Meconium aspiration syndrome
- Respiratory distress syndrome
- Pneumonia
- Pulmonary edema
- Pulmonary hemorrhage
- Pulmonary lymphangiectasia

Airway Abnormalities
- Choanal atresia/stenosis
- Laryngeal web
- Laryngotracheomalacia or bronchomalacia
- Subglottic stenosis

Developmental Abnormalities
- Lobar emphysema
- Pulmonary sequestration
- Cystic adenomatoid malformation
- Congenital diaphragmatic hernia
- Tracheoesophageal fistula
- Pulmonary hypoplasia

Mechanical Abnormalities
- Rib cage anomalies (e.g., Jeune syndrome)
- Pneumothorax
- Pneumomediastinum
- Pleural effusion
- Chylothorax

- Differentiating cardiac and respiratory causes of cyanosis (see Cardiology chapter)
  - Cyanosis w/o resp distress, O_2 sat <85% on RA and 100% O_2, likely dx intracardiac shunt
  - If O_2 sat ↑ >85% on 100% O_2, either intracardiac shunt vs. pulm cause of cyanosis. Need to perform a full hyperoxia test
  - Hyperoxia test: Obtain baseline right radial (preductal) ABG w/ neonate on RA, then repeat ABG after providing 100% O_2 for 10 min
    - A PaO_2 of >300 mm Hg is normal, >150 mm Hg suggests pulmonary disease, and 50–150 mm Hg suggests cardiac disease (or severe pulmonary HTN)

Respiratory Distress Syndrome (Hyaline Membrane Disease) (NeoReviews 2009;10:e351)

- **Definition:** Primarily dz of preterm infants, but 2° surfactant def seen in older infants w/ mec aspiration syndrome, pneumonia/sepsis, and pulmonary hemorrhage
- **Epidemiology:** Incidence is inversely proportional to GA and BW
  - 60% if <28 wk, 30% 28–34 wk, 5% >34 wk
  - Other risk factors: Male, maternal gestational diabetes, perinatal asphyxia, hypothermia, multiple gestations

- **Pathophysiology:** Surfactant deficiency leading to atelectasis is the primary cause, often complicated by an overly compliant chest wall
- **Clinical manifestations and diagnostic studies**
  - Resp distress develops w/i 6 hr of life, worsening distress over the 1st 48–72 hr
  - CXR: Characteristic reticular granular pattern ("ground glass") and air bronchograms
- **Management**
  - Resp support and routine eval for sepsis and electrolyte abn; other recs
  - Preterm infants at risk for surfactant deficiency (24–34 wk gestation) benefit from antenatal steroids
  - Surfactant given ASAP after intubation regardless of antenatal steroids or GA
  - Consider prophylactic surfactant replacement for extreme prematurity at high risk of RDS, especially those not Rx'd w/ antenatal steroids
  - Consider rescue surfactant for hypoxic respiratory failure 2/2 surfactant def
  - CPAP w/ or w/o exogenous surfactant may reduce need for additional surfactant and incidence of BPD w/o ↑ morbidity

Meconium Aspiration Syndrome (NeoReviews 2010;11:e503)
- **Definition:** Intrauterine stress resulting in the passage of meconium into the amniotic fluid in utero. May be aspirated by the fetus during gasping or deep breathing
- **Epidemiology:** Risk factors for meconium-stained amniotic fluid: Post-term, IUGR, and some maternal conditions (HTN, DM, preeclampsia)
  - 10–15% live births c/b mec-stained amniotic fluid; 4–5% of these develop MAS
- **Pathophys:** Direct toxicity of meconium causes chemical pneumonitis, surfactant inactivation, activation of complement, & vasoconstriction (can lead to pulm HTN)
- Also w/ airway obstruction by the thick meconium
- **Diagnostic studies:** CXR: Typically w/ patchy areas of atelectasis, +/– hyperinflation, +/– diffuse or local linear or patchy infiltrates
- **Management:** At delivery, depressed infant (not vigorous, decreased tone, HR <100 bpm) intubated and trachea suctioned w/ mec aspirator
  - Resp support w/ supplemental O_2, and in severe cases w/ mechanical ventilation
  - Surfactant therapy as well as inhaled nitric oxide may also be beneficial
  - In cases refractory to the above treatments, ECMO may be required

Neonatal Pneumonia
- **Definition:** May be acquired in utero, during delivery (perinatally) or postnatally. Is classified as early (<7 d of age) or late onset (>7 d of age)
  - **Intrauterine PNA:** Usually the result of maternal infection (TORCH infections)
  - **Perinatal PNA:** Often 2/2 GBS, but also by E. coli, Klebsiella sp., and C. trachomatis
  - **Postnatal PNA:** 2/2 resp viruses (adenovirus, RSV), Gram+ bacteria (Strep or Staph aureus), and gram-neg bacteria (Klebsiella sp., Proteus sp., Pseudomonas aeruginosa, Flavobacterium, Serratia marcescens, and E. coli)
- **Diagnostic studies:** CXR (classic patchy infiltrates) 2/3 cases w/ pleural effusion
- **Management:** Includes antibiotics, oxygen therapy, ventilatory support, +/– pressors

Transient Tachypnea of the Newborn (RDS Type 2) (Pediatrics 2008;121:419)
- **Definition:** Usually benign, self-limited dz w/ tachypnea that appears shortly after birth and usually clears w/i 1–5 d. Diagnosis of exclusion
- **Epidemiology:** Incidence 11 per 1,000 live births
  - M > F, infants born by C-section and those w/ perinatal asphyxia, umbilical cord prolapse, or certain maternal conditions (asthma, diabetes, or analgesia)
- **Pathophysiology:** Cause is unknown; though 2/2 delayed resorption of fetal lung fluid may be 2/2 ↑ CVP and delayed clearance of pulmonary liquid by lymphatics
- **Diagnostic studies:** CXR: Diffuse parenchymal infiltrates and fluid in the fissure
- **Management:** Usually benign and management consists of adequate oxygenation

Congenital Diaphragmatic Hernia (NeoReviews 2011;12:e439)
- **Definition:** CDH is a developmental abnormality of the diaphragm resulting in a defect that allows abdominal viscera to enter the chest. 85% are left sided, 13% right, 2% bilat
- **Epidemiology:** Incidence is 1 in 3,000 births. No sex association
  - 50–60% cases are isolated finding
  - 50–80% survival
- **Pathophysiology:** Classically, 1° defect thought to be in diaphragm and pulmonary hypoplasia 2/2 pressure from the abdominal viscera in the thoracic cavity
  - Recent studies suggest that proper formation of the diaphragm requires normal formation of the lung and that pulmonary hypoplasia is the 1° cause
- **Management:** Morbidity and mortality ↑ are 2/2 pulm hypoplasia and pulm HTN
  - Immediate Rx w/ intubation, mech vent, and NGT for gastric decompression
  - Surgery is generally delayed until patient is stabilized
  - Gentle ventilation w/ permissive hypercapnia and the use of ECMO are common

- Surfactant Rx has been used, but recent studies have shown no benefit
- Pulmonary HTN can be Rx'd w/ nitric oxide, can decrease need for ECMO

Chronic Lung Disease and Bronchopulmonary Dysplasia
- **Definition:** Any pulm dz resulting from neonatal resp disorder called CLD and BPD accounts for vast majority of cases of CLD
- **Definition of bronchopulmonary dysplasia** (N Engl J Med 2007;357:1946)
  - Diagnosis: Oxygen dependence for at least 28 d postnatally
  - Grading at 36 wk postpartum for pts born <32 wk, at 56 DOL if born ≥32 wk
    - **Mild:** FiO_2 0.21
    - **Moderate:** FiO_2 0.22–0.29
    - **Severe:** FiO_2 ≥0.30 or CPAP or mechanical ventilation required
- **Incidence:** (Pediatrics 2009;123:1562) Almost always in <30 wk GA & w/ BW <1,500 g
  - ~1.5% of newborns in US under 1,500 g and BPD develops in ~20% of them
- **Pathophysiology**
  - "Old" BPD: 1st described in slightly preterms w/ RDS before surfactant and were exposed to aggressive mech ventilation and high concentration of inspired O_2
    - Resulted in inflammation and fibrosis of the lung structures
    - Antenatal steroids, surfactant Rx, and conservative resp care have ↓ incidence
  - "New" BPD: "Developmental disorder" in those born at earlier gestational ages
    - Pts w/ mild RDS, but early GA and min exposure to injurious factors alter nml pulm microvasc growth/alveolarization, w/ fewer, larger alveoli
- **Treatment:** Corticosteroid Rx is controversial; rapidly improves lung mechanics, also assoc w/ ↑ risk of neurodev impairment, including cerebral palsy
  - Inhaled bronchodilators can improve short-term lung fxn, as can diuretics

Apnea of Prematurity and Periodic Breathing (NeoReviews 2007;8:e214)
- **Definition**
  - Apnea of prematurity: Cessation of breathing >15 sec, usually assoc w/ desat and bradycardia. Shorter if w/ signif hypoxemia or bradycardia
    - Traditionally classified into the following three categories
      - Central: CNS origin w/ total cessation of insp effort w/o evid of obstruct
      - Obstructive: Obstr airway w/ chest wall motion and resp effort w/o airflow
      - Mixed: Most common w/ obstructive resp effort following central pauses
    - Periodic breathing: Usually a benign condition w/ regular, recurring cycles of breathing of 10–15 sec interrupted by pauses of at least 3 sec in duration
- **Incidence:** Prematurity greatest risk: 84% in ELBW, 35% in those born <32 wk GA
- **Pathophysiology:** Immaturity in breathing reg w/ immaturity in resp responses to hypercapnia and hypoxia and exaggerated inhib response to stim of airway receptors
- **Management**
  - In addition to supp O_2 and occasional CPAP, caffeine is used as a 1st-line drug Rx
    - Loading dose of 20 mg/kg caffeine citrate (10 mg/kg caffeine base), followed by maintenance dose of 5–10 mg/kg per dose of caffeine citrate q24h

CARDIOVASCULAR

Patent Ductus Arteriosus
- **Definition:** Ductus open in all newborns at delivery, closure occurs rapidly after birth; closure in 90% of healthy FT infants by 48th hr of life
  - A ductus open beyond 72 hr is considered persistently patent
- **Epidemiology:** ↑ risk PDA w/ prematurity, RDS, excess fluid admin in 1st d of life, asphyxia, congenital syndromes (Trisomy 13), birth at high altitude, cong heart dz
- **Clinical manifestations**
  - Heart murmur (usually continuous, accentuated in systole, loudest at 2nd or 3rd intercostal space), bounding periph pulses (2/2 diastolic runoff through PDA), hyperactive precordium, resp deterioration may be gradual or rapid, HoTN
- **Diagnostic studies:** Ductus can be visualized directly by echocardiography
- **Management:** Indications to Rx controversial: Spontaneous closure in neonates born at >27 wk GA; however, ibuprofen not as effective in closure after ~DOL#5
  - **Ibuprofen** (NeoProfen): Nonselective COX-inhib; inhib prostaglandin prod vs. **Indomethacin (Cochrane Rev 2010;(4):CD003481)—same efficacy for closure**
    - Ibuprofen has fewer side effects compared to indomethacin: Does not reduce mesenteric and renal blood flow (N Engl J Med 2000;343:674)
    - Indomethacin has more neuroprotective effects than Ibuprofen (NeoReviews 2008;9:e477)
  - Fluid restriction as much as possible to decrease PDA shunt

- Surgery: Considered after failure of NeoProfen therapy, or w/ hemodynamically significant PDA, or a contraindication to the use of COX inhibitor

Persistent Pulmonary Hypertension of the Newborn (PPHN)
- **Definition:** Pulm HTN 2/2 ↑ pulm vasc resistance (PVR) and a Δ in pulm vasoreactivity leading to R-to-L extrapulmonary shunting across PDA and foramen ovale
- **Pathophysiology:** 2/2 underdeveloped vasc lung bed or maladaptation of pulm vascular bed to transition to extrauterine life
  - Vasodilatory & vasoconstrictive factors (leukotrienes & thromboxanes) regulate vascular tone during transition. Nitric oxide (NO) an important vasodilator
  - Assoc d/o (Pediatrics 2007;120:e272): Lung dz (meconium aspiration, RDS, PNA, pulm hypoplasia, cystic lung disease), systemic disorders (polycythemia, hypoxia, sepsis), congenital heart disease, perinatal factors (asphyxia, C-section, LGA, etc.)
- **Clinical manifestations**
  - Cyanosis, respiratory distress, lability in oxygenation within 1st 4–8 hr of life
  - Large A-a gradient leading to large decrease in arterial oxygenation
  - Pre- and postductal O_2 sats may demonstrate gradient (R-to-L shunt through PDA)
- **Treatment:** Supplemental O_2: Oxygen is a potent vasodilator; consider mechanical ventilation in infants w/ significant respiratory distress and CO_2 retention
  - Adeq SBP w/ vol support; consider dopamine to ↓ the R-to-L shunt by ↑ing SVR
  - Adequate sedation, minimize handling to avoid stimulation
  - Avoid acidemia, consider $NaHCO_3$ and mild hyperventilation
  - Inhaled nitric oxide: Start dose of 20 ppm; may improve PVR and oxygenation
  - ECMO may be indicated in those failing mechanical ventilation

GASTROENTEROLOGY

Gastric Aspirates
Checked by oral or NGT before feeding to see if feeds tolerated and digested
- **Issues to consider**
  - If bilious emesis → malrotation until proven otherwise
  - Prob w/ regimen: Interval btw feeds too short or delayed gastric emptying
  - Ddx: Constipation, bowel obstruct, NEC, meconium plug or ileus, Hirschsprung dz, malrotation, volvulus, ileus, factitious (tube in duodenum or jejunum), pyloric stenosis, infxn, bleeding disorder (DIC, congenital coagulopathy), stress ulcer, meds
- **Evaluation**
  - Assess volume and characteristics (bloody, bilious, undigested formula/milk) of aspirate, vitals, PE (distension, visible bowel loops, visible erythema)
  - Labs: CBC, Bld cx (?sepsis/bleeding), stool guaiac, blood gas (if ? met acidosis)
  - Radiology: KUB; check gas pattern, pneumatosis intestinalis or portal venous air, ileus, obstruction
    - Left lateral decubitus film: Check for air – fluid levels (obstruction) and for layering of air above liver (free air, perforation)

Necrotizing Enterocolitis (NeoReviews 2001;2:e103; NeoReviews 2001;2:e110)
- **Definition:** Death of intestinal tissue in neonate 2/2 combo of vascular, mucosal, metabolic, infectious, and other unidentified insults to relatively immature gut
- **Epidemiology**
  - Risk factors: Prematurity, asphyxia, acute cardiopulm dz, enteral feeds, polycythemia and hyperviscosity syndromes, exchange transfusions, enteric pathogenic microorganisms (*E. coli, Klebs, Enterobacter, Pseudomonas, Salmonella,* etc.), umbilical A-lines
- **Clinical presentation:** Modified Bell staging criteria for NEC

Stage	Systemic Signs	Abdominal Signs	Radiographic Signs	Treatment
IA – Suspected	Temp instability, apnea, lethargy, bradycardia	Gastric retention, abd distension, emesis, heme-positive stool	Normal or intestinal dilation, mild ileus	NPO, antibiotics × 3 d
IB – Suspected	Same as above	Grossly bloody stool	Same as above	Same as IA
IIA – definite, mildly ill	Same as above	Same as above, plus absent bowel sounds, w/ or without abdominal tenderness	Intestinal dilation, ileus, pneumatosis intestinalis	NPO, antibiotics 7–10 d

IIB—definite, moderately ill	Same as above, plus mild metabolic acidosis & thrombocytopenia	Same as above, + absent BS, definite abd tenderness, w/ or w/o abd cellulitis, or RLQ mass	Same as IIA, plus ascites	NPO, antibiotics × 14 d
IIIA—advanced, but intact bowel	IIB, plus HoTN, bradycardia, severe apnea, combined resp and met acidosis, DIC, neutropenia	Same as above, plus signs of peritonitis, marked tenderness, and abdominal distension	Same as IIA, plus ascites	NPO, Abx × 14 d, fluid resuscitation, inotropic support, ventilator Rx, paracentesis
IIIB—advanced, perforated bowel	Same as IIIA	Same as IIIA	Same as above, w/ pneumoperitoneum	Same as IIA, plus surgery

- **Diagnostic studies**
  - Early may resemble sepsis; but classically w/ triad of feeding intolerance, abd distension, and guaiac + stool
  - Labs: CBC/diff, (Plts <50,000/μL), bld cx, guaiac, ABGs, electrolytes
  - Radiology: Serial KUBs (assess for abn bowel gas patterns, ileus, portal venous or intramural gas [pneumatosis intestinalis], fixed sentinel loop of bowel). Lat decubitus (assess for pneumoperitoneum, indicates perforation)
- **Management**
  - Initial NEC protocol: NPO, NG tube for decompression
    - Abx coverage (ampicillin, gentamicin or cefotaxime; consider anaerobic Rx w/ clindamycin or Flagyl if pneumatosis or pneumoperitoneum seen)
    - F/u I/O, remove K from IVF if anuric, septic w/u, x-rays q6–8h in acutely ill
  - Surgical management: Resection of nonviable viscera with re-exploration later

Tracheal Esophageal Fistula and Esophageal Atresia (Am Fam Physician 1999;54:4:910)
- **Definition:** Abn communication btw esophagus and trachea; assoc w/ esophageal atresia (EA), where proximal and distal portions of esophagus do not communicate

Type A	EA without a fistula	8%
Type B	EA with proximal TEF	1%
Type C	EA with distal TEF	84%
Type D	EA with proximal and distal TEF	3%
Type E	Isolated TEF (H type)	4%

- **Pathophysiology**
  - 1° morbidity pulmonary. Esophageal obstruct w/ inability to clear secretions, drooling, aspiration/regurg of food/pharyngeal contents → pneumonia
    - W/ crying, straining, coughing, air enters stomach → abd distension, dilated loops of bowel, elevated diaphragm → basilar atelectasis and resp distress
- **Clinical presentation**
  - W/ esophageal atresia: Polyhydramnios in utero; excess salivation, choking, coughing, cyanosis; diff swallowing excess fluid need freq suctioning
  - ~1/2 of pts w/ EA/TEF have other assoc congenital anomalies (i.e., VACTERL), cardiac anomalies (VSD or tetralogy of Fallot), other GI anomalies
- **Diagnostic studies:** Inability to pass NGT & resistance 10–12 cm from nares
  - Imaging: Barium swallow may identify fistula, need caution and use nonionic contrast or dilute barium; +/– distal gas clue to presence and location of TEF; bronchoscopy is the most accurate procedure
- **Management:** Surgical correction is required
  - Presurgical management
    - Discontinue oral feedings, avoid bag-mask ventilation, and start IV fluids
    - Elevate head to limit risk of aspiration and NGT in pouch w/ continuous suction
    - Oxygen therapy if needed and mechanical ventilation if respiratory failure
    - Evaluation for other congenital anomalies, especially VACTERL
    - Repair delayed in VLBW infants and those w/ major concomitant anomalies
- **Surgical complications**
  - Stricture 2/2 gastric acid erosion of shortened esophagus, leak of contents at anastomosis, fistula recurrence, tracheomalacia, abn swallow & esoph dysmotility, GERD

Gastroschisis

- **Definition:** Centrally located full-thickness abd wall defect (a) w/o protective covering over extruded intestine, and (b) w/ intact umbilical cord. Typically, liver and spleen reside w/i peritoneal cavity. No syndromic association
- **Pathophysiology**
  - Unprotected intestine exposed to irritating amniotic fluid in utero → edematous, indurated, foreshortened appearance; w/ delay of peristaltic activity and effective absorption by several wk
- **Diagnosis:** Predominantly by prenatal U/S; differential dx: Ruptured omphalocele
- **Management:** Delivery at center equipped to provide definitive care
  - Debate if C-section vs. vag delivery ↑ mortality/morbidity w/ gastroschisis
  - Temperature regulation: Intestinal surface area exposed to environment puts infant at risk for hypothermia. Rx w/ protective covering: Saline-soaked gauze dressing and covering abdomen in plastic bag up to chest
  - Nasogastric decompression; antibiotic coverage; TPN
  - Surgical correction: Complete reduction of herniated intestine w/ 1° closure of wall or placement of unreduced intestine in prosthetic silo w/ staged reduction over 7–14 d

Omphalocele

- **Definition:** Herniation of abdominal contents into base of umbilical cord
  - Has protective covering enclosing malpositioned abd contents. Umbilical cord comes together over apex of sac to form a normal appearing cord
  - 24–40% assoc w/ other congenital anomalies including Beckwith – Wiedemann, trisomies, chromosomal abnormalities, CDH and various cardiac defects
- **Clinical presentation:** Vary in size; giant omphaloceles may contain liver and spleen
  - Peritoneal cavity underdeveloped as growth proceeded w/o solid organ in position
- **Diagnostic studies:** Typically picked up by prenatal ultrasound
  - Requires further evaluation for other anomalies
- **Management:** If ruptured sack, treat similar to gastroschisis w/ surgical correction
  - Intact sack: Less urgent surgery required, and may require period of time for daily dressing changes to dessicate/toughen sac

Hirschsprung Disease (Pediatr Rev 2006;27:e56)

- **Definition:** Congenital absence of ganglion cells of the myenteric and submucosal plexus of the intestines resulting in poor/dysfxnl intestinal motility
  - Begins at internal anal sphincter and variably extends proximally, may be patchy
  - Short-segment Hirschsprung: (75–85%) distal to splenic flexure
  - Long-segment Hirschsprung: (20%) aganglionic section extends past splenic flex
  - Total intestinal aganglionosis: Rare form involving all small and large bowels
- **Epidemiology:** Incidence: Highest in African-Americans and Asians, ~4:1 ♂ to ♀
- **Pathophysiology**
  - Craniocaudal migration failure of ganglion cells precursors during embryogenesis
  - Earlier arrest of migration results in longer segment involvement
- **Clinical manifestations**
  - Delay in passage of meconium (>48 hr) always concerning for Hirschsprung
  - Can p/w infreq BMs, abdominal distension, vomiting, diarrhea, refusal to feed
  - Exam w/ contracted anal sphincter, no stool in vault on rectal exam but explosive stool release w/ w/d of finger, abd distension
  - Isolated defect (70%) but 10× more common in pts w/ Trisomy 21
- **Diagnostic studies:** Gold std is rectal bx w/ staining for ganglion cells
  - Barium enema w/ transition zone btw contracted distal and dilated proximal bowel is very suggestive; but absence of transition does not r/o
  - Anorectal manometry to check reflex relaxation of anal sphincter (dx if no reflex)
    - Useful for controversial ultrashort segment dz w/ <5 cm involvement, (unclear whether this condition really exists)
- **Management:** Resection of aganglionic section (Am J Surg 2000;180:382)
  - Multi surgical approaches; most w/ 1° endorectal pull through (1-stage procedure)
  - Age when done & if staged approach used (w/ diverting colo in btw) varies
- **Complications**
  - Even w/ surgical Rx, 30% w/ cont constipation or never develop fecal continence
  - Major mortality/morbidity w/ Hirschsprung 2/2 enterocolitis (occurs in ~20% in one series) (Am J Surg 2000;180:382)
  - **Hirschsprung assoc enterocolitis:** Mostly pts <2 yo p/w abd distension, explosive watery stool, fever, and hypovolemic shock

Sepsis/Meningitis
- **Definition/Epidemiology**
  - Neonatal meningitis: Infection of meninges w/i 1st mo of life
    - Incidence 0.25–1.0 per 1,000 live births
    - Mortality high (20–50%) and neurodev morbidity is significant (often >50%)
  - Neonatal sepsis: Systemic illness with bacteremia at <30 d of life
    - Early onset: Defined as during 1st 7 d of life; majority p/within 1st 3 d of life
    - 1–10 per 1,000 live births, but preterm <1,500 g have ~2% incidence
    - Assoc w/ high mortality (up to 35% in very preterm) and morbidity (↑ risk for IVH, RDS, CLD, PVL in preterm neonates) (Pediatrics 2000;105:21)
    - Late onset: >7 d of life (Pediatrics 2002;110:285)
    - Incidence usually < early onset for term neonates, but preterm neonates <1,500 g have up to 20% incidence.
    - Mortality in preterm ~20%, and pts at ↑ risk for PDA, NEC, BPD
- **Risk factors**
  - Early-onset sepsis (vertical transmission): Prematurity, PPROM, GBS+, intrapartum maternal fever, meconium-stained amniotic fluid, chorio
  - Late-onset sepsis (horizontal transmission): Endotracheal intubation, Foley, central lines (UAC/UVC), exposure to broad-spectrum Abx
  - Meningitis: Similar as in sepsis; prematurity, VP shunts
- **Clinical manifestations, diagnostic studies and management**

Neonatal Sepsis/Meningitis					
Type	Course	Organisms	Signs/ Symptoms	Initial Workup	Management
Early onset	Up to 7 d of life • 85% w/i 24 hr • 95% w/i 48 hr	GBS, E. coli, Strep viridans, Enterococcus, Staph aureus, Listeria, Haemophilus	Typically fulminant presentation: Resp distress, szrs, lethargy, hypotonia, irritable w/ hyperreflexia, apnea, cyanosis, metabolic acidosis, hypo-/hyperglycemia, shock	CBC-diff, Blood Cx, lumbar puncture (do not delay Abx if suspicion is high), serial CRP, CXR (if resp sx). For late-onset sepsis workup, add UA/ Ucx	Ampicillin and Gentamicin IV • incidence of ampicillin-resistant E. coli increasing (up to 70%) • subsequent coverage should be based on culture results
Late onset	>7 d of life	Coag neg Staph, Klebsiella, Pseudomonas, E. coli, Candida	Typically gradual presentation: Increased O$_2$ req, feeding intolerance, temp instability, tachycardia		
Meningitis	1st mo of life	GBS, E. Coli, Listeria, Haemophilus, Klebsiella, Enterobacter, Serratia, Enterococcus	Similar to sepsis sx: Feeding intolerance, temp instability, vomiting, lethargy, irritability, apnea, seizures, purpuric rash		

From Pediatrics 2000;105:21; Pediatrics 2002;110:285; Pediatrics 2002;110:e42; N Engl J Med 2002;347:240; NeoReviews 2008;9:e571; NeoReviews 2010;11:e426.

Hepatitis B Virus (HBV) (Pediatrics 2003;112:193; RedBook 2009: Hepatitis B – Summaries on Infectious Disease)
- **Epidemiology**
  - Worldwide, 350 million people w/ chronic HBV; 1° transmission mother to child
    - E antigen + moms, neonatal transmission rate up to 90% (BMJ 2006;332:328)
  - In US, ~20,000 neonates born to mothers w/ HBsAg+ (Pediatrics 2003;111:1192)
  - Rates are highest among immigrant women, especially from Asia and Africa

Approach to Hepatitis B in Neonates

Maternal Status	Infant ≥2,000 g	Infant <2,000 g
HBsAg positive	Hepatitis B vac + HBIG (w/i 12 hr of birth); immunize w/ 3 vac doses at 0, 1, and 6 mo chrono age; check anti-HBsAb and anti-HBsAb at 9–15 mo, if infant HBsAg and anti-HBsAb neg, reimmunize w/ 3 doses at 2-mo intervals and retest	Hep B vac + HBIG (w/i 12 hr of birth); immunize w/ 4 vac doses at 0, 1, 2–3, and 6–7 mo of chrono age. Check anti-HBsAg and anti-HBsAb at 9–15 mo; if HBsAg, and anti-HBsAb neg, reimmunize w/ 3 doses at 2-mo interval and retest
HBsAg status unknown	Hep B vac (by 12 hr) + HBIG (w/i 7 d) if mom tests HBsAg+, test mother for HBsAg immediately	Hepatitis B vac and HBIG (both by 12 hr); test mother for HBsAg immediately
HBsAg negative	Hepatitis B vaccine at birth preferred; immunize with 3 doses at 0–2, 1–4, and 6–18 mo of chronologic age	Hep B vac dose 1 at 30 d of chrono age if medically stable, or at hospital d/c if before 30 d of chronologic age; immunize mo of chronologic age

HBsAg, surface antigen; HBIG, Hepatitis B immunoglobulin; HBsAb, surface antibody.

Herpes Simplex Virus (HSV)
- **Epidemiology** (Pediatrics 2001;108:223; Pediatrics 2011;127:e1)
  - Prevalence 1–3/10,000 deliveries; most (75%) are a result of HSV-2 (genital)
  - Most recent US data: 9.6 cases per 100,000 births, varies by region of US
  - Since advent of acyclovir in the 1970s, mortality has improved greatly
  - In 60% of cases, mother had no HSV symptoms at the time of delivery
  - Mortality extremely high in untreated neonates (up to 80% in disseminated HSV)
- **Pathophysiology**
  - Can be acquired while intrauterine, intrapartum (80% of cases), or postnatal
  - Virus enters usually through the skin, eyes, mouth, respiratory tract
  - Risk factors: Vag delivery, 1° HSV infxn in mom (up to 50% infxn to neonate vs. 5% w/ recurrent maternal infxn), high maternal # of sexual partners, low SES

Clinical Manifestations of Neonatal HSV

Type (% of HSV)	Time of Presentation	Signs/Sx	Mortality (with Rx)
Localized (~35% cases)	~10 d of life	Vesicles involving skin, mucous membranes. Can cause keratoconjunctivitis	Low (<5%)
CNS (~35% cases)	~2 wk of life	Can present with or without skin findings. Seizures, temp instability, tremors, lethargy, poor feeding, bulging fontanelle	~17%
Disseminated (~30% cases)	~10 d of life	Can involve the liver, adrenals, or any other organ system. Sx can include jaundice, rash, purpura, apnea, CV collapse, lethargy, fever, anorexia, vomiting	~55%

Adapted from Pediatrics 2001;108:223.

- **Diagnosis**
  - HSV PCR on CSF and/or blood
  - HSV DFA (Direct Fluorescent Antibody) of lesion
  - HSV viral cultures of lesion, nasopharynx, conjunctiva, urine, CSF, rectum
  - Avoid Tzanck smear as only 50% sensitive
  - CT/MRI/EEG can also be useful for evaluation for CNS involvement
- **Prevention:** C-section shown to reduce neonatal HSV in 1° infection of mother; risk also reduced w/ dec usage of invasive fetal monitoring (JAMA 2003;289:203)
- **Management**
  - IV acyclovir: 60 mg/kg/d × 21 d (Pediatrics 2001;108:230)
  - Ocular HSV drug of choice is trifluridine; 2nd line is vidarabine
  - Contact precautions; consider screening cultures
  - If mother has 1° infection in asymptomatic neonate; culture and empirically treat

Congenital TORCHs Infections

Infection	Common Clinical Findings	Prevalence per 1,000 Pregnancies	Mode of Infection	Diagnosis and Evaluation	Treatment
Toxoplasma	Retinopathy, cerebral calcifications, hydrocephalus, seizures, HSM, LAD	0.2–10	Cat feces, undercooked meat	Serologies, culture	Pyrimethamine, sulfadiazine, + leucovorin × 1 yr
Rubella	IUGR, cataracts, cardiac anomalies (PDA, pulmonary stenosis), deafness, blueberry muffin skin, HSM	0.7–1.7	Primary maternal infection of nonimmunized mother	Serologies (rising maternal IgG, cord blood IgM), PCR, Cx, echo, head US, eye exam	No treatment, supportive care only
CMV	Jaundice, HSM, thrombocytopenia, microcephaly, seizures, chorioretinitis, hepatitis, pneumonitis, deafness, cerebral calcifications	5–10 (<10% with sx)	Maternal primary or reactivation	Viral culture from urine, PCR of mucous membrane secretions, eye exam, CMV antigenemia	Congenital infection does not benefit from foscarnet/ganciclovir. Recent studies show effect of Rx of mother w/ CMV Ig
HSV	See neonatal HSV section				
Syphilis	Rash (hands, feet), bone abnml, HSM, hemolytic anemia, classic "snuffles" presentation	Varies (up to 25 in high-risk groups)	Vertical transmission high (50%) in primary maternal infection	Neonatal IgM, dark field microscopy of skin lesion, CSF PCR, RPR/VDRL	Benzyl penicillin, 30 mg/kg per dose 12 hourly

From Am Fam Physician 2003;67:2131; N Engl J Med 2005;353:1350; Pediatr Rev 2011;32:537.

ABO Incompatibility (Pediatrics 2004;114:297)

- **Definition:** Isoimmune hemolytic anemia 2/2 maternal sensitization to baby blood
  - 2/2 diff blood groups; most common, baby w/ A or B type born to type O mom
- **Epidemiology:** Incidence: 12–15% pregnancies but DAT (direct Coombs) + in only 3–4%
  - Symptomatic hemolytic dz in <1%; accounts for 2/3 of hemolytic dz of newborn
  - Risk factors: A1 antigen in infant has greatest antigenicity
    - 1st born have 40–50% risk for symptomatic dz and subsequent pregnancies without mod-to-severe dz, unlike Rh isoimmunization
- **Pathophysiology**
  - Active placental transport of maternal isoantibody, results in immune reaction w/ A or B antigen on fetal erythrocyte
  - Hemolysis balanced by compensatory reticulocytosis
- **Clinical manifestations:** Jaundice that evolves faster than nonhemolytic pattern
  - Anemia may occur until 8–12 wk of age
- **Diagnosis:** Blood type and Rh factor in mom and infant (usually from cord blood); Monitor HCT
  - Reticulocyte count: Elevated count (10–30%) support hemolytic anemia
  - Direct Coombs: May be weakly+ at birth as very little Ab on the RBC
  - Blood smear may demonstrate microspherocytes
  - Bilirubin: Indirect bili mainly, rapid rise suggests recheck freq (usually q4–8h)
- **Treatment:** Hydrate, eval for aggravating factors (sepsis, drugs, metabolic disturb)
  - Phototherapy: See section on indirect and direct hyperbilirubinemia
  - IVIG: Blocks neonatal reticuloendothelial Fc-R; ↓ing hemolysis of Ab-coated RBCs
  - Exchange transfusion: Removes Ab-coated RBCs, serum Ab and bilirubin; threshold level of hyperbili debated, see section on indirect and direct hyperbili

Rh Incompatibility (Clin Perinatol 1995;22:561)

- **Definition:** An isoimmune hemolytic anemia that occurs when the mother is Rh-negative and sensitized to Rh (D) antigen from a Rh-positive fetus
- **Epidemiology:** Incidence: RhoGAM prophylaxis has ↓ incidence of Rh sensitization to <1% of Rh-incompatible pregnancies
  - Risk factors: Fetomaternal hemorrhage, coexisting ABO incompatibility, male sex, Caucasian > African-American or Asian
- **Pathophysiology**
  - Mother exposed to Rh antigen w/ parturition, miscarriage, abortion, ectopic preg
  - Recognition of Rh antigen by immune system after initial exposure and subsequent re-exposure to Rh antigen induces maternal production of Rh IgG-Ab
  - IgG Rh-Ab crosses placenta and attaches to fetal erythrocytes, followed by sequestration in fetal liver and spleen and hemolysis
  - Compensatory reticulocytosis and shortening of the erythrocyte generation time are often unable to match the hemolysis, leading to anemia
- **Clinical manifestations:** Jaundice (unconjugated hyperbilirubinemia) usually w/i 1st 24 hr of life; anemia, which reflects severity of disease; hepatosplenomegaly
  - Hydrops fetalis has historical assoc w/ severe Rh disease
  - Nonimmune conditions are currently more frequently associated with hydrops
- **Diagnostic studies**
  - Blood type and Rh type in mom and infant
  - Reticulocyte count: Expected values 10–40% in symptomatic Rh disease
  - Direct antiglobulin test (Coombs) of neonate: Strongly+ DAT is diagnostic of Rh incompatibility w/ approp setup. If RhoGAM given at 28 wk GA, passive transfer of Ab across placenta will result in a false+ DAT
  - Indirect antiglobulin test (indirect Coombs) of maternal blood type can also be performed, although confounded by RhoGAM administration
  - Bilirubin levels: Unconjugated fraction will be elevated
- **Management**
  - Antepartum period, RhoGAM (Rh IgG) should be given at 28 wk's GA
  - Maternal antibody titers measured every 1–4 wk, depending on gestational age; ultrasound to assess for fetal scalp edema, ascites, or other signs of hydrops
  - Postpartum period: Severely anemic children should be resuscitated, monitored, and transfused if needed; blood bilirubin and hemoglobin, serial unconjugated bilirubin, phototherapy as indicated

Intraventricular Hemorrhage (IVH)

- **Definition**
  - Disorder of premature; periventricular subependymal germinal matrix bleed
  - Grade of IVH, determined by U/S, poorly predictive of mortality and neurologic prognosis, especially in ELBW neonates (J Pediatr 2007;151:500)

Classification of IVH	
Grade	Ultrasound Findings
I	Germinal matrix hemorrhage
II	IVH without ventricular dilatation
III	IVH with ventricular dilatation
IV	IVH with parenchymal involvement

- **Epidemiology**
  - Incidence and severity inversely proportional to gestational age
    - ~20% of neonates <1,500 g affected (<32 wk's gestational age)
  - Other risk factors: Birth asphyxia, rigorous resuscitation, seizures, rapid fluid admin, HoTN, PDA, hypothermia, early sepsis, PTX (Pediatrics 2003;111:e590)
  - 50% occur in 1st 12 hr of life, >90% occur within 1st 3 d of life
- **Clinical manifestations**
  - Sx usually subtle and nonspecific, and often is asymp
  - Can present w/ bulging fontanelle, change in level of consciousness, seizures, acidosis, bradycardia, apnea, drop in hematocrit
  - **Catastrophic syndrome:** Rapid bulging of fontanelle, coma, decerebrate posturing, fixed pupils, seizures, respiratory sx, paralysis (emergency)
- **Diagnostic studies**
  - Modality of choice: Cranial ultrasound
  - For GA <32 wk, screen at DOL #3, #10, #30 (controversial; institution specific), then qmo until discharge to eval for PVL (periventricular leukomalacia)
- **Prevention**
  - Avoidance of premature delivery, antenatal steroids shown to decrease IVH in premature neonates (Pediatrics 1993;91:1083)
  - Recent smaller study demonstrated delayed cord clamping in very preterm infants (average GA 28 wk) showed reduction in IVH (Pediatrics 2006;117:1235)
- **Management**
  - No known method to reverse IVH
  - Mainstay: Avoid fluctuations in BP, perform serial U/S to follow evolution, supportive care, and to Rx any subseq posthemorrhagic hydrocephalus

Hypoxic Ischemic Encephalopathy (HIE) (Pediatrics 2006;117:528; NeoReviews 2010;11.e85)

- **Definition:** Syndrome disturbed neuro fxn in term newborn, 2/2 perinatal insults
- **Clinical manifestations**
  - Can include abnormal respiratory drive, depression of tone and reflexes, subnormal level of consciousness, seizures
- **Epidemiology:** 1–6 per 1,000 live births, 15–20% mortality postnatal, and 25% survivors w/ long-term neurodevelopmental sequelae
- **Management**
  - Best evidence of benefit is for therapeutic hypothermia (proposed mech: ↓ neuronal metab demand, ↓ cytotoxin accum, prevention of apoptosis), now standard of care
  - Criteria: GA ≥36 wk, age ≤6 hr, evidence of hypoxia/ischemia (pH ≤7.0 or pH 7.0–7.15 + acute perinatal event + postnatal depression), sx of encephalopathy)
  - Protocol: Hypothermia to 33.5°C for 72 hr, then gradual re-warming. Before starting, obtain standard labs (chem 7, CBC, LFTs, coags, ABG, bld cx) and give antibiotics during cooling. Need a-line access. (MGH protocol)

PROPHYLAXIS IN CRITICAL ILLNESS

Ventilator-assoc PNA (J Pediatr 2009;154:582; Am J Infect Control 2006;34:84)
- **Prevention strategies:** Hand hygiene, HOB >30°, oral chlorhexidine bid, minimize narcotics, avoid unnecessary stress ulcer ppx (does not seem to ↑ VAP risk in PICU pts). Neuromusc blockers impair gastric emptying. Statistically significant ↓ VAP rate

Stress Ulcer (Pediatr Crit Care 2010;11:124; AACN Adv Crit Care 2007;18:158)
- Pathophysiology: Stress → splanchnic hypoperfusion → gastric mucosal breakdown and impaired gastric motility, leading to prolonged gastric acid exposure
  - pH has significant, nonlinear correlation w/ stress ulcer occurrence and bleeding
  - pH 7.0 protective, below w/ increased risk
  - After bleed, 50% ↓ in clot stability when pH dec from 7.4 to 6.5 (Crit Care Med 2002;30:S351)
- Generally during 3rd–7th ICU d; can cause signif bleed (up to 4× inc mortality)
- Prophylaxis indicated for high risk: Sepsis, shock, operative procedure ≥3 hr, trauma/ closed-head injury, status epilepticus, acute renal or hepatic failure, anticoagulation or coagulopathy, burns >35% BSA, concurrent steroids, parenteral nutrition (Crit Care Med 1992;20:1519)
- Regimens: Meta-analysis of available data failed to demonstrate ↓ mortality, ↓ ICU stay, ↓ rate ulcer, (Pediatr Crit Care 2010;11:124) did see ↓ erythema on EGD
  - Proton pump inhib: Preferred (though no benefit to any specific drug in meta-analysis)
    - Most potent (dose dependent, 99% achieve pH = 7), max effect not until 48 hr
    - Risks: CYP450 metabolism, poss assoc w/ C. diff infxn, acute interstitial nephritis
  - Histamine$_2$-receptor antagonists
    - Quicker onset of action but less effective. Maximum achievable gastric pH 4.0–5.0. After 24–48 hr, pH stabilizes at 3.0–4.0
- Risk of thrombocytopenia: Use PPI if Plt <50,000; cimetidine inh cytochrome P450

DVT Prophy (J Trauma 2010;68:52; J Pediatr Child Health 2010;46:288)
- See Pulmonary Embolism in Pulmonary section for details on treatment
- Incidence of DVT 10× lower for children compared to adults
- Major ICU risk factor is CVL (18–26% assoc w/ VTE in ICU). Others include prolonged immobility/paralysis, malignancy, sepsis, surgery/trauma, long-term TPN (up to 66%)
  - Peak incidence: Infants w/ CVL & adolesc s/p surgery, prolonged immobilization
- Dx: U/S most often used, but has low sensitivity (30–80%)
  - In ICU, a neg U/S does not rule out DVT. If high suspicion, treat until able to confirm w/ contrast U/S or venogram (gold standard)
  - Hypercoag workup recommended for all patients (same incidence as in adults)
- Prophy: EBM guidelines for ppx in long-term TPN use and complex cardiac patients w/ assoc procedures; extrapolation from adults difficult 2/2 diff in developmental hemostasis (varying levels/response of clotting cascade proteins) & pharmacokinetic/dynamic properties of anticoag agents in children
  - Methods: TEDs or pneumoboots, rarely LMWH
  - Pediatric evidence: No benefit of prophy in trauma pts <13 yo (J Trauma 2005;59:1345) or w/ warfarin in pedi-onc pts w/ CVL (Acta Paediatr 2006;95:1053)
  - **Bottom line:** Consider prophylaxis for adult-sized patients w/ significant risk factors (long-term immobilization, CVC, malignancy)

Catheter-related Blood Stream Infections (Pediatrics 2011;128:1077)
- Central venous catheters associated w/ ↑ risk nosocomial blood stream infection
- Rate of CRBSI ↓ 56% w/ CVC care bundle (5.2/1,000 line d to 2.3/1,000 line d)
- In one study, rate ↓ from 11.94/1,000 catheter d to 3.05/1,000 w/ efforts to ↓ insertion time and decreased use of parenteral nutrition
- Controversy exists about safety of chlorhexidine skin prep in children, use only if >6 mo

PICU · PROPHY 17-1

PAIN CONTROL AND SEDATION

- Pain & sedation scores should be followed for all receiving sedatives or analgesics

Equianalgesic Dosing		
	Oral (mg)	IV (mg)
Morphine	30	10
Fentanyl	N/A	0.1
Dilaudid	7.5	1.5
Codeine	200	N/A
Hydrocodone	20	N/A

- Commonly used analgesics and sedatives

Drug	Onset/ Peak (IV)	Duration (IV)	Relative Potency (IV)	Starting Dose (IV)
Morphine	20 min	3–5 hr	1	Infant/child: 0.05 mg/kg/dose. usual 0.1–0.2 mg/kg/ dose q2–4h prn (max 15 mg/dose)
Dilaudid	15 min	5 hr	7	Child: 0.015 mg/kg/dose q3–6h prn
Fentanyl	Immediate	30–60 min	100	Infants: Intermittent: 3 mcg/kg/dose q2–4h prn. Continuous: 1–2 mcg/kg load → 0.5–1 mcg/kg/hr; titrate upward. Children: Intermittent: 1–2 mcg/kg/dose; may repeat at 30–60-min intervals. Continuous: 1–2 mcg/kg load → 1 mcg/kg/hr; titrate upward (usual: 1–3 mcg/kg/hr)
Versed	1–5 min	2–6 hr	N/A	0.05 mg/kg IV × 1, repeat q2–3 min (max 0.4–0.6 mg/kg IBW); if vented cont at 0.5–1 mcg/kg/min titrate to effect
Ativan	15–30 min	8–12 hr	N/A	0.05 mg/kg IV (also IM) q4–8h, max 2 mg/dose

These are suggested doses & do not replace clinical judgment.
Follow institutional guidelines where available.

RESPIRATORY FAILURE

(Pediatr Rev 2009;30:470)
- **Definition:** Failure of oxygenation, ventilation, gas exchange or airway protection
  - Arterial O_2 tension <60 mm Hg, CO_2 tension > 50 mm Hg and pH <7.35
  - If w/ chronic resp insuff; acute hypercarbia = inc in PCO_2 20 mm Hg above baseline
- **Diagnostic eval:** ABG (VBG can be used to r/o hypercapnia), CXR (r/o PNA, edema)
  - Consider CBC (anemia), CT (if suspect PE), ECHO, BNP (if suspect shunt or CHF)
- **Interpretation of results**
  - **A-a gradient:** Alveolar–capillary gas exchange

$$PAO_2 - PaO_2 - (FiO_2 \times 713) - (PaCO_2/0.8)$$
$$\text{Normal value on RA} - 2.5 + (0.21 \times \text{age (yrs)});$$
$$PAO_2 = \text{partial pressure of } O_2 \text{ in alveolus, } PaO_2 = \text{oxygenation in artery}$$

  - Most useful in assessing etiology of hypoxia & progression of lung disease
  - **PaO_2/FiO_2 ratio (oxygenation index):** Measure of severity

$$\text{Normal >300; ALI: } PaO_2/FiO_2 \text{ 201–300; ARDS: } PaO_2/FiO_2 \leq 200$$

- **Hypercapnia ($\uparrow PCO_2$)**

$$\textbf{Paco}_2 = \frac{CO_2 \text{ production}}{\text{alveolar ventilation}} = k \times \frac{VCO_2}{RR \times VT \times (1 - V_D/V_T)}$$

- **Interpretation of blood gas**

Condition	pH	PCO_2	Base Excess
Acute respiratory acidosis	↓	↑	↔
Chronic respiratory acidosis w/ metabolic compensation	Slight ↓	↑	↑
Acute on chronic respiratory acidosis	↓	↑/–	↑
Acute metabolic acidosis w/ respiratory compensation	↓	↓	↓
Acute hyperventilation	↑	↓	↔

- **Etiology of hypoventilation (↑ $PaCO_2$)**

Cause	Pathophysiology	Clinical Scenario
Central	↓ resp drive	Metabolic alkalosis, CNS event/infection, sedation (med or toxin related)
Pulmonary	Lung/airway Musculoskeletal*	PNA, asthma, BPD, CF Obesity, kyphosis/scoliosis, pleural effusion. Neuropathy, botulism, myopathy (muscular dystrophy, hypophosphatemia)
Increased production	Increased CO_2 production from inc metabolic rate	Fever, sepsis, excess carb load

*Note: ↑ WOB may not be apparent; blood gas helpful.

- **Hypoxemia etiology (↓ PaO_2)**

Cause	A-a gradient	S_vO_2	Distinguishing Features	Clinical Scenario
Hypoventilation	Normal			Drug o/d (benzo's)
O_2 delivery/ consumption imbalance	High	Low		↑ demand (stress, infection) ↓ supply (hypoxia, ↓ CO, anemia)
	High	High		↓ demand (poor utilization – late shock) ↑ supply (high FiO_2)
True shunt	High	Low/ normal	Does not correct w/ O_2	R → L intracardiac shunt, AVM, alveolar collapse or filling
VQ mismatch	High	Low/ normal	Corrects w/ O_2	Airway (asthma), alveolar (PNA, CHF), vascular (PE)

- **Treatment:** Treat underlying cause, NPO (to prevent aspiration)
  - Hypoxemia: Supplemental O_2, consider CPAP or intubation
  - Hypercapnia: Consider BiPAP or intubation

MECHANICAL VENTILATION

Noninvasive Methods
- **CPAP:** Continuous PEEP. Useful for hypoxemia (atelectasis, edema, OSA, HMD)
- **BiPAP:** Pt-triggered PIP + CPAP. Useful for hypoventilation (CF, NM disease)

Invasive Methods
- **Support (PS/VS):** Spont breaths assisted to reach goal pressure (P) or volume (V)
  - No set rate, pt *must* initiate breaths. Pt determines I time. Less efficient if ETT leak
- **Assist/Control (AC):** Vent delivers minimum # supported breaths (synch to pt effort) with add'l pt-initiated breaths getting full assist to reach goal P or V w/ controlled I time
  - Downside: Uncomfortable, dyssynchrony and auto-PEEP (breath stacking)
- **SIMV:** Vent delivers minimum # supported breaths (sync to pt effort) but add'l pt-initiated breaths get no assist. May add PS to assist spont breaths (SIMV + PS)
  - Downside: Inc resp effort (pt must overcome circuit resistance during spont breaths)
- **HFOV:** Rapid oscillatory breaths given at set frequency (Hz); manipulate MAP and ΔP
  - Downside: Can easily hypervent. Vent Δ may take longer to equilibrate on blood gas
  - Used when conventional ventilation fails
  - Initial trials supporting HFOV over conventional vent strategies were done before ARDSNet low TV protocols, which appear to have the same mortality. They are likely equal, but HFOV may be an easier way to obtain the same result (Crit Care 2005;9:177)

Troubleshooting

- **Acute desaturation in pts w/ artificial airway on mechanical ventilator:** Think **DOPE**
  - **D**islodgement (ETT); **O**bstruction (mucus plug); **P**neumothorax; **E**quipment failure
- Oxygenation depends on mean airway pressure (MAP)
- Ventilation depends on minute ventilation and dead space

Vent Type	Parameter to Increase	pO_2	pCO_2
Conventional	RR	No effect	↑
	FiO_2	↑	No effect
	PEEP	↑	↓
	PIP	↑	↑
	I time (should not be 1st line)	↑	↓
HFOV	MAP	↑	
	ΔP		↑

Extubation Readiness Criteria (Ped Crit Care Med 2009;10:1)

- Pt awake w/ intact airway reflexes (cough, gag), hemodynamically stable, manageable secretions, acceptable gas exchange, O_2 requirement <40%
- Air leak: Used to predict upper airway obstruction (swelling) after extubation
  - Presence of audible leak around ETT @ <25 cm H_2O
  - Consider steroids if no leak (role unclear; may decrease risk re-intubation)
    - Decadron 0.5 mg/kg q6h × 6, 12 hr prior to extubate (Crit Care Med 1996;24:1666)
  - Negative inspiratory force: Strength of resp muscles in pts w/ neuromusc weakness
    - NIF > 30 mm Hg (not validated in children, unreliable)
- Spontaneous breathing trial (CPAP or PS + PEEP) prior to extubation

PEDIATRIC ECMO/ECLS

Definition

- Extracorporeal life support for lung &/or cardiac fxn

	Circuit	Indication	To ↑ O_2	To ↓ CO_2	Considerations
V–V	Blood returns to RA/central vein	Resp failure			Less efficient oxygenation (SaO_2 80–95%), watch for recirculation
V–A	Blood returns to aortic arch	Combined cardioresp failure	Inc FiO_2 HCT >35; inc flow; inc CO	Inc sweep	Carotid/IJ ligation, direct arterial emboli, renal nonpulsatile flow, inaccurate CVP, lower coronary artery O_2 supply, high LV afterload, cardiac stun

Pediatric Indications

- Death "imminent" with other treatment and
- Reversible lung disease (commonly PNA, burns/inhalation, acute chest, ARDS PPHN)
  - High ventilator support >7 d: PIP > 35, PEEP > 10, MAP > 18, OI > 40, PaO_2/FiO_2 > 150

$$OI\ (Oxygen\ Index) = \frac{FiO_2 \times MAP}{PaO_2}$$

  - No other significant organ dysfunction or
- Bridge for cardiac support (CHD postop, myocarditis, arrhythmias, bridge to transplant—must be at a transplant center, postresuscitation care for rapid cooling)
- Severe hypothermia, sepsis

Basic Management/Monitoring

- Lung rest: PEEP to keep lung open, FiO_2 21–30
- Goals
  - PaO_2 > 60, PCO_2 40–45
  - pRBC 20 cc/kg for HCT < 35, FFP 10 mL/kg for PT > 17, ACT 180–220, Plt >100 (>150 if bleeding), cryo 1 U/kg for fibrinogen > 150
  - MAP 45–65 (might need inotropic support, esp in VV)

- Sedation: Ativan, morphine, possibly intermittent midazolam; paralysis *not* routine
- Nutrition: Enteral feeds OK; frequent lyte repletion; Qwk LFTs; lipid <2 g/kg/d to avoid accumulation in circuit; total fluids 80–100 cc/kg/d
- ID: Antibiotic ppx (cannula)
- Neuro: Frequent assessment, screening U/S 24 hr post cannula, then ≥q48h
- Heme: Amicar avoided if possible (decreases life of ECMO circuit). Use if bleeding despite maintaining lower ACTs and adequate platelets
- Renal: Frequent volume overload, edema, may need diuretics/HD
- Pharmacokinetics/dynamics for many drugs altered on ECMO circuit: Hydralazine, nicardipine, furosemide, epinephrine, & dopamine can be used at regular doses, but esmolol, amiodarone, nesiritide, bumetanide, sildenafil, & prostaglandins require dose modification (J Cardiovasc Pharmacol 2011;58:126)

Prognosis/Course (Pediatr Rev 2009;30:470)
- **Complications:** Hemorrhage, hemolysis, clot in circuit, neuro (hemorrhage, szr, air emboli) renal dysfxn, infection, cardiac stunning (VA), equipment failure
- **Prognosis:** Survival rate for pediatric patients on ECMO for viral pneumonia ~64%
  - Neurologic: 72–91% no/mild disability, 6% cerebral infarction, 10% seizure
  - Rare chronic pulm disease
- **Post-ECMO monitoring:** Head U/S, CT scan, carotid Dopplers, auditory brainstem-evoked response testing, eye exam, follow BPs

VENTILATOR-ASSOCIATED PNEUMONIA (VAP)

Definition (Clin Infect Dis 2010;51:S136 PMID 20597664)
- National Health Safety Network definition: Pt w/o underlying dz w/ serial x-ray w/ 1 of following (2+ if underlying dz); new or progressive infiltrate, consolidation or cavitation in addition to 3 of the following (age >1, ≤12 yo) temp >38.4 or <36.5°C w/o cause, WBC < 4,000/mm^3 or ≥15,000/mm^3, new purulent sputum/Δ sputum/↑ secretions, new/ worse cough/dyspnea/apnea/tachypnea, rales / bronchial BS, worse gas exchange

Epidemiology (Clin Infect Dis 2010;51:S136; J Pediatr 2009;154:582)
- Rates 2.1–11.6/1,000 vent d; w/ ↓ to 0.3/1,000 w/ VAP prevention bundle (see later)
- 2nd most common nosocomial infxn in PICU (after bacteremia); VAP ~32% cases
- Risk factors: Immunosuppressant drugs, immunodef, NM blockade, genetic syndrome, transportation out of unit, reintubation, and transfusion. Other assoc include 1° bacteremia, trach, recent bronch, burns, TPN, steroids, H2-R blockers (Pediatrics 2002;109:758)
- Common pathogens: Gram-neg especially *Pseudomonas aeruginosa* (up to 44%) and *Klebsiella* species, *Enterobacter* species, nontypable *H. infu*. Most common GP: *S. aureus*

Clinical Manifestations/Workup (Clin Infect Dis 2010;51:S136)
- Sputum GS and cx can guide Rx and help distinguish infxn (high #polys, different organisms) in patients w/ chronic colonization (low # polys, similar organisms)
- ET aspirate 90% sens/40% spec, BAL GS 50% sens/81% spec, BAL cx 50% sens/80% spec

Treatment
- Empiric Abx should include broad coverage for gram-neg (PSA) and gram-pos
  - Vancomycin (coverage for MRSA) and Cefepime commonly used OR
  - Piperacillin/tazobactam 300 mg/kg/d div q6–8h (max 12 g/d) OR
  - Meropenem 60 mg/kg IV qd div q8h (up to 3 g/d)
  - Immunocompromised, may warrant coverage for unusual pathogens (PCP, fungus)
- Abx tailored by cx results, 7–10 d if uncomp; longer if *S. aureus* (by response if comp) or *Pseudomonas aeruginosa*
- Supportive care: Optimize vent settings (keep O$_2$ sat ≥95%, monitor for SIADH)
- Prevention bundle: Mouth care w/ chlorhexidine, HOB at 30–45° if possible, drain secretions from circuit q2–4h, hand hygiene (J Pediatr 2009;154:582)

Prognosis (Pediatrics 2009;123:1108)
- Complications: Lung abscess, ARDS
- VAP has risk up to ~2× longer PICU, ~2× longer hospital length of stay and higher mortality (10.5 vs. 2.4%) vs. other PICU pts. Early approp abx saves lives

ACUTE RESPIRATORY DISTRESS SYNDROME (ARDS)

Definitions (1994 American-European Consensus on ARDS)
- Acute lung injury (ALI): Acute onset of hypoxemia, bilateral infiltrates on CXR and noncardiogenic pulmonary edema w/ $PaO_2/FiO_2 > 200$ but <300
- ARDS: All of the above with $PaO_2/FiO_2 \leq 200$

Epidemiology (Intensive Care Med 2009;35:136)
- Incidence low (1–4%), onset generally within 72 hr after underlying disease onset
- Inciting illnesses: PNA, aspiration, sepsis, inhalational injury, near-drowning, meds

Pathophysiology (Pediatr Rev 1993;14:163)
- Pulm or systemic insult (e.g., sepsis) → injury to alveolar–capillary unit in 3 stages
  - Exudative (early): Lung endothelial + alveolar cell damage → microvascular thrombi and filling of airspaces with exudate
  - Proliferative (1st–3rd wk): Cellular proliferation converts intraalveolar hemorrhagic exudates into granulation tissue
  - Fibrotic (>3 wk): Remodeling and fibrosis
- Injury patchy, w/ airway collapse in dependent lung → V/Q mismatch and hypoxemia

Clinical Manifestations
- Hypoxia out of proportion to underlying dz, progress to dyspnea, tachypnea, diffuse rales

Treatment
- Rx underlying illness & ensure adequate O_2 (may require CPAP, BiPAP, or intubation)
- Protective ventilation strategy per ARDSNet: Adult data (N Engl J Med 2000;342:1301)
  - "Small lungs": 2/2 patchy involvement/collapse as little as 25% of lung tissue may participate in air exchange, but "normal" lung is at risk of overdistension
  - Maintain oxygenation: 100% FiO_2 during acute period, then increase PEEP to minimize O_2 while maintaining oxygen delivery
  - Minimize baro/volutrauma with $P_{plat} \leq 30$, small TV (6–8 mL/kg), extended I time (to allow more uniform ventilation) and permissive hypercapnia
  - If requiring escalating PIP/PEEP, consider switch to HFOV
- Eval: ABG, CBC/diff, CMP, BP (↑ MAPs needed for oxygenation compromise CO)
- Adjuncts: Surfactant may have mortality benefit (JAMA 2005;293:470), prone positioning, inhaled NO. Corticosteroids do not improve mortality except in PCP PNA

Prognosis (Intensive Care Med 2009;35:136)
- Complications: Ventilator-associated lung injury, oxygen toxicity, chronic lung disease from interstitial fibrosis, rare neurologic sequelae (Pediatrics 1981;67:790)
- Mortality 20–75%, 2/2 sepsis or other failure (↑ in near-drowning, heart dz, sepsis)
- Poor prognostic factors: Initial severity of hypoxemia, other organ failure, CNS dysfxn

SEPTIC SHOCK

Definitions (Pediatr Crit Care Med 2005;6:2; see ED chapter for Shock [general])
- SIRS (systemic inflammatory response syndrome): Required 2 of the following 4
  - T >38.5 or <36°C
  - HR > 2 SD > nml for age w/o other stimuli, or if <1 yo, HR <10th %ile for age
  - RR > 2 SD above normal for age
  - WBC <5 or >15, or >10% bands
- Sepsis: SIRS + suspected or proven infection
- Severe sepsis: Sepsis + end-organ dysfunction
- Septic shock: Sepsis + cardiovascular dysfxn (HoTN, oliguria, cap refill >5 sec, ↑ lactate)

Pathophysiology
- Endotoxin release, inflammatory mediators (TNF-α, interleukins) → vasodilation, ↑ capillary permeability → ↓ organ perfusion, lactic acidosis cytopathic hypoxia, mito dysfxn
- Dynamic process: Often evolves from "warm" shock (↑ CO, ↓ SVR) to "cold" shock (↓ CO, ↑ SVR) or mixed (↑ CO, ↓ SVR); many develop cardiac dysfxn (Pediatrics 1998;102:e19)

Diagnostic Studies
- Cx (blood, urine, sputum, CSF, as indicated) before Abx, do not delay Abx
- Imaging studies (CXR, CT scans) to identify source if the patient is stable

Management (see page 17-9 for treatment algorithm)
- **Early resuscitation:** Improve CV status; balance O_2 delivery and demand (Crit Care Med 2008;36:296)

- Aggressive volume resusc: 20 cc/kg × 3 w/i 1st hr (1st bolus w/i 5 min), may need up to 200 cc/kg total; titrate to improved MS, UOP, HR, cap refill (Crit Care Med 2009;37:666)
- Use crystalloid unless need for colloid (Hgb < 10, abnormal PT/PTT)
- Fluid refractory shock: >60 cc/kg volume or CVP 8–12 mm Hg w/ persistent signs shock; start vasoactive medications (see later)
  - Place CVL; goal SVC O$_2$ sat (CVO$_2$) > 70% (N Engl J Med 2001;345:1368)
  - **cVO$_2$ approximates SvO$_2$ (mixed venous O$_2$ sat):** ~O$_2$ demand/O$_2$ supply

$$cVO_2 - SvO_2 = SaO_2 - \frac{VO_2}{CO \times Hgb \times 13} \text{ [normal 70\% - 80\%]}$$

  - Think **COAL**
    - **C**ardiac output (CO); **O**$_2$ consump (VO$_2$); **A**mt of Hgb, **L**oading of Hgb (SaO$_2$)
  - If fluid refractory, pressor resistant → stress dose steroids (hydrocort 50 mg/m^2/d)

Definitive Therapy
- Broad-spectrum empiric antibiotics w/i 1st hr of recognition of sepsis/shock
- Consider source control: Remove lines, foreign bodies, débride/drain focal infections

Vasoactive Drugs
- Selected based on hemodynamic physiology; dopamine reasonable 1st choice

Shock Type	Drug	Mechanism	Dose
"Warm" shock (↑ CO, ↓ SVR)	Dopamine (may be less effective in age <12 mo, where stores of NE/Epi are low)	Low (D$_1$): ↑ renal, splanchnic blood flow (no evid of clinical benefit) Intermed (β$_1$): ↑ HR, ↑ SV (↑ CO) High (α$_1$): ↑ SVR	Low: 2–5 mcg/kg/min Intermediate: 5–15 mcg/kg/min High: 15–30 mcg/kg/min
	Norepinephrine	α$_1$, β$_1$ (↑ SVR, ↑ CO)	0.05–1 mcg/kg/min (max 40 mcg/min)
	Phenylephrine	α$_1$ (↑ SVR)	Bolus: 5–20 mcg/kg q10–15min Maintenance: 0.1–0.5 mcg/kg/min
	Vasopressin (adjunctive)	V1 (↑ SVR)	0.3–2 milliunits/kg/min
"Cold" shock (↓ CO, ↑ SVR)	Epinephrine	Low: β$_1$ + β$_2$ (↑ CO) High: α$_1$ (↑ SVR)	Low: 0.1–0.3 mcg/kg/min High: 0.4–1 mcg/kg/min
	Dobutamine	β$_1$ > β$_2$ (↑ CO, ↓ SVR)	2–40 mcg/kg/min
	Milrinone	PDE inhibitor (↑ CO, ↓ SVR)	Load: 50–75 mcg/kg IV over 60 min then 0.5–0.75 mcg/kg/min
	Nitroprusside	NO release, vascular smooth muscle dilator (↓ SVR and venodilation)	wt <40 kg: 1–8 mcg/kg/min wt >40 kg: 0.5–5 mcg/kg/min

Other Interventions
- Rx abs/relative adrenal insuff (pressor unresponsive shock, add hydrocort; defer cort stim until off hydrocort); felt to be highly prevalent in PICU pop w/ incidence ↑ w/ age
  - Use of steroids in this setting assoc w/ significant ↓ in vasopressor duration & dosage (Crit Care Med 2011;39:1145)
- Overly aggressive BS control associated with hypoglycemia (J Pediatr 2005;146:30; N Engl J Med 2008;358:125)
- Treat anemia: Goal Hgb >7 if SvO$_2$ <70%, conservative transfusion strategy not inferior to liberal (N Engl J Med 2007;356:1609)
- Consider IVIG in neonates or those w/ acquired or inherited IgG deficiency (hypogammaglobinemia, nephrotic syndrome)

Pediatric Shock Differs from Adults (Crit Care Clin 1997;13:553)
- $1/3$–$1/2$ children will change hemodynamics w/i 24 hr, requiring a re-evaluation of therapy

Choice of Cardiovascular Agents
- α_1 = vasoconstriction, ↑ duration of cardiac contraction
- β_1 = ↑ inotropy and chronotropy, β_2 = vasodilation, bronchodilation
- DA = renal, splanchnic, coronary, cerebral vasodilation
- PDEIII inhibition = ↑ inotropy, minimal chronotropy, vasodilation

Class	Name	Action	Use	Comments
Vaso-pressor Useful for: Nml CO ↓ SVR	Phenyl-ephrine	A	Obstructive shock, HOCM, sepsis	↑ afterload; constricts coronary, renal & pulm vessels; reflex vagal cardiac response; tissue necrosis
	Vasopressin	V_1, ↓ iNOS (deactivates K_{ATP} channel)	Sepsis	HypoNa; coronary and mesenteric ischemia at doses >0.04 U/min
Inotrope Useful for: ↓ CO Normal to high SVR	Dobut-amine	β_1, β_2	Sepsis	↓ SVR and splanchnic perfusion. Works best w/ dopamine
Inotrope + Pressor Useful for: ↓ CO ↓ SVR	Dopamine	DA < 2 β 2–5 α, β 5–15 α >15	1st line <12 yo sepsis	↑ PCWP, pulm shunting; renal dosing does ↑ UOP but no mortality benefit. ↓ pituitary and T cell fxn
	Nor-epinephrine	α, β_1	Sepsis	↑ afterload; constricts resistance = capacitance vessels; decreases splanchnic/renal flow; raises PAP; hyperglycemia and tissue necrosis
	Epinephrine	β 0.005–0.02 α > 0.02 Renal > 0.035	Anaphylaxis status asthmaticus Cardiogenic shock from ↓ HR, sepsis	Profound peripheral vasoconstriction (splanchnic + renal); increases mVO₂, arrhythmia, ischemia, RF, lactic acidosis
Inotrope + Dilator Useful for: ↓ CO in CHF	Milrinone	PDEIII inhibitor	Heart failure	Ventricular arrhythmias, $1/2$-life 2.5 hr

Table adapted with permission courtesy of R. Scott Harris, MD.

Adapted from Crit Care Med 2009;37:666.

INCREASED INTRACRANIAL PRESSURE

Pathophysiology/Etiology
- ↑ pressure if any intracranial compartment → displaces other structures
- Brain tissue: ICH, neoplasm, infarct, DKA (young and new dx ↑ risk)
- CSF: CNS infection, vasculitis, hydrocephalus, pseudotumor cerebri
- Blood: Hemorrhage (TBI, ruptured AVM, other vascular anomalies)
- Mixed: DKA → cerebral edema (cytotoxic, vasogenic, or interstitial), TBI (see TBI section)

Clinical Manifestations
- Neuro: ΔMS, irritability, bulging fontanelle, HA, lethargy → coma, retinal hemorrhage, dilated pupil (usually on side of lesion), CN palsy (esp III, IV, VI), incontinence, decorticate/decerebrate posturing
- Cardiorespiratory: Cushing triad (LATE – bradycardia, HTN, irregular respirations), Cheyne–Stokes breathing, apneusis
- GI: Vomiting

Diagnostic Evaluation
- Careful neurologic exam & fundoscopic exam; imaging: Head CT
- Labs: CMP (hypo- or hypernatremia), coags (bleeding can cause DIC, and for therapeutic intervention), CBC, and type and screen
- EKG: Cerebral T waves (deep T wave inversions)
- LP: Generally not recommended if concern for increased ICP. Treat empirically

- Goals: Minimize ICP and maintain CPP
  - Avoid 2° injury; avoid hypoxia, hypercarbia, HoTN, hypo/hyperglycemia, hyperthermia
- 1st-line therapy
  - ABCs: Intubate if needed (GCS <8 on presentation is absolute indication)
    - Thiopental or etomidate are drugs of choice; adequate sedation/analgesia
  - Keep PCO_2 35–40
  - HOB 30° (J Neurosurg 1992;76:207), midline. Avoid neck access (CVL)
  - Maintain normothermia (consider prophylactic Tylenol)
  - Avoid hypervolemia. TF = $^2/_3$–$^3/_4$ mntc isotonic fluid; may need diuresis
  - Treat underlying cause (Abx for infection, reduce IVF if DKA)
  - Prophylactic antiepileptics (phenytoin, Keppra; phenobarbital in infant) for sz risk are standard of care but not evidence based
- 2nd-line therapy
  - CSF drainage: Intraventricular drain w/ drainage and monitoring
  - Maintain CPP (MAP–ICP): In TBI, autoregulation lost; CPP ~ MAP, NE preferred
  - Muscle relaxants to reduce shivering
  - Suctioning adjuncts: Intratracheal lidocaine superior in preventing ICP spike (Intensive Crit Care Nurs 1996;12:303)
  - Hyperosmolar therapy: Hypertonic saline, mannitol
  - Therapeutic hypothermia (T 32–34°C): Reduces ICP but no ↓ mortality (adult data)
  - Dexamethasone (0.25–0.5 mg/kg q6h) only beneficial for tumor-related vasogenic edema. Do not use in cerebral edema assoc with TBI, anoxic brain injury, intracerebral hemorrhage, or pediatric meningitis
- 3rd-line therapy
  - Pentobarbital coma: For refractory cases
  - Decompressive craniectomy. Absolute indications: Refrac ICP, ICP >40 for >30 min

Treatments for Acute Herniation		
Treatment	**Mechanism**	**Notes**
Mannitol: 0.5–1 g/kg IV over 20 min q6–8h for goal sOsm 300–310 mOsm/L	↑ sOsm → net flow of water out of brain along gradient	Hyperosmolarity, profound osmotic diuresis → hypovolemia, abn lytes, ARF.
Hyperventilation	↓ P_aCO_2 → cerebral vasoconstrict → ↓ CBF	Risk of cerebral ischemia (↓ CPP)
3% normal saline Goal Na 155–160 Acute herniation: 2 cc/kg over 20 min or 50 cc of 23.4% saline if >40 kg	↑ sOsm → net flow of water out of brain along gradient	Risk of hyperosmolality, central pontine myelinolysis
Pentobarbital coma (refractory cases)	↓ cerebral metabolic rate → dec CBF	Risk of HoTN, need continuous EEG
Decompressive craniectomy		Abs indications: Refractory ICP or ICP >40 for >30 min.

Dosages are suggestions and do not replace clinical judgment. Follow institutional guidelines where available.

Prognosis (J Pediatr 2002;141:793)
- Mortality: Severe TBI ~8%, severe TBI w/ either HoTN, hypoxia, or hypercarbia ~55%
- Other poor prognostic signs: Hyper-/hypoglycemia (TBI), ↑ BUN, GCS ≤ 7, PCO_2 < 22 (DKA), hypoxia, hypercarbia, each episode of HoTN leads to worse neurologic disability

Pediatric Brain Death Criteria (Crit Care Med 2011;39:2139)
- Definition: Absent neurological fxn w/ known irreversible cause of coma and apnea
- Prerequisites: HoTN, hypothermia and metabolic abn corrected; sedatives, NM blockers, anti-convulsants d/c'd for reasonable duration prior to exam. Exam 24–48 hr after resuscitation or acute brain injury
- Criteria
  - 2 neuro exams (2 diff attendings) 12–24 hr apart w/: Coma (LOC, unresponsive to noxious stim, no purposeful mvmt), absent brain stem reflexes (no pupillary resp [CNII], absent corneal resp; Absent gag, cough, sucking, rooting reflexes (CN IX, X), absent oculovestibular reflex (CN XIII; cold water caloric testing w/o eye deviation or nystagmus), absent facial mvmt (CN VII, no grimace w/ deep pressure at supraorbital ridge), flaccid tone (w/ exception of spinal cord reflexes)
  - Apnea testing ×2 (can be the same provider); begin by ventilation/oxygenation to nml parameters. Cease support and PaCO₂ must rise 20 mm Hg (>60 mm Hg abs) w/o resp effort; terminate test if desat or pt destabilizes. Can sub ancillary testing for apnea
  - Ancillary testing: Not necessary; EEG, NM scan, cerebral blood flow, angiography; these can be substituted for apnea testing but does not replace neuro exam

RAPID SEQUENCE INTUBATION

Preparation
• SOAPME: **S**uction, **O**xygen, **A**irway equipment, **P**harmacology, **M**onitoring **E**quipment

ETT Size (mm) = (age in yr/4) + 4

Age	Birth	6 mo	1 yr	2 yr	3 yr	4 yr	5 yr	6 yr	8 yr	10 yr	12 yr	14 yr	Adult
Average weight (kg)	3.5	7	10	12	14	16	18	20	20	30	40	50	70
Blade	0–1 Miller	1 Miller	1 Miller	2 Miller	2	2	2	2	2–3	2–3	2–3	3	3
ETT size	2.5–3.5 uncuffed	3.5–4 uncuffed	4 uncuffed	4.5 uncuffed	4.5–5 uncuffed	5 uncuffed	5–5.5 uncuffed	5.5 uncuffed	6 Uncuffed	6–6.5 uncuffed	7	7.5	8
ETT length at lip (cm)	1 kg = 7 cm 2 kg = 8 cm 3 kg = 9 cm	10	11	12	13	14	14.5	15	16	17	18	19	20
LMA size	1	1.5	2	2	2	2	2	2.5	2.5	3	3	4	4
LMA Max cuff volume (mL)	4	7	10	10	10	10	10	14	14	20	20	30	30

Adapted from 2002 Broselow Pediatric Resuscitation Tape, modified from Hazinski MF, ed. Manual of Pediatric Critical Care 1999.

- **Premedication:** Oxygen, lidocaine, atropine, defasciculating dose NM blocker, sedation, analgesia = fentanyl, NM blocker

Pretreatment Medications

Agent	Dose	Useful in	Adverse Events
Lidocaine	1.5 mg/kg IV	TBI (blunts ICP response, cough, dysrhythmia)	Seizure, brady/HOTN
Fentanyl	2–5 mcg/kg IV	TBI (may blunt ICP response)	Resp depression, ↓ HR. laryngospasm, rigidity, N/V
Atropine	0.02 mg/kg IV min: 0.1 mg; <0.1 mg assoc paradox ↓ HR	Blunts bradycardia + secretions (all children <1 yr)	Anticholinergic contraindications: Closed-angle glaucoma, myasthenia gravis
Defasciculation Vecuronium Rocuronium	(¹/₁₀ usual dose)	Prevent fasciculations and ICP/IOP response before succinylcholine	
Midazolam	0.05–0.2 mg/kg IV	Amnestic, sedative	HoTN
Etomidate	0.2–0.3 mg/kg IV	CV neutral TBI drug of choice (↓ ICP)	Myoclonus, adrenal suppression (increased risk in sepsis)
Thiopental	1–6 mg/kg IV	Sedative TBI (lowers ICP)	HoTN (avoid in myocardial dysfxn/trauma), asthma; no analgesia
Ketamine	1–1.5 mg/kg IV 2–5 mg/kg IM	Analgesic amnestic Asthma drug of choice (bronchodilator + preserves resp drive) CV neutral	Emergence rxn, laryngospasm, tachy/HTN contraindications: Increased ICP/TBI, pheochromocytoma, hyperthyroid
Propofol	1–3 mg/kg IV	Sedative, amnestic, neuroprotective, rapid on/off	Brady, HoTN, lactic acidosis, prop infus synd contraind: Egg allergy

Sedation Paralysis					
Agent	Onset	Duration	Dose	Useful in	Adverse Events
Succinylcholine	30–60 sec	10–30 min	1–2 mg/kg IV 5 mg/kg IM	Rapid on/off	Bradycardia, cardiac arrest, HoTN, ↑ ICP/IOP, malignant hyperthermia, bronchospasm, myoglobinemia contraindications: Hyper K-prone (crush/burn, renal failure, myopathy, rhabdo, severe infection)
Rocuronium	30–60 sec	26–40 min	0.6–1.2 mg/kg IV	Renal failure, hemodynamically very stable	Rare HoTN and bronchospasm
Vecuronium	60–180 sec	30–40 min	0.1 mg/kg IV	Renal failure	Liver metabolism Bronchospasm
Pancuronium	120–180 sec	40–60 min	0.1–0.15 mg/kg IV test dose: 0.02 mg/kg × 1	Useful in hepatic failure (renally excreted)	Vagolytic, tachycardia, wheezing

Cisatracurium	120–180 sec	35–45 min	0.1–0.2 mg/kg IV	Hoffman degradation: Useful in renal or hepatic failure	Histamine release, wheezing, laryngospasm

Protection
- Cricoid pressure to reduce aspiration

Postintubation Management
- Confirm placement (color change, auscultation, CXR), sedation and pain control, avoid further NM blockade unless necessary

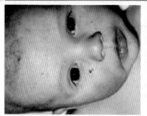 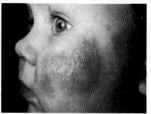

Atopic Dermatitis – Pruritic dry erythematous skin or erythematous papules usually w/ associated excoriations. Develops scaling, lichenification w/ accentuation of skin lines. Pts generally w/ hx of atopy, family hx atopy. **Dx:** Clinical dx. See Allergy & Immunology chapter. Left image from Goodheart HP, MD. *Goodheart's Photoguide of Common Skin Disorders.* 2nd ed. Philadelphia, PA: Lippincott Williams & Wilkins; 2003. Right image from Sauer GC, Hall JC. *Manual of Skin Diseases.* 7th ed. Philadelphia, PA: Lippincott-Raven; 1996.

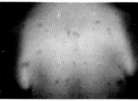 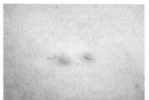

Varicella – Vesicle on erythematous base ("dew drop on rose petal"), with all stages of lesions present at once (papule, vesicle, pustule, crust; unlike small pox w/ all lesions of same stage), if systemic illness, whole body involved w/ crops of lesions, ↓ incidence 2/2 vaccination, if dermatomal distribution then "zoster," reactivation of prior varicella infection raising concern immune suppression/deficiency. **Dx:** Clinical dx, can use DFA of vesicle base scraping. Both images from Goodheart HP, MD. *Goodheart's Photoguide of Common Skin Disorders.* 2nd ed. Philadelphia, PA: Lippincott Williams & Wilkins; 2003.

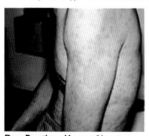 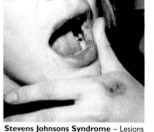

Drug Reaction – Many possible patterns but 95% maculopapular w/ presentation 1–4 wk after exposure. Common offenders: β-lactams, sulfa drugs, NSAIDs, AEDs, etc. **Dx:** Based = on history exposure. From Goodheart HP, MD. *A Photoguide of Common Skin Disorders: Diagnosis and Management.* Baltimore: Lippincott Williams & Wilkins; 1999.

Stevens Johnsons Syndrome – Lesions begin on face & trunk, irregular purpuric macules w/ occasional blistering. Most w/ extensive mucosal involvement; often medication related. **Dx:** Skin biopsy. See Allergy & Immunology chapter for detail. From Goodheart HP, MD. *Goodheart's Photoguide of Common Skin Disorders.* 2nd ed. Philadelphia, PA: Lippincott Williams & Wilkins; 2003.

A **B**

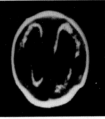

Congenital Cytomegalovirus Infection – Most common TORCH infection in US; **A:** Severe congenital CMV w/ petechial rash, microcephaly, jaundice. **B:** CT head in CMV congenital infection w/ severe periventricular calcification and hydrocephalus. For details on evaluation of TORCH infections including CMV see NICU chapter for details. Images from Engleberg NC, Dermody T, DiRita V. *Schaecter's Mechanisms of Microbial Disease.* 4th ed. Baltimore: Lippincott Williams & Wilkins; 2007.

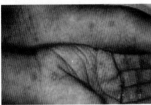
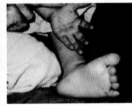

Hand, Foot, and Mouth Disease – Due to infection w/ enteroviruses (most commonly Coxsackievirus A16), generally affecting children <5 yo but can affect all ages. P/w fever, blister-like sores in mouth (herpangina) and rash w/ erythematous papules primarily involving palms of hands and soles of feet. Image on left from Fleisher GR, MD, Ludwig W, MD, Baskin MN, MD. *Atlas of Pediatric Emergency Medicine.* Philadelphia, PA: Lippincott Williams & Wilkins; 2004. Image on right courtesy of Philip Siu, MD.

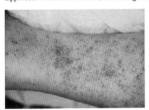
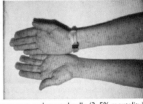

Rocky Mountain Spotted Fever – Most common and most deadly (3–5% mortality) rickettsial infection in US; 2/2 *Rickettsia rickettsii* transmitted by *Dermacentor* tick. P/w sudden onset of fever, HA, muscle pain followed by rash usually on days 2–5 of illness w/ centripetal (inward) spread w/ non-pruritic macules staring classically on wrists & ankles that blanch w/ pressure. Eventually become papular. By day 6 can see characteristic petechial rash. 10–15% may not develop rash. Treat immediately w/ doxycycline if suspected. (Pediatr Rev 2005;26:125). Image on left courtesy of Steven Manders, MD; on right Courtesy of Sidney Sussman, MD.

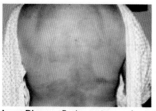
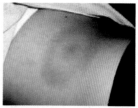

Lyme Disease – Erythema migrans rash seen in 80% of cases of proven Lyme disease. Initially p/w annular macular lesions at site of tick bite w/ central clearing that can be 6–40 cm in size. Subsequently develop multiple similar lesions anywhere on skin. Can be seen in early localized or early disseminated disease. **Dx:** Based on serology. See Infectious Disease chapter section on Lyme Disease for further details. From Goodheart HP, MD. *Goodheart's Photoguide of Common Skin Disorders.* 2nd ed. Philadelphia, PA: LW&W; 2003.

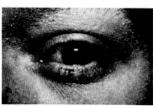
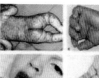
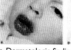

Kawasaki Disease – Acute self-limited vasculitis. Dermatologic findings include polymorphous exanthem, mucosal erythema w/ cracked lips and "strawberry tongue," bilateral bulbar conjunctival injects w/ limbic sparing, acute erythema of palms and soles w/ edema of hands and feet, periungual peeling of fingers and toes (2nd and 3rd weeks of illness). See Rheumatology chapter section on Vasculitides subheading Kawasaki Disease. Image on left from Goodheart HP, MD. *Goodheart's Photoguide of Common Skin Disorders.* 2nd ed. Philadelphia, PA: LW&W; 2003. Images on right from Circulation 2001;103:335.

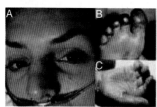
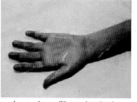

Toxic Shock Syndrome – Diffuse confluent macular erythema (like sunburn) w/ involvement of the palms and soles often w/ conjunctival injection. Blanches when pressed and non-tender. Associated with fever and hypotension and may result in end-organ underperfusion. Eventually involved skin desquamates, especially over soles and palms. Associated with *Staphylococcus aureus* & *Streptococcus pyogenes*. **Dx:** Clinical history & exam and isolated source of infection with above etiologies. Consider ribosomal suppression of toxin production w/ clindamycin in addition to appropriate antibiotic therapy. Limited data to support IVIG. Images on left from Engleberg NC, Dermody T, DiRita V. *Schaecter's Mechanisms of Microbial Disease.* 4th ed. Baltimore: LW&W; 2007. Image on right from Sweet RL, Gibbs RS. *Atlas of Infectious Diseases of the Female Genital Tract.* Philadelphia, PA: LW&W; 2005, Fig 9-2.

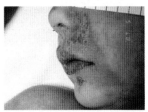 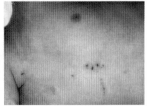

Staphylococcal Scalded Skin Syndrome – Begins w/ erythematous and tender rough ("sandpaper-like") rash, often in the flexural areas progressing to large flaccid bullae (+ Nikolsky sign) w/ exfoliative desquamation. Often w/ associated honey-colored crust at nares or lips as this condition is often secondary to impetigo. **Dx:** By skin bx which can be used to distinguish it from toxic epidermal necrolysis which is more severe, but rare in infants & children. Consider cultures of eyes, nose, & throat as well as bullae to isolate *Staphylococcus*. Images from Fleisher GR, MD, Ludwig S, MD, Baskin MN, MD. *Atlas of Pediatric Emergency Medicine*. Philadelphia, PA: Lippincott Williams & Wilkins; 2004.

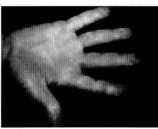 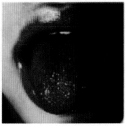

Scarlet Fever – Diffuse macular erythema with rough texture ("sandpaper-like") which blanches on compression and generally follows a *Streptococcus*-related pharyngitis or skin infection. Rash generally begins on face or neck and then spreads to trunk, arms, and legs. Also classically w/ "strawberry tongue." Can see petechiae in axillary or antecubital folds called Pastia's lines. **Dx:** Can check anti-streptolysin O & anti-DNAse B if no + cx for *Strep*. Image on left from Goodheart HP, MD. *Goodheart's Photoguide of Common Skin Disorders*. 2nd ed. Philadelphia, PA: Lippincott Williams & Wilkins; 2003. Image on right from Neville BW, Damm DD, White DK. *Color Atlas of Clinical Oral Pathology*. 2nd ed. Baltimore: Williams & Wilkins; 1998.

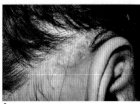 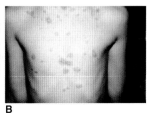

A   **B**

Psoriasis – Inherited skin d/o affecting 2% of US population w/ 25–45% pts w/ first clinical signs prior to age 16. **A:** Classical psoriasis w/ round erythematous plaques w/ silver scale. Scale attached at center and w/ removal left w/ punctate bleeding (Auspitz sign). Commonly involve scalp, elbows, knees, and gluteal crease. Diaper area is commonly involved in infants & toddlers with an appearance similar to candidal diaper rash. Can also see associated nail pitting. **B:** Gutate psoriasis w/ 2 mm to 1 cm diameter lesions symmetrically distributed, 2/3 w/ URI or streptococcal infection in the preceding 1–3 wk. **Dx:** Generally clinical. (Pediatr Rev 1998;19:106). Images from Goodheart HP, MD. *Goodheart's Photoguide of Common Skin Disorders*. 2nd ed. Philadelphia, PA: Lippincott Williams & Wilkins; 2003.

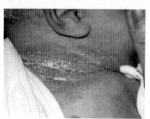 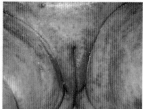

Seborrheic Dermatitis – Erythematous patches w/ greasy scale. Commonly involves hair-line, behind ears, external ear canal, base of eyelashes & eyebrows, nasolabial folds, chest, umbilicus, groin. Can be assoc w/ systemic illness; DM, malabsorption, & obesity. **Dx:** Clinical. Images from LW&W Image Library.

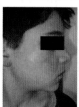 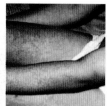 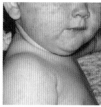

Fifth disease (Erythema infectiosum) – Infection with parvovirus B19. Results in "slapped cheek" rash, sparing of periorbital areas and nasal bridge. Also w/ "fishnet" pattern, lacy rash involving extremities, trunk, and buttocks. Generally self-limited. **Dx:** Clinical. Image on left from Stedmans, middle image from LW&W Image Library, far right image from Dale Berg and Katherine Worzala, Atlas of Adult Physical Diagnosis. Philadelphia, PA: LW&W; 2006.

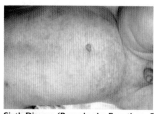 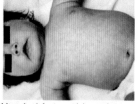

Sixth Disease (Roseola aka Exanthem Subitum) – Infection with human herpes virus 6 or 7. Usually seen in children <3 yo. P/w sudden onset of high fever w/o other symptoms. Fever breaks in 2–3 days and with defervescence patient develops blanching maculopapular rash on trunk which spreads to neck and extremities. **Dx:** Clinical. Image on left from Goodheart HP, MD. Goodheart's Photoguide of Common Skin Disorders. 2nd ed. Philadelphia, PA: Lippincott Williams & Wilkins, 2003. Image on right courtesy of John Loiselle, MD.

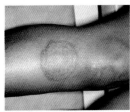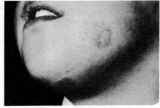

Ringworm (tinea corporis) – Scaly, raised, erythematous, annular lesions w/ central clearing. Often pruritic and with hair loss in areas of infection. Due to dermatophyte infection which can be spread from direct person to person contact, fomites, and pets. **Dx:** KOH preparation of skin scraping. Can be treated with topical anti-fungals. Image on left from Goodheart HP, MD. *Goodheart's Photoguide of Common Skin Disorders.* 2nd ed. Philadelphia, PA: Lippincott Williams & Wilkins; 2003. Image on right from LW&W Image Library.

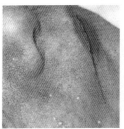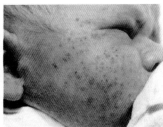

Milia – White pearly bumps on a neonates nose, chin, or cheeks. **Dx:** Clinical, self resolving. Image from O'Doherty N. Atlas of the Newborn. Philadelphia, PA: JB Lippincott, 1979.

Erythema Toxicum – Rash w/ yellow to white papules w/ surrounding erythema on face and trunk appearing in 50% of eonates in first 2 wk of life. **Dx:** Clinical, self resolving. Image from Fletcher M. *Physical Diagnosis in Neonatology.* Philadelphia, PA: Lippincott-Raven Publishers, 1998.

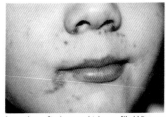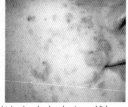

Impetigo – Single or multiple pus-filled blisters which when broken leaving reddish raw base with honey yellow crust generally involving face, lips, arms, or legs. Can spread to other areas if scratched. **Dx:** Clinical; culture of lesion usually grows *Streptococcus* or *Staphylococcus* but rarely done unless MRSA suspected. Images from Goodheart HP, MD. *Goodheart's Photoguide of Common Skin Disorders.* 2nd ed. Philadelphia, PA: LW&W, 2003.

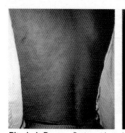 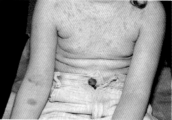

Pityriasis Rosea – Begins with single large patch (herald patch) followed by multiple smaller lesions, in a "Christmas tree" pattern, often pink or pale red, oval in shape w/ most attacks lasting between 4–8 wk. Can be scaly and pruritic. **Dx:** Clinical, rarely biopsy; in sexually active adolescents should rule out syphilis. Image on left from Fleisher GR, MD, Ludwig S, MD. Baskin MN, MD. *Atlas of Pediatric Emergency Medicine.* Philadelphia, PA: Lippincott Williams & Wilkins; 2004 and image on right from Goodheart HP, MD. *Goodheart's Photoguide of Common Skin Disorders.* 2nd ed. Philadelphia, PA: Lippincott Williams & Wilkins; 2003.

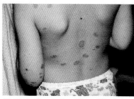 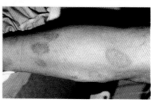

Guttate Psoriasis – Generally <1 cm scaling papules and plaques on trunk and extremities, often 1–2 wk after Strep pharyngitis. **Dx:** Clinical. Can check anti-streptolysin O (ASLO) titer. From Goodheart HP, MD. *Goodheart's Photoguide of Common Skin Disorders.* 2nd ed. Philadelphia, PA: LW&W; 2003.

Nummular Eczema – "Coin-shaped" patches and plaques involving arms and legs, sometimes involving the trunk, often in patients with history allergies, asthma, or atopy. **Dx:** Clinical; avoid trigger. From Goodheart HP, MD. *Goodheart's Photoguide of Common Skin Disorders.* 2nd ed. Philadelphia, PA: Lippincott Williams & Wilkins; 2003.

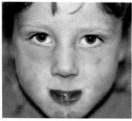 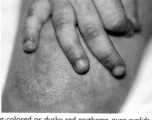

Dermatomyositis – Characteristic violet-colored or dusky red erythema over eyelids often with periorbital edema as well as erythema involving area around nails and/or knuckles (Grotton's rash). Can be sole symptom in up to 40% of cases at onset. See Rheumatology section. Images from Fleisher GR, MD, Ludwig S, MD, Baskin MN, MD. *Atlas of Pediatric Emergency Medicine.* Philadelphia, PA: Lippincott Williams & Wilkins; 2004.

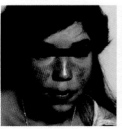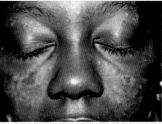

Systemic lupus Erythematosis – Image on left with classic "butterfly" rash associated with SLE, fixed erythema, flat or raised over malar eminences, spares nasolabial folds. Image on right with discoid-lupus rash, raised erythematous patches w/ adhered keratotic scale. **Dx:** ANA testing. Both images from Goodheart HP, MD. *Goodheart's Photoguide of Common Skin Disorders*. 2nd ed. Philadelphia, PA: Lippincott Williams & Wilkins; 2003. See Rheumatology chapter for details.

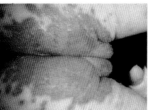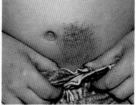

Candida Dermatitis – Erythema with fragile satellite pustules, sharply demarcated with raised rim and often white scale at border. **Dx:** Clinical, rarely scrapings & culture. From LW&W Image Library.

Contact Dermatitis – Erythema, edema, vesicles in geometric pattern of exposure. From Goodheart HP, MD. *Goodheart's Photoguide of Common Skin Disorders*. 2nd ed. Philadelphia, PA: LW&W; 2003.

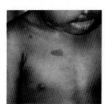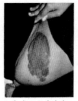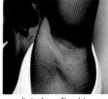

Neurofibromatosis – Diagnostic findings include but are not limited to café au lait spots (far left; well demarcated uniform brown macules), plexiform neurofibromas (middle; drooping soft doughy loose lesion color of skin, "bag of worms"), and axillary freckles (far right). See Neurology chapter for details. Left-most image from Fleisher GR, MD, Ludwig S, MD, Baskin MN, MD. *Atlas of Pediatric Emergency Medicine*. Philadelphia, PA: Lippincott Williams & Wilkins; 2004. Middle and right-most image from Goodheart HP, MD. *Goodheart's Photoguide of Common Skin Disorders*. 2nd ed. Philadelphia, PA: Lippincott Williams & Wilkins; 2003.

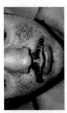 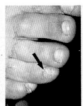 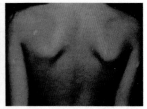

Tuberous Sclerosis – Diagnostic findings include but are not limited to adenoma sebaceum (far right image; red- and skin-colored papules/nodules generally on face), peri/subungual fibromas (middle image; same pathology as face papules, arise late in childhood), and ashleaf spot (far left image; hypomelanotic macules). See Neurology chapter for details. Far right and middle images from Goodheart HP, MD. *Goodheart's Photoguide of Common Skin Disorders.* 2nd ed. Philadelphia, PA: Lippincott Williams & Wilkins; 2003. Far left image from Gold DH, MD, and Weingeist TA, MD, PhD. *Color Atlas of the Eye in Systemic Disease.* Baltimore: Lippincott Williams & Wilkins; 2001.

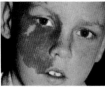 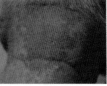

Port-wine Stain – Macular vascular stain composed of ectatic dermal capillaries. Present at birth & persists lifelong. Grow proportionally & asym w/ pt. Majority w/o other assoc, can be seen in Sturge–Weber & Klippel–Trénaunay syndrome. Far left image from G. C., Hall JC. *Manual of Skin Diseases.* 7th ed.. Philadelphia, PA: Lippincott-Raven; 1996. Middle and far right images from Stedmans.

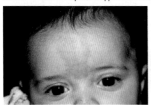 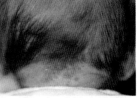

Salmon Patch (Nevus Simplex) – Dull pink to red macule on head or neck. Most common benign vascular lesion in infants. Facial salmon patches fade w/ time, nuchal ones can persist but asympt. Do not require further eval or treatment. Image on left from Goodheart HP, MD. *Goodheart's Photoguide of Common Skin Disorders.* 2nd ed. Philadelphia, PA: Lippincott Williams & Wilkins; 2003. Image on right from Fletcher M. *Phyical Diagnosis in Neonatology.* Philadelphia, PA: Lippincott-Raven Publishers; 1998.

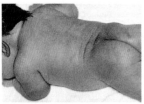 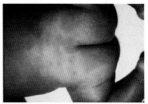

Mongolian Spot – Large blue-black macular lesions characteristically located on buttocks/lumbrosacral area in Hispanic, Asian, and dark-skinned populations. Benign congenital lesion, present at birth and fades in first 1–2 yr or life. Asymptomatic and most noticable at birth. **Dx:** Clinical. Image on left from O'Doherty N. *Atlas of the Newborn.* Philadelphia, PA: JB Lippincott; 1979. Image on right courtesy of Sidney Sussman, MD.

INDEX

Note: Page numbers in *italics* denote figures; those followed by t denote tables.